PRAISE FOR THE LI

"This book is gold! It is a science-based, effective solution to the rampant chronic health problems that plague millions today. It is easy to understand, simple to implement, and most importantly, will be a guiding light for so many who are out of answers and are desperately searching for a path home to health."

Dr. Mindy Pelz, DC
Bestselling author of *The Reset Factor, The Reset Factor Kitchen,*
and *The Menopause Reset*

"Building on the valuable information shared in the first two volumes of The LDN Book, book three is an equally important and authoritative treasure trove of documented research furthering our understanding of naltrexone. Essential reading for clinicians and patients alike!"

Larry Trivieri, Jr.
Author and Health Freedom Advocate

"Praises to Linda Elsegood through the LDN Research Trust for once again compiling such a comprehensive, informative book on LDN and its multitude of uses, filled with so many practical and relevant usages of LDN! I would highly recommend it to all who are interested in the potential of LDN's efficacy in today's integrative world. This book contains current clinical research, up-to-date protocols, and appropriate dosing for LDN. I cannot speak more highly of such a pertinent book regarding LDN!"

Lisa Hunt, DO, DOH
Specializing in strengthening the immune system, anti-aging, etc

"The LDN Book 3 Is an invaluable resource for all clinicians that treat patients suffering from chronic inflammatory conditions. The book offers detailed references, protocols, insight, and information on how to use low dose naltrexone to treat CIRS, latent viral infections, autoimmune conditions, refractive depression, and many other challenging conditions. Like the previous two books, Book 3 is a must-have for any physician."

Alina D Garcia, MD
Specializing in fibromyalgia, chronic fatigue, Lyme and CIRS, etc

"Rarely does a naturopathic doctor consider any medicine to be a "miracle drug," but LDN has been a life-altering medicine for my patients. Kudos to Linda Elsegood for once again offering a resource for patients worldwide."

Dr. Nancy L. Evans, ND
Specializing in HRT and thyroid disorders

"A wonderful resource to build upon patients' and clinicians' knowledge of LDN by addressing current research and new applications of the medication."

Dr. Jennifer Rickner, PharmD, RP
Compounding Pharmacist and LDN Specialist

"The LDN Books continue to be a treasure chest of information. We recommend them to our patients and practitioners. Book 3 carries on this tradition of being a timely and valuable resource on the many conditions that benefit from LDN."

Steve Hoffart, PharmD
Compounding Pharmacist

"The LDN Book 3 gives valuable insight into the drug of the decade. The immense knowledge within can change and improve the quality of life. For many, it's a game changer."

Nat Jones, R.Ph. FAPC
Clinical Compounding Pharmacist

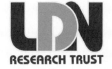

The
LDN
Book 3

-Low Dose Naltrexone-

The Lastest Research on:

Viral Infections,Long COVID,
Mold Toxicity,Longevity,
Cancer, Depression and more.

EDITED BY LINDA ELSEGOOD

Printed in the UK
First printed October 2022

ISBN: 978-1-7391070-0-0

Published by LDN Research Trust
PO Box 1083
Buxton
Norwich
NR10 5WY
UK

www.ldnresearchtrust.org

To my hero, Dr. Mark Mandel

CONTENTS

PREFACE

In 2000, at the age of 44, I was diagnosed with relapsing-remitting multiple sclerosis (RRMS). With hindsight, I can see I had been having minor relapses for thirty years after Epstein-Barr virus almost killed me and kept me from school for nearly a year when I was thirteen. In 2003, I was diagnosed with secondary-progressive MS. I was unable to function and had poor quality of life. When my neurologist said he could do nothing more for me, I started researching alternative treatments. That's when I learned about low dose naltrexone (LDN), a safe, non-toxic, and inexpensive drug that helps regulate a dysfunctional immune system. Just three weeks after being prescribed LDN by Dr. Bob Lawrence in Wales, I regained clarity of mind, and slowly my symptoms started to recede.

My success with LDN led me to found the LDN Research Trust, a UK-registered, non-profit charity intended to help and support other people whose lives have been taken away from them. Since 2004, our long-term goal has been for the effects of LDN to be tested in gold-standard clinical trials so that ultimately the drug can be made available worldwide to anyone who might benefit from it. We are assisted in this work by a team of medical advisers, who give their time and expertise freely. The Trust is run by volunteers; we receive no funding and rely on donations to operate. Every contribution, however small, is greatly appreciated, and you can access more information, resources, and educational materials (including conference presentations, podcasts, interviews, and more) on our website: www.ldnresearchtrust.org.

This book provides the latest research on the benefits of LDN for treating many different conditions, along with clinical experiences and up-to-date dosing protocols. There is a wealth of quality information from LDN experts in their fields who have generously shared it with us.

An important caveat to LDN is that it isn't a miracle drug or a cure. However, it has helped me, and millions of others worldwide improve the quality of our lives, which is why it's well worth researching further.

LINDA ELSEGOOD
FOUNDER, LDN RESEARCH TRUST

FOREWORD

After almost 44 years in practice, as an emergency room physician and as a precision medicine specialist, as well as an internationally known author and lecturer, if I could select only a few medications that have been able to change the lives of my patients the most, one of them would be low dose naltrexone (LDN).

The body's inflammatory response can be provoked by physical, chemical, and biologic agents, including mechanical trauma, exposure to excessive amounts of sunlight, x-rays and radioactive materials, corrosive chemicals, temperature extremes, or by infectious agents such as bacteria, viruses, and other pathogenic microorganisms. It is all about balance. A small amount of inflammation heals. When you run a temperature after catching a cold or have bronchitis, when you have a cough or other symptoms, all of these are related to the body's inflammatory process setting up a healing response. Excessive inflammation, however, is linked to the development of almost every major illness.

Chronic inflammatory diseases are complex to treat and have an impact on many individuals. In low doses, naltrexone can regulate the immune system by exerting its immunoregulatory activity by binding to opioid receptors in or on immune cells and tumor cells. LDN also operates as a novel anti-inflammatory agent. It binds and blocks toll-like receptors, which release inflammatory cytokines, thereby reducing inflammation.

The following are some examples of diseases related to inflammation for which LDN can effectively be used as an adjunct therapy.

- Allergy
- Alzheimer's disease and other forms of cognitive decline
- Asthma
- Diabetes
- Cancer
- Candida infections
- Canker sores and mouth ulcers
- Cardiovascular disease (heart disease)
- COVID-19
- Depression
- Epilepsy
- Food addictions and eating disorders
- Headaches
- Heartburn
- Hypertension
- Hypoglycemia
- Inflammatory bowel disease
- Kidney disease
- Lyme disease
- Obesity
- Parkinson's disease
- Periodontal disease
- Respiratory diseases
- Rheumatoid arthritis

The great news is that inflammation can be balanced using many modalities from traditional medications, to changing eating habits, to adding nutrients and herbal therapies, along with the newest treatment, low dose naltrexone. LDN is a prescription compounded medication that very effectively reduces inflammation.

Low dose naltrexone has been shown to be one of the keys to the future of medicine for many disease processes that are inflammatory in nature. It is also an efficacious pain control agent.

It is my hope, and the hope of the world-class authors of this book, that you begin your medical journey toward healing by learning more about this wonderful medication.

PAMELA W. SMITH, MD, MPH, MS

ONE

Pharmacology and Best Clinical Practices

J. Stephen Dickson

BSC (HONS), MRPharmS

L ow dose naltrexone (LDN) has been used to treat a wide range of diseases, and many clinicians may find it difficult to understand how one drug can have a positive effect on pathologies ranging from multiple sclerosis to various cancers. The mechanism of action of LDN has been clearly elucidated and described in both volumes of The LDN Book, edited by Linda Elsegood, but the first thing to understand is that naltrexone—the drug in LDN—comes in a 50:50 mixture of two different shapes (called isomers). It has been recently discovered that one shape binds to immune cells, whilst the other shape binds to opioid receptors. Although consisting of the same components, the two isomers appear to have different biological activity. To summarize the past ten years of research, LDN is effective because levo-naltrexone is an antagonist for the opiate/endorphin receptors, leading to increased endorphin release.

The purpose of this chapter is to give a clinical refresher to the pharmacology as applied in practice and to examine the current uses of LDN in a wider population, with reference to the best practices in real world scenarios.

Pharmacology of LDN in Summary

To understand how LDN works requires a grasp of three fundamental biological principles.

First, opiate receptors are present in multiple biological systems in the human body, as they regulate a great number of biological functions via the central release of natural opiates (endorphins/met-enkephalins).[1][2]

Second, a class of proteins called toll-like receptors (TLRs) are part of the immune system, providing a first line of defense against microbial invasion and possessing the ability to recognize and be activated by not only pathogens, but also endogenous signaling molecules.[3]

Lastly, naltrexone, when given at a low dose, has antagonistic activity in both of these areas, and is able to modify biological functions of these receptor groups by suppressing unwanted immune reactions, or by stimulating disease-suppressed immune activity.[4]

Naltrexone, taken at the full dose of 200mg daily, has been licensed for use for the treatment of addictions since 1984.[5] It is currently used for both opiate and alcohol addiction, as a full dose is able to completely block endogenous (endorphins released by the brain) and exogenous (recreational drugs such as heroin) opiates. In the licensed dose it is used as an oral tablet, a long-acting injection, and as an additive in painkillers to prevent them from being abused.[6]

As have many drugs that have been widely used for an extended period, naltrexone has been found to have different actions when used in lower doses than originally intended. These in part are due to the chiral nature of the molecule and the different, dose-dependent effects of the levo and dextro isomers of naltrexone.

The concept of chirality is not new, (chiral chemistry was discovered by Louis Pasteur in 1848), as all drugs when synthesized are produced as a racemic mixture of 50:50 left- and right-handed molecules.[7] Half of the mixture synthesized is a left-handed shape and the other half is a right-handed shape. Although consisting of the same components, and being chemically identical, they have different shapes (as with left and right hands), enabling the different isomers to interact with different groups of receptors the body.

In general, most drugs only have biological activity in the human body in levo (left) handed shape, as this is how most of the receptor groups in the human body are arranged. Common examples of these drugs—such as levothyroxine, levocetirizine, levobutanol—are manufactured as racemic mixtures of 50:50 levo and dextro isomers; however, the manufacturer discards the dextro isomer and presents the medication in the levo-only form, sometimes because the dextro isomer carries unwanted side effects, or is not active on the intended target receptor.[8]

In the case of naltrexone, the levo isomer interacts with the commonly understood opiate (endorphin) receptors group and the dextro isomer interacts with the toll-like receptor group.[9] [10]

The basic effects of LDN can be summarized as follows:

DEX-Naltrexone
- Blocks (antagonizes) some TLR receptors
- Reduces production of pro-inflammatory cytokines
- Suppresses cascade inflammation
- Central and system effects as TLR receptors are present on microglial cells, mast cells, and macrophages

LEVO-Naltrexone
- Blocks opiate receptors for a brief period
- Increases natural production of anti-inflammatory endorphins
- Upregulates opiate receptors
- Has direct effect on some cell proliferation rates

Again, these mechanisms are fully elucidated in both volumes of *The LDN Book*, but the main point is that LDN is extremely useful in the treatment of many poorly managed autoimmune and oncological conditions.

Clinical Use of LDN

A poorly functioning immune system is the root cause of a vast number of long-term, debilitating conditions. The LDN Research Trust maintains a research base on its website, as well as list of conditions for which LDN seems to benefit. Though the list is not exhaustive, it is clear that LDN's ability to modify the immune system and support normal function can have a dramatic and long-lasting effect in conditions when standard therapies are suboptimal.

The clinical uses of LDN are extremely extensive, including but not limited to the conditions and diseases featured in all three LDN books. However, the first step in treating a patient is making the decision to prescribe the medicine. The resources listed are helpful, but all prescribers should be aware of the legal framework surrounding using this medicine in an unlicensed (off-label) way.

Unlicensed (Off-Label) Use

When LDN is used clinically in patients, the first hurdle faced by prescribers is the unfortunate fact that LDN has not yet obtained a pharmaceutical license for any of the conditions listed by the Research Trust. The reasons for this are many and varied; however, the fundamental problem with repurposing such an old drug is that it is available generically—relatively inexpensively—and even if a drug company were to invest millions in a clinical trial, there would be very limited protection for an end-product, therefore no way to recoup the cost of the trial.

Another critical issue with LDN, as a licensed product, is that the number of conditions it can be used for is extensive. Even if a licensed product were created for one condition (for example, Crohn's disease), the drug would still have to be used for all the other conditions in an unlicensed/off-label way. This is a fundamental problem with the way drugs are licensed: the focus is on the specific condition and not the overall mechanism of action.

Over the last 20 years, a significant number of clinical effectiveness studies, or "pre-clinical trials," have been conducted by researchers. For any other drug, or for a new compound (not a repurposed generic drug), these studies would have quickly resulted in drug development and a push to licensure. At the time of this writing, there are 57 recent clinical trials available to view on clinicaltrials.gov, showing that work is continuing and the use of LDN is widespread all over the world. Both the size of the trials, and the number of patients for each trial are limited due to the constraints of university and hospital funding. Even when the results are spectacular, as they have been in a number of cases, moving the current clinical trial designs into a multi-centered, placebo-controlled study that could lead to licensure is still financially prohibitive.

Prescribers must therefore be comfortable with using this medication without all the legal and ethical protections of a product license and be aware that liability (dependent on country) is either 100% personal to the prescriber or shared 50% with the dispenser. This is seen by many prescribers as a massive challenge; however, risk can be carefully mitigated and the lack of any significant adverse effects from LDN in the last 20+ years of extensive clinical use should give prescribers confidence to try this medication where standard therapies have failed.

Overcoming the Unlicensed (Off-label) Barrier

Prescribers often supply treatments to patients in an unlicensed way without giving it a second thought.[11] [12] In the UK, for example, the NHS spends hundreds of millions of pounds every year providing pharmaceutical specials. The UK has one of the most stringent drug licensing frameworks and, due to there being a nationalized health service with central oversight of prescribing, has extensive data on the prescribing and dispensing of medicines in an unlicensed way.[13]

Medicines are commonly prescribed off-label for children. Almost every medicine in pediatric wards is used off-label, as very few clinical trials focus specifically on a pediatric population. In general practice, doctors have for many years prescribed anti-depressants such as amitriptiline for back pain, or liquid versions of medicines for people with swallowing difficulties, without really understanding that these are in the same legal category as prescribing LDN.

When prescribing a medicine that does not have a license, it is important for the prescriber to consider the patient first. There are great resources provided by the regulatory compliance association for each country outlining how to best comply with legal and ethical standards when provisioning an unlicensed medicine to a patient. In the UK, which has some of the most stringent standards in the world, the General Medical Council, the Royal Pharmaceutical Association, the General Pharmaceutical Council, and the MHRA all have guidance around the use of these sort of medicines. Any prescriber embarking on their LDN journey should be aware of the guidance for their local area; however, most guidelines are based on sensible precautions and a risk assessment.

Mitigating Prescriber Risk

As discussed, the responsibility for any side effects or problems with an unlicensed medicine like LDN fall directly to the insurances held by the prescriber, and not to the drug company. Though there are very few risks to prescribing of LDN, there are some simple processes to follow which significantly ameliorate any/all risks to the prescribing from potential litigation, however unlikely.

Step 1: By prescribing LDN, are you compliantly meeting an "unmet need"?

- Is the patient self-directed?
- Have they exhausted standard licensed therapy options?
- Have they had ample resources to complete their own research?
- Do they understand that no guarantee can be given for any effect from an unlicensed medicine?
- Has the clinician had a direct conversation with the patient in order to make a joint clinical decision that LDN is the best way forward? Has this been recorded?
- Has the effect on other medicines been considered?
- Has a review period been formally decided?

Step 2: Has a Risk:Benefit review been completed?

- What is the expected benefit to the patient by prescribing LDN?
- Are there any risks (pregnancy for example)?
- Can those risks be mitigated against?
- How will these risks be reviewed?

Step 3: Has adequate consent been obtained?

- Patients receiving an unlicensed medicine like LDN must be able to give informed consent.
- Informed consent, where practicable, should be formally documented.
- Consent is an ongoing process and should be reviewed as still appropriate at least annually.

Step 4: Is the clinical decision to prescribe an unlicensed medicine clearly not made under duress, or financially beneficial for the prescriber?

- The patient, if paying for therapy, should not be able to "click and order" something like LDN.
- Any provision of LDN should come from a consultation, in which there is no significant financial incentive for the prescriber to write a prescription.

The Importance of Patient Education

Patients starting on LDN must be willing and able to give a full medical history for the prescribing clinician. Often, due to the specialist nature of this medicine, the first place a patient will come into contact with LDN is an autoimmune or specialist holistic clinic dealing with oncology or hormone therapy.

Patients must be fully educated in the use of LDN; the best way is generally to refer them to the LDN Research Trust website and then ask them a series of questions during the consultation.

The Importance of Follow Up and Review

Historically, unlicensed medicines are generally used for short periods of time. One of the most important differences between a short term "special" for a specific unlicensed need and LDN, however, is that LDN is likely to be a long-term chronic treatment.

There are significant differences between how clinicians should manage acute and chronic illnesses, the most important one to consider for LDN is the duration of treatment and what follow-up will be required. There are very few reported incidences of long-term side effects, or massive pharmacokinetic drug interactions. There are, however, pharmacodynamic and holistic considerations to be taken into account when initiating LDN.

When obtaining LDN from a private specialist service, the patient should be encouraged to discuss their therapy with their standard primary care physician. Even if initially hesitant, patients who respond well to LDN will often be happy to discuss this with their normal doctor. This will allow the doctor to make informed decisions when prescribing other medicines (painkillers, for example).

Patients should also be made aware that taking LDN has impacts on things like dental surgery (taking the LDN right before dental surgery may stop the pain medication working correctly). In general, patients should stop taking LDN 1-2 days before any surgery.

Follow-up with chronic patients on LDN can sometimes be time-consuming but is often quite simple provided they have used some sort of tool to assess their progress. There are a number of internationally recognized scales for pain diaries, or for symptom recording in various disease conditions. Clinician and patient should decide on which (if any) of these they are going to use and have a review at least three times a month for the first six months then annually thereafter. In the case of oncology patients, the reviews should be tailored to meet their individual needs.

What to Expect When Initiating a Patient on LDN

Different disease groups respond differently, and there are various dosage charts available; a whole chapter in this book is dedicated to them. However, as a general rule, "low and slow" is a good place to start. For patients with leaky gut, consider starting on sublingual LDN drops. The usual starting dose is 1mg, increasing weekly until at 4.5mg. However, with chronic fatigue patients it is often better to start at 0.5mg. For patients with very significant multiple chemical sensitivities, ultra-low dose LDN (ULDN, 0.04mg/dose) is also an option.

During the first week of treatment, patients will generally not experience much in the way of side effects, a mild headache or GI upset is the most common. As the doses increase over the coming weeks, mild, flu-like symptoms often present in chronic fatigue patients (if they become unmanageable, halve the dose and start titrating up again). Multiple Sclerosis (MS) patient often feel an immediate boost, but then experience a worsening of symptoms after a few weeks; this is quite common, and often a good predictor for a better long-term outcome. If this is the case, as with CFS, halve the dose and start titrating up again.

When initiating a patient on LDN, it is likely that they will have read somewhere that they should take it at night, as this is when the body produces the most endorphins. In clinical practice, which has been frequently reaffirmed by clinicians at the regular LDN conferences, time of day of dosing is not very relevant to long-term outcome. Taking LDN at night often results in disturbed sleep and vivid dreams so most patients in the UK take LDN in the morning.

Commonly Asked Questions

Finally, here are some answers to questions I receive a lot, but whose answers haven't yet been addressed in the literature on LDN.

Q: Can I put LDN through a PEG tube?

A: Yes, when in liquid form. Capsules can generally be opened and dispersed in an acidic liquid such as orange juice. Flush the tube after.

Q: Can I take LDN with my other medications?

A: In general, yes, as long as they are not opiate-containing painkillers.

Q: Should I have something to eat before taking LDN?

A: This probably makes no difference, but a higher peak blood level will be achieved when on an empty stomach. The main thing is to be consistent.

Q: What do I do if I miss a dose of LDN?

A: Miss it entirely and start again at the usual time next day on the same dose.

Q: What if I miss a few days of LDN when I am titrating? Do I need to go back to the start?

A: As long as it has not been longer than a week, you can take the highest previously tolerated dose when restarting. After a week, go back to the start.

Q: Can I take my LDN with my chemotherapy?

A: This varies dependent on chemotherapy. In general, LDN is safe along with most traditional chemotherapy drugs, but should be stopped a few days before some of the newer immunologics. When in doubt seek advice from a competent pharmacist or a colleague who has done this before.

Q: Is it safe to take during pregnancy?

A: LDN is used widely to help support fertility and pregnancy and championed by NeoFertility in Ireland. This is, however, a specialist indication and not enough information is available for pregnancy or breastfeeding advice, unless this is the specific clinical specialty of the prescriber.

- TWO -

Drug-Resistant Depression

DR ELIZABETH LIVENGOOD, NMD

Depression represents the number one cause of disability worldwide and is often fatal.[14]
—Eléonore Beurel, Marisa Toups, and Charles B. Nemeroff,
"The Bidirectional Relationship of Depression and Inflammation: Double Trouble"

By the time a person with depression reaches my integrative medical practice, their story has developed a common thread shared with thousands of other people who experience chronic depression. It usually goes like this: *I've been dealing with depression since I was a teenager. I was put on an anti-depressant but then I felt so numb I couldn't enjoy life, so I was given a different drug. I gained a lot of weight on that and felt even worse about myself, so they switched me to another medication. That didn't help at all and at this point I've tried seven or eight different medications that either don't work or I can't tolerate. I'm still depressed, and I don't want to live like this.*

The details change from patient to patient, of course, but certain variables raise a red flag for me. The onset of depressive symptoms can start surprisingly young and is sometimes accompanied by an injury, illness, or other trauma. A detailed family history often reveals a form of depression or other mental health issues. Interestingly, the personal and family reproductive history is an important area to ask about as well. Low energy is ubiquitous but difficult to tease apart from other diagnostic criteria for depression such as anhedonia and low motivation. However, the singular commonality among all the stories is that multiple medications have failed to provide an amount of relief that outweighs the side effects.

In Western medicine, the standard of care is essentially a litany of anti-depressant medications which we tick off in specified order until we find one that helps and is tolerable. Fortunately, or not, there are many medications to choose from and the newer ones usually have less bothersome side effects. However, "monotherapy with either an antidepressant or psychotherapy results in remission in … 28% of 'real-world' patients."[15] So why does the usual regimen fail 72% of the time? Are there clues that could help save a patient time, money, and unwanted side effects when they are not a good candidate for the typical standard of care in the first place? The answers are important for any doctor or patient who faces this challenging situation. Most importantly, there are other ways to treat patients who do not respond to the typical anti-depressant protocols.

I stumbled onto this common phenomenon in a roundabout way. Though I am not a psychiatrist, as a holistic practitioner I always address my patients' mental health. I minored in psychology and took all the psych electives I could during medical school, including some excellent clinical rotations. During my residency, my supervising doctors used an off-label medication to treat depression, bipolar, anxiety and other mental health issues with great success. That was my introduction to LDN, which led me into my specialty area treating autoimmunity. Over the years, I noticed how depression and chronic illness often overlapped and how LDN usually helped with both conditions.

It became clear that chronic illness, autoimmunity, and depression often share a common etiology and physiological mechanism. In contrast, the pharmacological standard of care assumes that depression is always and only caused by low serotonin and/or norepinephrine. While this is based on valid science, we now know that there are many other causes and mechanisms that can trigger acute or chronic depression. To make the identification of accurate treatment even more complex, depression often involves more than one causative factor or biochemical change. Some of these variables, which should be addressed in a thorough patient intake, include:

- Family and personal history of any mental health issue or reproductive issue
- Family or personal history of poor outcomes on anti-depressant medications

- Family or personal history of severe fatigue, chronic fatigue syndrome or autoimmunity
- Family or personal history of cardiovascular disease or atherosclerosis
- Personal history of chronic illness, allergy or other immune deficit
- Injury, chronic pain or trauma prior to onset of depressive symptoms
- Tendencies towards OCD, ADD, ADHD, high reactivity or low tolerance to stress
- Sleep deprivation, sleep disorders or long-term shift work
- Gastrointestinal issues, dysbiosis or food sensitivities
- Adrenal insufficiency
- Hormone imbalances
- Atypical Depression (mood temporarily lifts in positive events, increased appetite or weight gain, sleeping too much but still feeling sleepy in the daytime, heavy feeling in arms or legs >1 hour daily, sensitivity to rejection or criticism, which affects your relationships, social life or job)

By investigating these potential triggers and comorbidities, we can effectively provide our patients with shortcuts to more effective treatments that target the actual cause of depressive symptoms. The first four topics involving family and personal history point to issues related to the very common genetic SNP (single nucleotide polymorphism) on the enzyme that activates folate, which plays a crucial role in inflammation and neurotransmitter formation.[i] Without folate, homocysteine (an inflammatory marker) will accumulate while methionine decreases; low methionine limits our production of glutathione which is the major antioxidant in our body, therefore reducing our ability to eliminate free radicals and other damage. This vicious cycle results in increased systemic inflammation, which needs to be addressed with anti-inflammatory measures and in the case of an MTHFR SNP, methylated folate and B vitamins.

Low methionine also leads to low SAM-e, which is a required precursor to dopamine and serotonin production.[16] Note that an SSRI (selective serotonin reuptake inhibitor) may be helpful briefly but if

i   Methylenetetrahydrofolate reductase (MTHFR)

the body does not have the ingredients to make more serotonin, then this drug will eventually fail.

Also: "Elevated homocysteine levels have been shown to be a risk factor for cardiovascular disease (CVD) and may play an etiologic role in vascular damage by promoting oxidative stress, systemic inflammation and endothelial dysfunction."[17] Finally, low folate can lead to neural tube defects or miscarriages as well as extraordinary fatigue and depression. Because the SNP is a genetic change, family history with any of these issues may indicate that it was passed down. Keep in mind, a genetic SNP may be de novo and therefore free of an incriminating family history.

And this is just the tip of the folate iceberg, as there are 1,821 folate-related genes that affect neurons, development, and brain health.[18] On the other hand, a lack of MTHFR cofactors could produce similar results, so check the nutrient status of B1, B6, and B12 if the MTHFR genes are the normal wild type (C677 and A1298). Nutrient deficiencies can lead to clinical symptoms within four months and are often caused by pregnancy, poverty, alcoholism, and medications such as metformin, oral birth control, proton-pump inhibitors, and anti-convulsants.

Next, we need to investigate the personal medical history of chronic illness, autoimmunity, or other immune deficits including the atopic triad of allergy, asthma, and eczema. The singular long-term effect of all these conditions is chronic inflammation. "Inflammatory processes have been implicated in the pathophysiology of depression. It is now well established that dysregulation of both the innate and adaptive immune systems occur in depressed patients and hinders favorable prognosis, including antidepressant responses."[19] Therefore, we need to recognize the signs of inflammation:

1. Pain: Low grade persistent pain or bouts of stronger pain levels
2. Labs: CRP > 1 mg/L predicts poor response to SSRIs and indicates inflammation; homocysteine > 15 nMol/L, Sedimentation Rate (ESR) > 13 mm/hour, Plasma Viscosity (PV) > 1.72 mPa.s, Omega 6: Omega 3 > 4:1, elevated cytokines e.g. TNF, IL6.

3. Musculoskeletal: Joint pain/stiffness, myalgias, fibromyalgia / ME
4. Allergies or sensitivities: Congestion, rhinitis, injected sclera or conjunctiva, rash, pruritus
5. Skin: Red skin/visible capillaries on cheeks, easy bruising, petechiae, bleeding gums, dark circles under the eyes, Dennie Morgan lines, dermatographia, eczema
6. Swelling: Scalloped tongue edges, indicating swollen tongue, edema or B12 deficiency, bloating, distension, swollen joints

Systemic inflammation will affect the brain if prolonged to subacute or chronic durations. Signs of brain inflammation have been described by renowned psychiatrist Dr. Mark Shukman, who first described "Tired Brain Syndrome." Symptoms include:

- Mood decline
- Anhedonia
- OCD spectrum
- Cognitive decline
- Inattention
- Fatigue
- Cravings
- Sleep changes

Inflammation in the brain occurs when "excess or prolonged inflammatory cytokine activity perturbs multiple neuronal functions, including impairment of neurotransmitter signaling, disruption of the synthesis, reuptake, and release of neurotransmitters."[20] The inflammatory cytokines, including CCL 5 and 11, and most of the Interleukins, can enter the brain when the Blood Brain Barrier (BBB) is "leaky," similar to a "leaky gut" or intestinal permeability. The breakdown in the BBB is not entirely understood but has links to injury, psychological and physical stress, EMF exposure, autoimmunity, and many other environmental insults. Dr. Tom O'Bryan elucidated many of these in his book, *You Can Heal Your Brain*. The individual cytokines have even been linked to specific symptoms. For example, sleep and appetite disturbances along with dysbiosis are all linked to elevated IL6 and CRP, while anxiety and difficulty concentrating are linked to TH17, IL17a and TNF.

Increased inflammatory markers have also been associated with atypical symptoms of depression, listed above.[21]

The good news is that blocking peripheral cytokines has been shown to "tighten the BBB and that blocking BBB disruption is sufficient to exhibit antidepressant actions."[22] Fortunately, LDN effectively modulates these cytokines from the top of the inflammation cascade to keep the immune system alert but not over-reactive. Therefore, LDN should be a cornerstone in any treatment protocol targeting systemic and central inflammation. Even mildly elevated CRP can indicate low-grade systemic inflammation which is correlated to drug-resistant depression.[23] Conversely, elevated IL6 and TNF are linked to greater chronicity and severity of depression symptoms and therefore indicate the need for longer-term LDN use and more aggressive and consistent anti-inflammatory treatments. Another study showed that Major Depressive Disorder (MDD) and inflammation were tightly linked in children who experienced specific adverse events.[24] This finding warrants a review of the ACE's questionnaire "Adverse Childhood Experiences," which could lead to life-changing root cause therapies such as EMDR.

When multiple inflammatory signs and symptoms are present, these must be addressed if we expect any depression protocol to be effective. While general anti-inflammatory measures (such as diet, LDN, and supplements) provide an immediate stopgap, the source of inflammation should be pursued and identified. This is the art and science of medicine: noticing which systems are primarily involved, identifying contributing lifestyle habits and triggers, and properly diagnosing inflammatory conditions. One example of an effective stopgap measure is to implement an anti-inflammatory diet. While there are numerous cookbooks, research articles, and online resources available on this topic now, it is only in the last decade that nutrition has been widely recognized by Western doctors as a contributing health factor. I still have patients report that their GI doctor told them they can eat whatever they want because food has no bearing on their condition. In contrast, I have witnessed patients who reversed their chronic symptoms in a matter of days by eliminating the offending food sensitivity or allergy from their diet. For 35 years, researchers have noted the effects of Red Dye #40 on brain activity and other behaviors. Excitable changes in electroencephalographic beta-band power, otherwise known as "mind storms" or bursts of brain electrical activity, have been directly connected to red dye #40 and cause symptoms such as aggression, anxiety, depression, upset stomach, migraines, jitteriness, nervousness, and inability to concentrate.[25] Long term effects of red dye #40 include allergies, notable for their chronic contribution to the inflammatory cycle. When the process is more complex than a food sensitivity, it becomes even more imperative that we continue our search for the cause of inflammation.

Injury, trauma, and chronic pain can also trigger depression due to the inflammatory responses described above. Trauma "promotes the formation of a neuroimmune pipeline in which inflammatory signaling between the brain and periphery is amplified," which could explain why depression is linked to decreased pain tolerance and increased sensitivity to stressors.[26] This is not to say that all sources of inflammation can lead to depression. Inflammation is the necessary and natural response to injury, but when it is prolonged, aberrant, or ineffective, and then combined with genetic predisposition, poor nutrition or lifestyle habits, dysbiosis, etc., unwanted sequelae can occur.

We begin to see how many psychiatric disorders are tied to inflammation which in turn responds to numerous stimuli both inside and outside of the physical body. Hence, obsessive compulsive disorder/spectrum disorder (OCSD), attention deficit disorder (ADD), and low stress tolerance may be further indications of both peripheral and central inflammation. These same behaviors are also linked to disrupted sleep cycles. Sleep-related symptoms of depression include sleep fragmentation, early morning awakening, decreased rapid eye movement (REM), sleep latency, increased REM density, and more negative dream content; therefore, a reversal of these symptoms indicates positive response to therapy.[27]

Deep sleep, also known as slow-wave sleep, is accompanied by a "pro-inflammatory endocrine milieu [of] high growth hormone and prolactin levels and low cortisol and catecholamine concentrations."[28] This occurs just before REM sleep when we have our most vivid dreams and process events of the day. We need a regular and complete 24-hour sleep cycle to promote all forms of immune cells, create a balanced immune system, and restore brain function for the next day. The numbers of undifferentiated naïve T cells and pro-inflammatory cytokines peak during early nocturnal sleep whereas circulating numbers of immune cells like cytotoxic natural killer cells, as well as anti-inflammatory cytokine activity peak during daytime wakefulness. Therefore, even one night of shift work, jet lag, or pulling an "all-nighter" can have detrimental effects on the immune system. While it is possible to "catch up on sleep," regular exposure to sleep deficits will negatively impact the immune system and increase inflammation. Assessing and treating patients for insomnia, sleep apnea, and sleep hygiene issues is another cornerstone in an effective long-term treatment plan. Short-term sedatives or melatonin may be necessary to obtain sleep while other, slower processes are implemented to reset the circadian rhythm. These might include sleep hygiene correction, herbal medicine, meditation, sleep studies, or weight loss. LDN is traditionally given at night due to the increased effects on the endogenous opioid system. This can help alleviate anxiety that keeps some people awake at night. It can also help with restless legs syndrome (RLS), possibly due to the positive effects on dopamine. Approximately 10% of LDN patients experience vivid dreams which may indicate increased levels of serotonin and dopamine or more intense and longer REM sleep.[29] All of these are positive indications of improved immune function. Restoring sleep will allow the brain to store new memories and improves its ability to collect and recall information. Deep sleep provides rest and recovery from a day of thinking, filtering, and processing. Glucose levels are restored for the next day. Deep sleep also plays a role in keeping the hormones balanced. The pituitary gland secretes human growth hormone during this stage, which helps tissues in the body grow and regenerate cells.[30]

On the topic of hormones, a lack of progesterone can create insomnia for both males and females and is easily tested with a blood sample. Sleep can also be disturbed by estrogen surges or elevated cortisol. Menopause and andropause are associated with mood changes, particularly depression, due to hormonal changes and imbalances that occur during these years. While antidepressants are often prescribed for menopausal symptoms, they may not be effective because they are not addressing the cause of the mood changes. Hormones can be balanced with bioidentical replacement, liver-supporting foods and supplements, increased exercise, meditation, and other lifestyle changes.

Thyroid hormone also has a direct relationship with mood, which is why hypothyroidism is tightly linked to depression. However, TSH is not our best indicator for mood issues due to hypothyroidism. TSH is tightly controlled by the brain and one of the last biochemical markers to indicate thyroid issues. Neither TSH levels nor treatment with T4 (levothyroxine) were associated with improvement in the Beck Depression Inventory or the Hamilton Depression Rating Scale. Interestingly, T3 has been shown in many different studies to be a viable, safe, inexpensive, and effective treatment in euthyroid patients with depression, where TSH was still within a normal range.[31] A massive meta-analysis from Israel supports the use of T3 (liothyronine) in the augmentation of tricyclic antidepressants and SSRI's. It is also effective in a specific subgroup of thyroid patients who are euthyroid but with low T3 (32% of patients) or low-normal T3 (70%). There also was a significant clinical improvement in women having lower T3 that was correlated to repletion rates. The authors noted that the conversion rate of T4 to T3 in males tends to be more efficient than in females, so the greater recovery rate in males may be a secondary effect of their metabolism. No correlation was found between free T4 levels and depression severity or recovery. Less evidence is available to support the use of T4 for depression or, when it was included in the trials, it was not as effective.[32] The abundance of research on thyroid hormones and depression indicates that free T3 testing should always be included in an initial workup for patients experiencing low mood. I also add free T4, looking for a respective ratio of 1:3, along with autoimmune antibodies and Reverse T3. If RT3 is elevated, adrenal support, stress management, anti-inflammatory protocols, and sleep hygiene correction are all warranted. If antibodies are present, LDN and ashwagandha can help reduce the overactive immune response of those antibodies. In my experience, many patients undergoing T3 repletion will require a sustained release formula to mitigate a potential spike of anxiety, tachycardia, and nervousness due to the immediate bioactivity of T3.

Another often overlooked hormone is vitamin D, which is activated internally and then circulated to specific cells and tissues to produce a specific action. It helps up-regulate the immune system, providing defense against everything from viruses to cancer cells. Deficiency is linked not only to bone loss, but also to sleep disruption. People with clinically low vitamin D (< 20 ng/ml) had a significantly increased risk of poor sleep quality, short sleep duration, and daytime sleepiness.[33] We have already seen the detrimental effects of poor sleep on the immune system, brain function, and inflammation. Patients who are clinically low in vitamin D will benefit from a series of high dose injections followed by oral D3. In my experience, these patients usually feel an improved sense of well-being within a week or two.

Nutrients obviously play a significant role in every facet we have discussed, from neurotransmitter production to the activation of folate and vitamin D. Therefore, an assessment of gut health, food intake, and micronutrient status via testing is another vital step in creating an effective treatment plan for drug-resistant depression. Food sensitivities by definition cause inflammation from the B-cell mediated humoral immune response, usually in the form of IgG or IgA antibodies. Suspect food sensitivities if symptoms come and go with unexplained triggers. Symptoms range from brain fog and nasal congestion to joint pain and digestive upset. The difficulty in identifying the cause is that sensitivities have a delayed response up to 72 hours after intake of the offending item. The most efficient way to determine sensitivities is to take a blood test for IgG, IgA, and C3D responses to a large list of foods. While this can be a costly test, it is simple, quick, and accurate.

We know how to assess for nutrient status, inflammation, and the offending proteins. The last frontier is the microbiome of the gut, whose ailments are the subject of prolific research and literature on topics ranging from SIBO and IBS/IBD to a lack of biodiversity and the benefits of each strain of bacteria. A poor microbiome has been correlated to diabetes, dementia, depression, and cancer—and we know that the gut houses about 70% of our immune cells. So, if it's not healthy, our immune system is not healthy. Additionally, the gut bacteria produce the neurotransmitters serotonin, dopamine, and GABA, all of which play a key role in mood regulation. Gut health can be assessed clinically for non-infectious issues and treated with amino acids, herbs, and nutrients known to heal the gut and tonify function. For more obvious or severe gastrointestinal issues, lab testing is warranted. Even if GI symptoms are not overtly present, be aware of medical history red flags such as abdominal surgery, chronic constipation, or frequent antibiotic use. Any of these situations indicates a need for a proven gut healing protocol. Some of my most-used supplements include zinc carnosine, aloe vera, slippery elm, cat's claw, l-glutamine, marshmallow, colostrum, and probiotics. Of course, IBD was one of the early recipients of positive research on LDN and gut health.

The plethora of contributing factors to drug-resistant depression can be overwhelming. Start by listening to the patient and identifying fragile body systems and possible inflammatory triggers. Investigate root causes. Eradicate superfluous inflammation. Heal the gut. Make sure they sleep. Show them how to obtain adequate nutrition. While most medications are not helpful in the cases described here, remember the value of liothyronine, vitamin D, hormone replacement (or restoration), and LDN. All of these can directly treat the root cause of drug resistant depression and likely spare your patient significant expenditures of time, money, and suffering through side effects of medications that won't work for them anyway.

THREE

Treating Virally Damaged Tissues with LDN

SARAH J. ZIELSDORF, MD, MS

The origins of the Great Influenza of 1918 are still being studied. As a physician and microbiologist interested in the history of infectious diseases, I integrate research findings on pandemics of the past with those of emerging infectious diseases. Simply put, an important way to anticipate the future is to understand the past. In this chapter, I will briefly compare and contrast (a) viral illnesses, (b) their damage to cells and tissues, as well as (c) the use of LDN to help promote healing of virally damaged cells, tissues, and organs. Throughout, I will provide a set of therapeutic goals, which I use to treat acute, progressive, and long-term viral illnesses, as well as their autoimmune sequelae. In addition, I have highlighted in bold type several key concepts for clinicians to consider. At the end of the chapter, I provide a list of commonly used antiviral therapeutics.

In 2002, Severe Acute Respiratory Syndrome Coronavirus 1 (SARS-CoV-1), a novel zoonotic infection (animal-to-human) emerged in China. Countries were able to successfully contain this viral pathogen in 2004, because nearly all known CoV-1 patients were symptomatic (e.g. high fever and cough), during its period of transmission.[34] This made individuals infected with CoV-1 easy to identify, and isolate.

Over 8000 individuals died from CoV-1, a virus found in certain bat colonies as well as in civet cats. However, bats are not typically harmed by CoV-1 (an epidemiologic term known as a "reservoir"). The main mode of transmission in the 2002 SARS-CoV-1 outbreak was via respiratory droplet inhalation. However, there were documented super-spreader events of CoV-1 involving fecal-oral or even fecal-aerosol transmission.[35]

During my graduate training in public health in 2006, highly pathogenic avian influenza emerged. The expected pandemic of H5N1 bird flu never materialized, however. Large poultry culls helped curb the transmission of the virus into human populations.[36] During this time, I participated in pandemic preparedness tabletop exercises, which were undertaken in Washington, D.C. The Strategic National Stockpile in the United States became a focus for adding personal protective equipment (PPE) including over 52 million surgical masks and 104 million N95 air-filtration masks during this time.

A subsequent severe influenza, the 2009 H1N1 swine flu pandemic, resulted in a tremendous demand for N95 respirators and face masks among health professionals; subsequent disparity between supply and demand resulted in a nearly three-year backlog, as well as pervasive shortages in the marketplace. Due to this, significant supply chain analyses and strategies for understanding the complexities in the manufacturing, distribution, and ordering for PPE, were undertaken. It was understood that supply of PPE involved many manufacturers and distributors. However, these supply distribution problems were never clearly addressed or solved, though they were occasionally revisited in the intervening decade (such as during the heightened intensity of PPE demand during the 2014 Ebola virus disease response).[37]

During 2020, it was unsettling to witness health care workers without appropriate PPE during SARS-CoV-2 (COVID-19), thus dramatically increasing their risk of occupational exposure. Since 2020, my clinical practice interests have been focused on finding ways to reduce viral attachment and colonization through use of the prophylactic nasal sprays, mouthwashes, or liquids, for health care workers and other high-risk populations.

Once-in-a-Century Plague

For as long as human civilization has existed, people have congregated into communities, increasing the risk of widespread epidemics. Virologists trained in the 20th century knew that a clock was ticking. They anticipated that a new scourge of biblical proportions would eventually appear. We were exceedingly lucky for 102 years. We know that the description of COVID-19 as being a "once-in-a-century plague" is fundamentally flawed. Human societies are increasingly vulnerable to "traveler-borne" pandemics. Rapidly moving and closely interacting, humans are the primary vector of modern human pandemics.

Deadly pandemics occur frequently. Rapid implementation of public health measures helps stop their spread. Comparison of the COVID-19 pandemic with the four waves of the 1918-1920 influenza pandemic has been overly politicized by governments as well as oversimplified in various media. It is well-known that humans have experienced multiple flu pandemics during the last 100 years. During this time, the world has gotten smaller and smaller. Humans now share an immune bubble with all other humans, which is hours wide. A major catalyst for the horrific mortality rate of the 1918 influenza was World War I and the United States' shipment of many thousands of soldiers to fight in Europe, who helped to spread the virus throughout the world at an unprecedented rate.[38] In my hometown of Chicago, Illinois, over a million people are only one non-stop flight away from potential animal reservoirs harboring the next hemorrhagic fever virus in Africa, a zoonotic pathogen in an open market in Asia, or a new COVID variant arising somewhere in the Americas.

During most of my adult life, the threat of a coming pandemic has never been far from my mind. As a microbiology graduate student at The George Washington University, I researched how to improve laboratory emergency preparedness in the wake of the 2001 anthrax attacks in the United States.[39] I helped to train microbiology laboratory staff at The GWU Hospital on potential bioterrorist (BT) agent identification, as well as helped develop protocols for BT identification and containment.

The other major reason for the deadliest flu pandemic in recent history was its ability to rapidly kill the strongest, healthiest population: young adults. This is because of the ability for the virus to set off a dramatic reaction leading to the massive systemic inflammatory response known as "cytokine storm" by the affected persons' immune system, and secondary bacterial infection of the lungs which lead to people in the prime of their lives unable to breathe and drowning on dry land. Cytokines are small cell signaling proteins that are directly responsible for modulating the immune system. The H1N1 "Spanish flu" of 1918 was also an avian influenza. Previous and most subsequent flu pandemics have had a U-shaped mortality curve (most deaths occur in the very young and very old), while 1918 yielded a W-shaped mortality curve. Upwards of 50 to even 100 million deaths have been cited worldwide, a figure dwarfing the up to 40 million killed during "The War to End All Wars," as reported by the US Department of War in 1924 and amended by the Office of the Secretary of Defense in 1957.

The four genera of influenza viruses (A-D) in the family Orthomyxoviridae include the influenza A and B varieties that are associated with the annual seasonal epidemics. Emergence of radically different viruses, which have periodically been responsible for other significant worldwide flu pandemics (1957, 1968) are because of the different combinations of surface proteins on the influenza virus, called hemagglutinin (HA) and neuraminidase (NA). Influenza pandemics occur when combinations of HA and NA subtypes affect large populations of humanity whose immune systems have never seen this virus. Regarding influenza viruses, there are two major processes responsible for the recombining and mutations that are constantly occurring. The first is antigenic drift, whereby frequent point mutations in the viral genome cause minor changes in the RNA, which can alter the genes in regions of the HA and/or NA proteins. This does cause reduced immunity in previously exposed populations. The more significant process is antigenic shift: the complete exchange of HA and/or NA genes. This only occurs in influenza A viruses because of the more extensive known animal reservoirs for the virus, namely swine and avian sources, to incubate antigenically distinct viruses (antigens are substances that cause immune system responses). When antigenic shift occurs, a pandemic can occur due to a population's complete immunologic naivety toward the virus, with devastating results.[40, 41]

History Repeats Itself

"Those that fail to learn from history are doomed to repeat it," is a quote often attributed to Winston Churchill that may actually be a misquotation of philosopher George Santayana's comment, "Those who cannot remember the past are condemned to repeat it." [42] The unfolding of the last twenty months (December, 2021 at the time of this writing) of the COVID-19 pandemic has illustrated this phrase on a nearly daily basis by the actions of people, institutions, governing bodies, and the leaders of most countries and major cities worldwide.

The game changer of SARS CoV-2 lies in its transmission during an asymptomatic or pre-symptomatic infectious period. Emerging variants have yielded ever more infectivity and questionable reduction in burden of disease as time has passed. The true magnitude of the sequelae of the pandemic will not be revealed for decades to come. The questions that must be asked include which cocktails of "hard pharma" therapeutics (agents with major side-effect profiles) and "soft pharma" (neutraceutical supplements, vitamins, minerals, etc.) are effective in reducing infectivity, viral carriage, viral transmission, morbidity, and mortality, for a complicated and poorly understood foe.

Failures to Diagnose and Treat Chronic Viral Infections

Medicine in the twentieth century frequently ignored many chronic infections. The procedure known as differential diagnosis in medicine became inappropriately focused on diagnosing physiologic versus psychological conditions. Only recently have we begun to piece together how a chronic inflammatory and immunologic response to a pathogen (virus or bacterium, for example), can be responsible for illness, even decades after the initial infection.

Encephalitis lethargica (also known as chronic fatigue syndrome, or CFS), was one of the greatest medical mysteries of the twentieth century. CFS is now recognized as being a consequence of many long-term infectious diseases, as well as their autoimmune sequelae. We now know that cerebrospinal fluid contains pro-inflammatory cytokines IL-1, IL-6, and TNF-alpha. These individual cytokines are responsible for the classical "sickness behaviors" of fatigue, malaise, and weakness omnipresent in CFS.[43, 44]

The neurological syndrome known as encephalitis lethargica was recognized in 1916 but likely emerged in 1915 in Romania, spread by soldiers in WWI. It spread from that time through the 1930s and is thought to affect over a million people worldwide.[45]

This condition has been classified into acute and chronic phases, including an influenza-like prodrome, hypersomnolence, wakeability, ophthalmoplegia (palsy of cranial nerves affecting the eye muscles and pupillary reflexes), and psychiatric changes. In the past, patients that survived were left with permanent neurologic disorders including the near complete loss of movement in some cases (akinesis). The chronic phase, best described as a form of Parkinsonism, was marked by a latent period of months or even years. The acute and chronic forms could overlap and be rapid in occurrence, leading to death for some patients. During the epidemic period, about 9,000 academic papers were published describing the overlapping psychiatric and neurological conditions, which, while varied, often included marked and persistent lethargy. In 1918 the British epidemiologist F.G. Crookshank identified several historical epidemics that resembled encephalitis lethargica, including the English sweats (England, 1529), *mal mazzuco* (Italy, 1597), *Kriebelkrankheit* (Germany, 1672–75), *Rafania* (Sweden, 1754–57), and *nona* (Italy, 1890–91).[46]

Using encephalitis lethargica as a broader example of a syndrome with varied but discrete presentations, we have a model for how other epidemics may have caused other chronic disease states formerly thought to be psychological or termed "functional disorders." Acute encephalitis lethargica's most common form was known as "somnolent-ophthalmoplegic," whereby patients would experience a gradual onset of flu-like symptoms (malaise, low-grade fever, headache, vertigo, and vomiting), followed by delirium, a sign of meningitis. Cranial nerve palsies and pupillary abnormalities were common, and then patients would sleep for abnormally long time periods. However, they were easily awakened and were aware of everything that had occurred during their semi-catatonic state. The next most common presentation was the hyperkinetic form: an initial manic phase consisting of abnormal movements (chorea), vocalizations, and involuntary muscle movements (myoclonus), followed by restlessness, weakness, and fatigue. A hypomanic phase followed consisting of neuralgic pain in the face and extremities, hallucinations involving vision and touch, and circadian rhythm dysfunction. The least common type of encephalitis lethargica was the amyostatic-akinetic form, whereby patients developed rigidity and inability to move without known weakness. There were no mental deficits, though they could not show emotion on their faces (masked faces).[47]

The chronic phase was best characterized as Parkinson-like, but there was a prevalence of sleep disturbances, ocular abnormalities, involuntary movements, respiratory problems, and speech and psychiatric disorders. Up to 30 years following the Great Influenza pandemic, it was estimated that up to 50% of Parkinsonism occurred after inflammation of the brain (postencephalitic).[48]

The brilliant neurologist and humanist Dr. Oliver Sacks, whose book Awakenings (1973) was made into the 1990 film starring the late Robin Williams and Robert De Niro, called postencephalitic patients living in a New York nursing home "extinct volcanoes," which illustrated the chronic effects of encephalitis lethargica many decades after the initial infection. The movie beautifully depicts the "extinct volcanos" who "erupted into life" with L-DOPA treatment after they had "long been regarded, and regarded themselves, as effectively dead."[49]

The search for the specific cause of encephalitis lethargica has been without clear evidence for one pathogen, including influenza. However, the influenza strains that caused the H1N1 pandemic of 1918 disappeared from circulation prior to 1933, which is a plausible reason for the disappearance of the condition. During the pandemic, animal experiments were undertaken to inject bodily tissues and fluids from encephalitis lethargica patients; no recognized strain of virus was found, though a theory was put forth that it was either a herpes virus or a focal brain infection from streptococcal bacteria.[50]

Encephalitis lethargica as a model of a post-infectious autoimmune disorder gained traction in the twenty-first century. One model of post-infectious autoimmune disease resembling the hyperkinetic form of encephalitis lethargica is anti-NMDA receptor encephalitis, which begins in the same way with a flu-like illness. It can happen that due to molecular mimicry, viral components mimic human tissues—in this case, the NMDA receptors in the brain. Another example are antibodies against cellular water-channels which affect ability to control pressure and fluid balance in the brain (antibodies against aquaporin-4 in the hypothalamus). Epidemiologic case reports affirm these hypotheses with the observation that during the 2009 H1H1 influenza pandemic there were increases in cases of narcolepsy following influenza infection or influenza vaccination.[51] The overall hypothesis is that chronic neuro-inflammation post-infection, tissue-specific antigen-antibody mediated destruction, and, after a latent period, neurodegeneration, occurs leading to a specific central nervous system diagnosis such as Parkinson's disease, multiple sclerosis, or amyotrophic lateral sclerosis (ALS). Will we have millions of chronically affected, critically neurologically compromised individuals due to chronic autoimmune-mediated inflammation in the next several decades post COVID?[52]

Non-Predictive vs. Predictive Clinical Epistemologies

"Long-COVID," or "post-infectious COVID," is facing a broken epistemology of differential diagnosis and therapeutic assessments. Epistemology is asking the question: "how do we know what we know?" I have treated many patients suffering residual effects of their COVID-19 infection, as well as others who have sustained flare-ups of either known autoimmune conditions or new immunologic dysfunction post-vaccination. These "long-haulers" have faced a veritable gaslighting by some members of the medical community, who initially labelled many long-COVID conditions as functional, psychological disorders, never considering immunologically mediated mechanisms for long-COVID symptoms. This is only one of the barriers to treating these patients.

It is human nature not to accept new evidence. In the past, the medical community was exceptionally cruel. Take for instance the case of Dr. Ignaz Semmelweis (1818–1865), a Hungarian obstetrician who showed that nearly all cases of childbed fever (puerperal fever) were caused by bacteria introduced to the birth canal by the medical attendant. In those days physicians would go directly from an autopsy performed with unwashed and ungloved hands to delivering a mother. After a friend, the forensic pathologist Professor Kolletschka, died after a student accidentally cut Kolletschka's finger during an autopsy, Semmelweis observed that Kolletschka's autopsy findings were identical to those of the mothers that died from childbed fever, and that the cause must be due to "cadaveric particles." The solution became clear to him to require physicians and midwives to wash their hands in a chlorine solution, which was found to be the most efficient way to remove the smells that were left on the hands. Semmelweis showed that mothers had a much higher mortality rate in the First Division because medical students/ physicians participated in autopsies but the midwives in the Second Division did not. When he required staff to use the chlorine solution and employed strict handwashing protocols for the obstetrics wards, maternal mortality fell in the hospital he ran to less than one percent compared to the 10-15% childbed fever mortality rates at other hospitals in Prague and Vienna in the 1850s. He was met with strong resistance from administrators and colleagues alike and was refused further development of his career. He died having not been professionally vindicated for his theories of aseptic technique after admission to an insane asylum. He was likely beaten while trying to escape and succumbed to his infected wounds at the age of 47.[53]

Original thinkers often must weather the storms previously faced by those like Semmelweis. We are on the precipice of another revolution of original thought in chronic disease medicine, which as the German philosopher Arthur Schopenhauer stated, goes through three stages of truth:

1. It is ridiculed
2. It is systematically opposed
3. It is accepted as being self-evident

A landmark study from July 2021 illustrates the profound shift in scientific understanding of the pathophysiology of chronic conditions such as fibromyalgia, which is a pain syndrome characterized by widespread tender points, profound sleep disturbance and fatigue, chronic musculoskeletal pain, and often cognitive dysfunction. It has been shown that there is an inflammatory component and there was a theory of autoantibody formation against components of the central nervous system and the peripheral nerves. This study showed that antibodies (IgG) from fibromyalgia patients injected into mice produced hypersensitivity reactions by sensitizing nociceptive (pain-sensing) neurons. This means that the mice became more sensitive to mechanical and cold stimulation, with the corresponding nerve fibers also showing heightened responsiveness to cold and mechanical stimulation. In addition, these mice did not move as well, had decreased grip strength, and underwent changes in the nervous system wiring of their skin cells.

The objective findings after passive transfer of serum from fibromyalgia patients to mice show that an autoimmune-mediated process underlies the characteristic tenderness and thermal hypersensitivities experienced by patients.[54] Fibromyalgia is real, and is physiologic in etiology. It has never been a psychosomatic illness. How can we distinguish between physiological maladies: infectious, inflammatory, autoimmune?

Polymicrobial Infections During COVID

Since the start of the pandemic in 2020, clinicians have noted the highly variable presentation of cases, depending on viral load, age, comorbidities, and the variant causing the infection itself. We have seen a variety of viral-mediated reactivations associated with COVID infections, such as oral cavity lesions and inflammation of fingers and toes, and skin rashes (due to a variety of latent herpes viruses).[55, 56] My colleagues and I now look at COVID infections as "COVID+ A, B, C,...", a reference to the myriad potential infections influencing a patient's clinical course with their illness. We have coined these conditions "Polygenic-CytoPathologies," cellular pathologies that affect the expression of many different genes.

How then, are we to treat COVID (or chronic viral infections/ reactivations) utilizing this point of view? We must take an "Organelle-Centric Medicine" stance, and even get to sub-cellular components. We must address chronically inflamed and potentially auto-reactive cells. It all boils down to this: virally impacted organelles.

Aberrant Cytoarchitectures in Virally Impacted Cells

Profound cellular injury occurs due to a severe case of COVID-19. As the central component, we have DNA damage that can occur. Evolutionarily speaking, there is an important protective mechanism known as chromatin to allow cells to withstand genotoxic stress. Chromatin is the fiber that makes up a chromosome and consists of DNA and protein. DNA is responsible for the cell's genetic instructions. Histones are the proteins in chromatin, which act to package the DNA in a highly compact way so that it fits in the cell's nucleus (brain of the cell). Chromatin structure changes according to needs for replication of DNA and gene expression. The term heterochromatin refers to more highly condensed chromatin, which is unable to be accessed for transcription of the DNA to RNA. Euchromatin is loosely structured chromatin that is considered active for transcription, the first part of active DNA replication. We now know that chromatin will dramatically change its structure in response to DNA damage not only if it is local, but also if it occurs anywhere in the genome. Nucleosomes are the basic repeating unit of chromatin, and equal about 150 base pairs of DNA wrapped around a core of eight histone proteins.[57] These nucleosome-histone complexes come in many different varieties, due to many variants and modifications to the structure, which enables much more genetic (how genes affect us) and epigenetic (how environmental triggers affect gene expression) individuality. Different signals can be added to the "tails" of histones, which stick out from the nucleosome, much like the flags on a mailbox. These modifications are considered "post-translational," that is, they occur after DNA is transcribed to RNA and RNA is translated to an active message: protein. These involve adding small organic compounds including acetylation, methylation, phosphorylation, and ubiquitination to the histone tails. Histone modification is paramount for chromatin remodeling and gene expression.[58]

Episomes are circular genetic components inside the host cell's nucleus that are closely associated with, but not integrated into, the host cell's chromosomes.[59] Insulators are DNA-protein complexes, which have been defined experimentally as having the ability to block enhancer-promoter interactions and/or serve as barriers against the spreading of heterochromatin's effect to silence gene expression.[60] Enhancers and silencers (also known as insulators), are regulatory sequences that, as their name suggests, are short amino acid sequences which, respectively, activate their target genes and/or silence gene expression/confine gene expression within defined boundaries of chromatin.[61]

Methylation is the process whereby genes are turned on or off. Viral infections, including COVID-19, have been shown to significantly affect methylation signaling, thereby acting as epigenetic controls of gene expression. Research is ongoing to identify methylation signals, which can portend severe disease, hospitalization, and death due to COVID-19.[62] Practically, methyl groups (or "methyl donors") come from B vitamins including B6 (pyridoxine), B9 (folate), and B12 (cobalamin). Over 50% of the human population has single nucleotide polymorphisms, or SNPs, which can hinder a person's ability to effectively provide methyl donors in the folate cycle, and may require specific supplementation to optimize.[63] Herpesvirus genomes exist and replicate as episomes inside the host cell nucleus during latent infection. Chiu et al.[64] find that unlike Epstein–Barr virus, which partitions viral genomes faithfully during cell division, Kaposi's Sarcoma–associated herpesvirus clusters viral genomes into loci that are distributed unequally to daughter cells.

Due to any insult, injured organelles (the subcellular organ components of the cell) will be poorly functioning and may be threatened. With respect to viral infections, membrane-bound organelles are targeted individually and specifically, and are themselves required for viruses to survive in cells. Viruses are parasitic pieces of genetic material (DNA or RNA), and thus, cannot survive on their own. The steps of a viral life cycle utilize different organelles of the cell by hijacking the host's own cellular machinery, starting with cellular reorganization and alteration of many host proteins. The viral life cycle includes entry, translation, replication, assembly, and egress. Organelles including the mitochondria (energy producers), endoplasmic reticulum (some functions include protein and lipid synthesis, calcium regulation), and peroxisomes (involved in fatty acid metabolism and metabolism of toxic reactive oxygen species) are important for the innate immune system (first responders) against viral infections.[65]

Thus, a taxed immune system due to successful viral infection in the setting of injured cellular components and systemic inflammation leads to further impairments. In the central nervous system, the correlates include injured neurons and non-neuronal cells called glia. One kind of glial cell is the microglia, or the specialized macrophages (cell-eating immune cell) in the central nervous system. Low dose naltrexone (LDN) is an important target for microglial immunomodulation. The concern is that when microglia are activated due to a chronic inflammatory process, it cannot be stopped. The microglia burn hotter and brighter until they die, a process that can lead to neurodegenerative conditions as previously discussed. An important study by Dr. Jared Younger on fibromyalgia patients using LDN showed that greater pain relief/benefit correlated with higher erythrocyte sedimentation rate (ESR) levels, showing that patients with more inflammation have more improvement given LDN's mechanism of anti-inflammatory and immunomodulatory effects.[66]

The pathogenesis of fibromyalgia has shown altered brain activity patterns, chronic glia activation in the brain, impairment-conditioned pain modulation and widespread hypersensitivity to a variety of stimuli. This underscores the neuroplasticity achieved in this chronic condition leading to pervasive altered central nervous system functioning. Of note, the peripheral nervous system is also altered via autoimmune processes, i.e., small-fiber nerve changes and altered cytokine levels.[67] How can we attenuate this vicious cycle of tissue injury and proinflammatory cytokine production? Answer: Utilize the anti-inflammatory metabolites of vitamin D.

Calcifediol Therapy (25 hydroxyvitaminD) for COVID

A tremendous difficulty during the COVID-19 pandemic has been the reliance on meta-analyses and randomized controlled trials, which are considered the gold standard in peer-reviewed scientific research and evidence-based medicine. Meta-analyses often fail to account for the pleomorphic nature of viral infections, which requires a multifaceted and individualized approach.

Vitamin D is a steroid hormone that binds to VDR (vitamin D receptor), a steroid/thyroid hormone nuclear receptor, which has been identified on many immune cells. The immune benefits of the active form of vitamin D—1,25(OH)2D3, or calcitriol (CTR)—are innumerable. Thousands of genes are upregulated from calcitriol, and powerful immune modulation and regulation has led to the study of using active vitamin D metabolites in the treatment of immune dysfunction, such as autoimmune diseases or cancer. Much of what we know from animal models has previously involved renal disease, since calcitriol plays a central role in the regulation of calcium and phosphorus.[68]

Of significant note is that several independent researcher-clinicians have shown that chronic renal failure patients have a survival benefit in their risk of hospitalization and death from COVID, likely due to their treatment with calcitriol for secondary hyperparathyroidism and hypocalcemia. A Spanish study determined that calcitriol use, prior to COVID infection, statistically reduced risk of severe COVID-19, as well as COVID-19 mortality, in patients with advanced chronic kidney disease (CKD). It also found an inverse association between the mean daily calcitriol dose and COVID-19 severity or mortality in treated patients, independently of renal function.[69]

The active immune hormone, calcitriol, is fundamentally different from the nutrient Vitamin D (cholecalciferol). Critics of vitamin D supplementation for COVID often discuss the failure of vitamin D3 (cholecalciferol) supplementation to show improvements in COVID-19 morbidity and mortality. Vitamin D3 must be activated in the liver to calcifefiol (25-hydroxyvitamin D), which is then converted in the kidney to the active form, calcitriol. The crux of the argument to use active vitamin D metabolites (calcifidiol does not have the same risk of hyperparathyroidism as sustained calcitriol supplementation in a non-end stage renal failure or late-stage chronic kidney disease patient) is that the virus hijacks the immune system's ability to convert to the active metabolites of vitamin D. The key intervention is to attack the dysfunction on VDRs in COVID and autoimmune patients, which lies downstream of regular over-the-counter vitamin D3 supplementation. Up to half of patients hospitalized with COVID-19 have acute kidney injury (AKI). Interventions with calcitriol have shown improvement in glucose tolerance and lipid metabolism in CKD patients as well.[70] The mechanism for this is that patients with kidney disease or an acute infection have reduced activity of the enzyme 1-alpha hydroxylase, which converts the intermediate 25-OH D3 (calcifediol) to its active form (1,25(OH)2D3, calcitriol).[71] To summarize: a deficit in calcitriol plus inhibition of calcitriol conversion is a huge problem. Herein lies the rationale for active vitamin D metabolite therapies, including an easily procured over-the-counter calcifediol supplement. The inhibitor of calcitriol is fibroblast growth factor-23 (FGF-23), which inhibits 1-alpha-hydroxylase gene expression. This causes metabolic shunting of the active forms of vitamin D to the inactive metabolites (24,25D and 1,24,25D), by increasing a different enzyme, 24-hydroxylase, which is induced by FGF-23.[72,73]

More studies demonstrate that calcitriol upregulates VDR expression in the lungs of mice infected with influenza.[74] There are many additional potential benefits of calcitriol therapy for COVID patients. Antimicrobial peptides (AMPs), small pieces of immune boosting proteins are secreted from cells in response to VDR-activation.[75] Calcitriol also mediates the activation of defensins, which are naturally produced antimicrobial agents including LL-37 (Human cathelicidin), beta-defensin 2, and hepcidin.[76]

The role of the microbiome has been neglected in COVID treatment. Calcitriol improves gut innate immunity, which has secondary benefits for the CNS, enteric, and autonomic nervous systems.[77, 78] We are dealing with multiple infectious agents in COVID-immunocompromised patients. Multiple organelles are malfunctioning. Hormones are not being secreted and thus, there are major endocrine imbalances. Active vitamin D metabolites such as calcifediol and calcitriol prevent latent viral gene reactivation and re-silence those that are reactivated. COVID-19 is really a case of polymicrobial sepsis—multiple infections that can lead to an acute systemic inflammatory response and multi-system organ failure. As active vitamin D metabolites can also modulate the adaptive immune system (improving activation of T cells), this is exceptionally important to advanced cancer patients undergoing immunotherapy, autoimmune patients, and those battling an acute infection.[79] In order to treat the patient we must simultaneously neutralize multiple viral and bacterial toxins.

CoV-2 Spike-Protein Has Multiple Cytotoxic Actions

High levels of serum FGF-23 and spike protein S1-fragments are two key pathogenic agents that will depress the calcitriol/VDR-signaling axis, leading to hyper-inflammation and immunodeficiencies in COVID infection. Clinical research needs to shift focus to suppressing/mitigating the endocrine/immunologic impacts of high levels of FGF-23 and S1-fragments in COVID-infected patients. Spike-protein (also known as S-protein, or "Spike") promotes hyper-inflammation via ACE-2 receptor (angiotensin-converting enzyme) binding and inactivation, which normally acts in an anti-inflammatory way.[80]

Pathogenesis of COVID-19 is associated with a hyper-inflammatory response. Recent studies have demonstrated that spike (S) protein potently induces inflammatory cytokines and chemokines including IL-6, IL-1ß, TNFa, CXCL1, CXCL2, and CCL2, via activation of the NF-κB pathway (a major pro-inflammatory response). This activation was found not to happen in toll-like receptor 2 (TLR2)-deficient macrophages. Toll-like receptors are proteins that act to recognize pathogens. Together these data reveal a potential mechanism for the "cytokine storm" during severe SARS-CoV-2 infections and suggest that TLR2 inhibition could be a potential therapeutic target for COVID-19.[81] It is known that TLR2 and TLR4 are both blocked by LDN. Experimental rat models of multiple sclerosis (induction of experimental autoimmune encephalopathy, or EAE) demonstrate hippocampal neuro-inflammation and associated paralysis, pain, and cognitive deficits. These effects were ameliorated by using naltrexone (clinical correlation: LDN), which is a relevant blood brain barrier (BBB)-permeable TLR2/TLR4 antagonist. Targeted TLR blockade prevents autoimmunity-mediated pathology. TLR4 is a potent mediator of lipopolysaccharide (LPS), also known as endotoxin in the gut, the most immune-reactive/systemic inflammation driving antigens in existence.[82, 83] Spike protein fragments binds to LPS and potentiates its highly pro-inflammatory activity.[84] Spike protein components also induce hyper-coagulation and microclotting in the lungs and vasculature of COVID-19 patients. We can call the S1 component an inflammagen, and it may interfere directly with blood flow. Spike protein-S1 fragment can cause structural changes in proteins related to the complement cascade (process whereby blood clots) including fibrinogen, complement 3, and prothrombin when added to platelet-poor plasma, as well as prevent the dissolution of clots (a process called fibrinolysis).[85] Finally, spike proteins are superantigenic. This may cause an accelerated and excessive immune response due to directly binding to T cell receptors, a hyper-inflammatory syndrome resembling toxic shock syndrome (TSS) in pediatric severe COVID-19 patients called MIS-C (multisystem inflammatory syndrome in children).[86]

The spike-protein S1-fragment can be viewed as a pleiotropic, "viral exotoxin." The S1-toxin (S1x) has cytotoxic actions similarities to the cytotoxicity of certain snake venom proteins. Immunity to S1x has two primary sources: Nabs (neutralizing antibodies) and AMPs. People with adequate calcitriol levels will likely have a larger pool of AMPs in the serum and tissues and will be better equipped to neutralize the S1-toxin (S1x). AMPs (e.g. LL-37, defensins) that bind S1x will become depleted, owing to the high concentration of S1x that can be generated in progressive COVID. Depletion of AMPs could set the stage for secondary opportunistic bacterial and fungal infections. The key to reduced S1x pathogenesis may be to boost AMPs early in COVID infections, using calcifediol and/ or calcitriol supplements with the goal of boosting innate immune defenses (particularly increasing levels of neutralizing AMPs).[87] While there is no major sex difference in viral or bacterial toxins, there is a major sex difference in the sequelae of viral and bacterial illnesses, and that connects to autoimmunity.

Sex Differences in Viral Reactivation and Autoimmune Expression

COVID infection reactivates dormant viruses. In female mammals with two X chromosomes, one of the X chromosomes in a cell will be inactivated, and the chromatin condensed into what is known as a Barr body. Barr bodies may accumulate more dormant viruses because they contain great masses of heterochromatin. Viruses integrate near heterochromatin sites to become latent. Research is focused on understanding whether Barr bodies are prevalent in certain breast and ovarian cancers. Errors in cellular replication can cause the loss of the inactive X chromosome, but the compromise of Barr body heterochromatin in some cancers may signal broader deficits of nuclear heterochromatin. Viral infections can drive heterochromatic instability, which may lead to widespread genomic dysregulation and the evolution of some cancers.[88]

Studies have looked at the genetics of fruit flies but found no evidence that X chromosome or sex determination pathways are controlling the regulation of autosomal (non-sex chromosomes).[89] A conjecture for yet another reason why women are more susceptible to autoimmunity is the presence of the Barr body itself. A small population of women with autoimmune disease may carry autoantibodies against one or more components of the Barr body.[90] This is highly significant as it pertains to the reactivation of dormant viruses such as Epstein-Barr.

Epstein-Barr Virus and other Herpes Virus Reactivations

Epstein-Barr virus (EBV), a gamma herpes virus known as human herpes virus-4 (HHV-4) and the causative agent of infectious mononucleosis, is one of eight human herpes viruses. It is known that herpes viruses are ubiquitous in the human population. Over 95% of all adults have had EBV. All herpes viruses establish lifelong latency and can reactivate and also infect others. Maintaining a latent infection is extremely complicated and requires multiple steps including:

    a. Maintaining the herpes viral genome in the nucleus of the cells.

b. Ensuring the herpes viral genomes are divided appropriately to dividing cells known as daughter cells.

c. Limiting protein expression so as not to attract recognition by the host immune system.

d. Suppression of lytic gene expression (active virus that would kill host cells during replicative cycles) by producing non-coding viral RNA.

e. Epigenetic modulation of the viral genome to regulate viral gene expression.

f. Reactivation opportunistically to infect other hosts.

Prescription antiviral therapies reduce active infection by preventing viral replication but do not eliminate latency. The future of latent herpes viral infections and/or reactivations depends on mechanisms of latency itself. Novel approaches to destroy latently infected cells or inhibit reactivation from latency involve fundamental understanding of the mechanisms involved in development of this complex process.[91]

At least a third of COVID-19 patients continue to be affected by long-term symptoms after recovering from acute infection. I have correctly observed this phenomenon in my own clinic. These symptoms vary from chronic fatigue or brain fog, to sleep difficulties, joint and/or musculoskeletal pain, chronic sore throats, headaches, intermittent fevers, gastrointestinal abnormalities (bloating, constipation, diarrhea), and a variety of skin rashes and evidence of viral reactivations in oral mucosa or skin. Each long-COVID patient has a completely unique presentation all their own. Of note, each symptom of long-COVID is also a symptom of EBV reactivation. Because EBV infects both epithelial cells and B cells, it efficiently causes skin eruptions/rashes and exacerbations or flares of underlying autoimmune conditions. It is tricky to detect a true reactivation of EBV, and multiple serologic tests are often required. EBV can switch between lytic and latent phases of its life cycles often in the same patient. The unique viral antigen, EBV early antigen-diffuse (EA-D) IgG or EBV viral capsid antigen (VCA) IgM suggest an active infection but may represent abortive replication of viral components. One must draw quantitative DNA real-time polymerase chain reaction (PCR) viral titers to determine whether whole virus replication is occurring. EBV EA-D antigen is a harbinger of chronic EBV infection, and EBV VCA IgM may only be detected during the early acute stage or a primary or reactivated infection. There has been a statistically significant correlation between positive titers for EBV EA-D IgG or EBV VCA IgM and presence of long-COVID symptoms. In the cited study, only EBV EA-D IgG demonstrated a significant relationship with the number of reported long COVID symptoms observed.[92]

Acute stress has been linked to the duration, intensity, and level of viral expression in reactivated infections. A Wuhan, Chinese study in early 2020 found that EBV reactivation was highly prevalent (95 vs 84%) in medical intensive care units versus surgical ICU patient. They also demonstrated that EBV reactivation is associated with longer median ICU stays (15 days versus 8 days). Many manifestations of COVID-19 overlap with EBV reactivation, including Raynaud's phenomenon of the hands or feet, which resembles COVID toes. EBV has also been associated with hives (urticaria), tinnitus, and other neurologic, hematological, and cardiovascular complications, including myocarditis, inflammatory cardiomyopathy, and acute myocardial infarction (heart attack). While there are no standard of care antiviral protocols for reactivated EBV, the authors of this review and myself have used long-term (at least 6 months but up to 18 months of administration) of valacyclovir to reduce the rate of EBV-infected B cells and sometimes with the addition of Valganciclovir to block replication of EBV, especially in the case of multiple concomitant herpes viral infections.[93] In addition, cytomegalovirus (CMV, a beta-herpes virus also known as human herpes virus 5 or HHV-5) also exhibits reactivation, but there usually is no concern for disseminated infection unless there is significant immunodeficiency, such as in a transplant patient.[94]

In my practice I frequently see reactivations of viruses presenting with sore throats or spots on the palate, cold sores of human herpes virus (mainly HSV-1), and a variety of skin rashes.[95] This is especially important for understanding the progression of COVID.

Herpes Simplex Virus (HSV 1 & 2)

HSV reactivations are often triggered by psychological stress, acute illness, exposure to sunlight, fever, menstruation, or surgery. It is thought that reactivations are a multifactorial process in an immunocompetent host. It likely requires both signals acting directly on latently infected neurons in addition to suppression of immune responses that usually prevent reactivation, as well as the clearance of replicating virus.[96]

Varicella-Zoster Virus

Other herpes viruses have been known to reactivate as well. During the COVID-19 pandemic I have seen many severe reactivations of human herpes virus 3 (HHV-3), varicella-zoster virus, an alpha herpes virus whose primary infection is chicken pox, in which latent infection in nerves presents as zoster (shingles), and significant post-herpetic neuralgias—pain that occurs along distinct dermatomes of the skin, which do not cross the midline. A dermatome represents an area of the skin supplied by a single spinal nerve.

I have also observed other vague/poorly localizable neuropathic pain, often severe and migratory, which is associated with reactivated EBV infection. In addition, it is now concluded that the observation of a varicella-like papulovesicular rash often described as the "dewdrop on a rose petal" rash of chicken pox is a specific COVID-19-associated skin presentation. In Europe, researchers have found that COVID patients often have multiple reactivating herpes viruses in the fluids tested from the skin eruption. The susceptibility to reactivation of all herpes viruses including varicella-zoster may be due to the decrease in absolute lymphocytes from infection, as well as immune system dysfunction in general from acute COVID infection, and stress of an inflammatory response.[97]

Key Clinical Concept: Viral reactivations should always be included in the differential diagnosis of "non-dermatomal pain."

Human Parvovirus B19 (B19V)

Parvovirus B19 prefers infecting erythroid progenitor cells (EPCs), which produce different types of blood cells in the bone marrow or the fetal and is usually a mild illness in early childhood. It is primarily transmitted via aerosol droplets to the respiratory tract and is mainly associated with erythema infectiosum (also known as fifth disease, or "slapped-cheek disease"). B19V infection can also lead to more severe clinical diseases because of the blocked blood cell production in predisposed individuals. Parvovirus can cause fetal loss if transmitted from the mother to her infant in utero. More recently B19V has been associated with autoimmune diseases including the development of rheumatoid arthritis or vasculitis, meningoencephalitis, and hepatitis. In addition, acute and chronic inflammatory cardiomyopathies have also been linked to B19V infection.[98]

Rounding out the herpes virus infections are HHV-6 and HHV-7, which present in young children with fever and rash and known as roseola. Also associated with HHV-6 and HHV-7 are other conditions, especially pityriasis rosea (PR). PR begins with a single, oval, erythematous scaly plaque (also known as a herald patch) that is followed within two weeks by a secondary eruption, which consists of smaller scaly flat and raised patches distributed along the cleavage lines of the trunk, which makes the back look like a Christmas tree. This eruption may last from 2 weeks to a few months (45 days on average). Lesions on the oral mucosa have been described in about 30% of patients with PR following the course of the skin eruption, disappearing with skin eruption of PR or a few days later.[99]

Of note, I have seen more of the mainly childhood viruses expressed either nearly the same time as an acute COVID infection, or immediately following their illness. These include enteroviruses and coxsackie viruses, which may present with hand-foot-and mouth disease. There have also been other mainly gastrointestinal manifestations and conjunctivitis in addition to mild respiratory symptoms from adenovirus infections or other nondescript mild viral illnesses.[100] How do herpes viruses reactivate in their host cells?

Epstein-Barr (EBV) Episome Regulation
After they first infect cells, many herpes viruses establish a latent lifecycle with the viral genome existing as circular genetic elements called episomes inside the host cell's nucleus that are closely

associated with, but not integrated into, the host DNA.[101] EBV is associated with different cancers, and its carcinogenic properties are linked to its ability to persist in a latent form for the entire host's lifetime.[102] EBNA-1 is a DNA-binding protein consistently expressed by EBV-transformed cell lines (tumors) and it is the only viral protein that is required in order to maintain the virus's episome during latent infection.[103]

During latency, the EBV genome associates with repressive, heterochromatin compartments of the nucleus, then associates with active compartments during reactivation.[104] During COVID, high levels of IL-6 is a reactivator of EBV.[105]

IL-6 Levels, EBV, and COVID-19 Infection

Chronic EBV infection is associated with nasopharyngeal carcinoma (NPC). It has been shown that the activation of STAT3 (signal transducer and activator of transcription 3) is common in human cancers including NPC. It has an important role in pathogenesis and progression. Interleukin-6 (IL-6), one of the major pro-inflammatory cytokines, is a powerful activator of STAT3. IL-6 receptor overexpression paired with enhanced IL-6/STAT3 signaling may enable the malignant transformation of EBV-infected premalignant NPE cells into cancer cells and enhance malignant properties of NPC cells.[106]

An Austrian retrospective case series revealed the first systematic report of EBV viremia in critically ill COVID-19 patients, and elucidated two important findings:

1. COVID-19 patients have a higher prevalence of EBV viremia compared to non-COVID-19 patients.
2. The levels of EBV viremia correlate with IL-6 in COVID-19 patients but not in non-COVID-19 patients.

It is theorized that because EBV viral infections can induce immune dysregulation and expression of IL-6 in peripheral blood mononuclear cells (PBMCs), that EBV is an additional inflammatory trigger in critically ill COVID-19 patients.[107] It is theorized that there is a finite window for treatment with anti-IL 6 immunomodulatory agents and steroids: intervention at the start of hyper-inflammation but before critical illness causes irreversible tissue damage. One way to define this clinically is by elevated biomarkers of systemic inflammation, such as C-reactive protein (CRP) levels higher than 75 mg/L in the case of one study.[108] VitD-metabolites offer a safe and effective way of reducing production of these inflammatory mediators.

Clinical Goal: Attenuate IL-6 Production Using VitD-Metabolites

Biologically active vitamin D3 metabolites affect immunomodulatory changes on immunological and inflammatory responses, which are reflected by altered levels of pro-inflammatory chemokines. Nasal polyposis (NP) is a chronic inflammatory process of the upper respiratory system. A study reviewed the ability of calcitriol and tacalcitol on the secretion of pro-inflammatory cytokines IL-6 and IL-8 by fibroblasts derived from NP. The study found a potential therapeutic application of topical active vitamin D metabolites in NP. This warrants further investigation.[109] The relationship between prostate cancer and modulation of IL-6 signaling via calcitriol has also been linked.[110] And again, active vitamin D metabolite calcitriol shown to inhibit esophageal squamous cell carcinoma progression via reduction in IL-6 signaling.[111]

Calcifediol and Calcitriol Reduce COVID Morbidity and Mortality

In an observational cohort study conducted in Barcelona, Spain on 838 COVID-19 patients, 447 were given calcifediol (532 µg on day one plus 266 µg on days three, seven, fifteen, and thirty), whereas 391 were not treated at the time of hospital admission. ICU admission was required by 102 (12.2%) of the participants. Out of 447 patients treated with calcifediol at admission, twenty (4.5%) required the ICU, compared to 82 (21%) out of 391 non-treated. Overall mortality was 10%. In the intention-to-treat analysis, 21 (4.7%) out of 447 patients treated with calcifediol at admission died compared to 62 patients (15.9%) out of 391 nontreated; calcifediol treatment significantly reduced ICU admission and mortality in patients hospitalized with COVID-19.[112] A companion survival study on a retrospective cohort of 15,968 patients was performed and comprised all COVID-19 patients hospitalized in Andalusia between January and November 2020. The effect of prescription of active vitamin D metabolites for other indication previous to the hospitalization was studied with respect to patient survival. Kaplan–Meier survival curves and hazard ratios show an association between prescription of these powerful active hormone metabolites and patient survival. This finding was stronger for calcifediol (hazard ratio, HR=0.67, with 95% confidence interval, CI, of [0.50–0.91]) than for cholecalciferol (HR=0.75, with 95% CI of [0.61–0.91]), when prescribed 15 days prior hospitalization.[113]

Key Clinical Goal: Rapidly boost serum calcifediol levels (25-OH D3) to treat COVID induced polymicrobial infection.

Bacterial and Fungal Co-Infections

Viral pneumonias increase a patient's susceptibility to bacterial and fungal superinfection. One example includes invasive pulmonary aspergillosis (IPA). Influenza-associated pulmonary aspergillosis (IAPA) has been known to complicate the clinical course of many critically ill patients with acute respiratory distress syndrome (ARDS). The onset of the COVID-19 pandemic also brought with it a wave of COVID-19-associated pulmonary aspergillosis (CAPA), raising concerns that this superinfection could be an additional contributing factor for mortality. These fears were validated in a prospective cohort of 108 critically ill patients with ARDS: higher 30-day mortality was observed in patients with CAPA than in patients without aspergillosis (44% *vs.* 19%). The association of COVID-19-associated fungal disease with mortality was also supported by another study. Yet another poor prognostic factor for CAPA patients is that there have been more reports of antifungal resistant infections, which may be more invasive, thereby causing direct damage to the epithelial cells in the airway. Meanwhile, the initial viral infection interferes with ciliary clearance and leads to immune dysfunction/dysregulation, either locally or systemically. Finally, some COVID-19 patients develop pronounced immunosuppression, which directly enables bacterial and fungal superinfection. There is a decrease of T cell populations, especially in patients with severe disease.[114] When T cells are deranged, self-tolerance is lost, and increases the risk of autoimmunity.

Autoimmunity Workup

Molecular workups will be needed to gauge individualized therapies. A full complement of autoantibody titers should be drawn commensurate with the patient's story and their symptomology. Autoimmune therapy requires individual cocktails, so physicians and patients need to be informed that successful remission require permutations, and often polypharmacy. This perspective often conflicts with people who expect rapid and sustained results from single treatments (monotherapies). Shifting long-lived plasma cells (B cells, which produce antibodies) from autophagy (damaged cells being eaten) to apoptosis (programmed cell death), is key to obtaining autoimmune remissions.

The treatment of post-infectious COVID will need to draw from the soft pharma toolbox, to curb recurring flares of potentially dangerous hypercoagulable pathology due to the development of antiphospholipid syndrome (APS) via autoantibody generation, a common autoimmune phenomenon in COVID survivors. Autoantibodies and immune complexes are known disruptors of the endocrine system (endocrine disruptors).

Hormone Workup

Because COVID infections (can also extrapolate this to a general model of polymicrobial sepsis) affects every organ-system in the body, there are a multitude of endocrine concerns to address post infection. Two of the greatest risk factors for morbidity and mortality in COVID-19 include diabetes and Cushing's syndrome, an endocrinopathy of hypercortisolism and immune deficiency. Screen for diabetes including new onset autoimmune mediated if clinically suspicious, be aware of stress hyperglycemia and sick euthyroid syndrome due to recent infection, and screen for adrenal insufficiency including autoantibodies, again, if concerned. Optimize immune function via glucose control and stress management.[115] The concept of "epigenetically-rebooting" the immune system and the inflamed nervous system is a solid premise. These physiologic states are complex, combinatoric, but comprehensible. In short, these are assessments I utilize to design therapeutic interventions for individual patients.

Therapeutic Strategies for Treating Viral Illnesses

We acquire pathogens throughout our lifetime. Some of these infections are eliminated, thus helping to build a strong immune response. However, these infections can leave scars. Take the literal deep pockmark scars on the skin of smallpox survivors. In polio, the anatomical scars are deep within the body: lifelong peripheral nerve damage leading in some cases to paralysis. In the 1950s, thousands of polio victims were placed in iron lungs after motor neurons to their breathing muscles were destroyed during their primary polio infection.[116]

Key Clinical Concept: Left untreated, long-lasting tissue damage can occur during acute viral infections.

Other infections become chronic but in the case of many, latent (i.e., dormant). We harbor an individual microbial load of bacteria, viruses, fungi, protozoa, prions, and other parasitic infections, which can be re-expressed under times of physiologic stress. COVID infection represents a brew of virus, toxins, and a battleground of cytokines, which weaken the immune system leading to an acute immunodeficiency.

Key Clinical Concept: Virologists define this as viral toxemia, which involves the systemic circulation of viral toxins.[117]

In the case of progressive COVID infection, we are dealing with a much more complex clinical presentation. Damage to the gut epithelium, as well as damage to the pulmonary epithelium results in novel portals of entry for bacteria and bacterial toxins to enter the bloodstream.

Consider the evolving battleground in the first (upper) part of the small intestine, the duodenum, during a SARS-CoV-2 infection. This directly leads to polymicrobial sepsis. One of the key molecular agents that will ignite a cytokine storm in the gut is LPS. This is the cellular and molecular battleground site: the microvillus. LPS, the endotoxin, enters and causes activation of the innate immune system in the gut. This is analogous to inflammatory bowel disease, increased permeability and holes in the epithelial lining of the gut. This becomes self-sustaining (a vicious cycle). It involves toll-like receptors, especially TLR4 in COVID.[118]

Clinical Goal: Attenuating TLR4 with LDN

LPS, the endotoxin from gram-negative bacteria such as *Escherichia coli,* activates TLR4, hyperactivation of which sets off a cytokine storm. This endotoxin is a sugar (polysaccharide), which is recognized by TLR 4. The spike protein of COVID also contains surface sugars (glycans), that also activate TLR4. The net result is hyperactivation of innate immune cells and immune attack involving CD8 killer T cells and the vicious cycle of damage and poration of the gut epithelium. This is the genesis of polymicrobial sepsis. The goal is to attenuate this immune response, and the power of LDN is to attenuate TLR4 hyperactivation without making the person immunocompromised. This treatment is safe, available, inexpensive, and scalable. We know from our treatment of autoimmune diseases such as Hashimoto's thyroiditis, multiple sclerosis, Lyme disease and rheumatoid arthritis that there are no increases in chronic viral infections from the use of LDN. In short, LDN attenuates the hyperactive immune response without causing immunodeficiency. Loading LDN into endosomes of the gut epithelium and the endosomes of the innate immune cells in the microvillus protect them from being poisoned by viral toxins or endotoxin itself.

When I take LDN, it passes through the stomach, is dissolved rapidly as a tablet or capsule, and then coats my gut epithelium. A very small amount of naltrexone (20 times less a therapeutic dose for opioid overdose or alcohol abuse) goes a long way. In the case of COVID, protecting the gut epithelium is a prime target of this therapeutic, and in my view, a key clinical target in my practice. The endosome is a storage site where the battle takes place. In progressive infection we have to load endosomes with Nabs (IgAs, IgGs) and AMPs (LL-37, beta-defensin), LDN, active hydroxylated metabolites of vitamin D (calcifediol, calcitriol). The endosome is a key volume-of-distribution for these pharmacological agents.[119]

It is important for people to recognize the endosome as a key battleground in viral infection. Neutralization of viruses, as well as neutralization of viral toxins takes place in endosomes. For that reason, it is important to load endosomes with neutralizing agents. By doing this, the physician has strengthened the mucosal immunity of the gut. It is now generally recognized that a lack of mucosal immunity makes an individual susceptible to severe and progressive viral infections. It is imperative for twenty-first century clinicians to recognize the endosome as the target to strengthen the mucosal immunity of the gut, the nasopharynx, and the lungs.[120]

We know from the work of Dr. Bruce Patterson and his colleagues that long-COVID is characterized by a population of aberrant, invasive, non-classical monocytes. Monocytes are leukocytes, which normally only circulate. Here again, the importance of endosomes controlling immune cell behavior is illustrated. We have spike-protein laden endosomes in these atypical monocytes, which cause them to have uncharacteristically aggressive and invasive behavior. These aberrant monocytes can invade multiple tissues and organs, contributing to a Pandora's box of pathology, consisting of an array of over 200 debilitating, long-COVID symptoms.[121]

Neutralizing virions, viral toxins, and other viral products within endosomes is critical to healing virally injured cells and tissues. These non-classical monocytes can potentially survive for months, as can increased active mast cells, which are also long-lived cells causing increased histamine/inflammatory symptoms.[122]

Key Therapeutic Concepts
   a. Viral illnesses lead to viral toxemia.
   b. Injury to gut epithelium and injury to pulmonary epithelium lead to polymicrobial sepsis.
   c. Hyperactivation of toll-like receptors leads to cytokine storm.
   d. Attenuating TLR4 is central for treating COVID. The targets are the gut and lung epithelia.
   e. Loading of LDN occurs in the endosomes of gut epithelial and immune cells.
   f. Endosomes are a storage compartment for neutralizing agents Nabs, AMPs, vitamin D metabolites, and LDN.
   g. LDN is the most well studied and well-established attenuator of multiple toll-like receptors.

h. LDN is currently being used by a number of practitioners for the treatment of acute, progressive, and long COVID (see chapter "- Eight -") as well as other viral infections.

Immediate Interventions to limit Tissue Damage during Initial COVID Infection Primarily Prevents Gut-Mediated Polymicrobial Sepsis

How can we prevent Pandora's box of pathologies from ever opening? We already have parts of the answer. Spanish physicians have found an 85% reduction in ICU progression and mortality in patients who have been treated with high-dose calcifediol. In my practice, my patients are routinely maintained on 1-4.5mg of LDN for inflammatory and autoimmune disorders. I also maintain my patients with immune optimal levels of 25-OH D3, calcifediol. During the past two plus years, in a clinic of nearly 2,000 patients, I have had very few hospitalizations of any of my patients that have contracted COVID, many of whom are older patients with multiple comorbidities including autoimmune conditions, nor am I aware of any of them developing long-COVID. This is my clinical experience in treating patients with COVID.

Pre-Infection

The following is a list of therapeutics and assessments that I use both to prevent and treat viral illnesses:

- Boost active vitamin D metabolites with the goal of 50-60 ng/mL for non-autoimmune patients and 60-80 ng/mL for autoimmune patients. For acute COVID, 80-100 ng/mL. No risk of hypercalcemia unless sustained high-dose use achieving levels over 150 ng/mL. I am unaware of any documented cases of hypercalcemia in the current medical literature using high dose vitamin D supplementation. Caveats to high dose active vitamin D metabolite supplementation: caution in CKD patients; do not use in sarcoidosis, any autoimmune conditions marked by elevated active vitamin D levels, and not for patients with hyperparathyroidism. Both sarcoid and hyperparathyroidism can cause hypercalcemia.
- Take LDN.

- Exercise, sleep, anti-inflammatory diet (you cannot out-supplement a bad diet).
- Epsom salt baths (transdermal magnesium absorption); magnesium is a critical cofactor for energy production.
- Tailored supplementation of any known vitamin or mineral deficiencies.

Selected Integrative Polypharmacy Therapies

Once someone has been infected, the following treatments are how I aim to reduce the severity of COVID.

LDN

A consensus from all medical advisors to the LDN Research Trust is that LDN is an absolute good with regard for its ability to enhance proper immune response toward vaccines, support immune system modulation, and cool chronic inflammation. Dosing for acute COVID is low, about 1mg nightly unless already taking a higher maintenance dose. LDN is very promising for treating neuro-inflammation and neuro-autoimmunity because it can cross the blood-brain barrier and permeates the tissues of the central nervous system and can enter neuro-inflammatory lesions. LDN use is an excellent strategy for the prevention of long-COVID manifestations.

Zinc

Zinc plays a crucial role in the function of all immune cells. Zinc deficiency increases susceptibility to a variety of infections. Increasing intracellular zinc concentrations in cell culture has shown the impairment of replication of a variety of RNA viruses including SARS-CoV-1. In vivo evidence for zinc's antiviral role comes from a Cochrane review that found zinc intake significantly reduced the duration of the common cold. Many of the studies showing benefit when taken during the course of an infection were in the form of a zinc lozenge. Therefore, it does make sense to use this type of delivery system during the acute phase. Additionally, zinc suppresses Th17 cell development, which is implicated in the development of autoimmunity and an inflammatory feedback loop because IL-17 is made by Th17 cells and induces IL-6 in the process. Zinc requirements increase for older adults, and one of the hallmark symptoms of COVID infection is loss of smell or distorted taste (anosmia and dysgeusia, respectively). While it is being shown that COVID causes damage to the neurons in the olfactory bulb responsible for smell, zinc deficiency also may be a cause or effect in this case as well.[123]

Nicotinamide Adenine Dinucleotide (NAD⁺)

NAD^+ is a molecule responsible for many cellular reactions involved in the generation of energy and maintenance of cellular function, including proper immune responses to viral infections. The hyper-inflammatory response that sometimes occurs with COVID infection is associated with high mortality. A hypothesis suggests that an NAD^+ deficiency may be the primary factor related to the SARS-Cov-2 disease spectrum and the risk for mortality due to subclinical nutritional deficiencies, which may be unmasked by any significant increase in cellular oxidative stress. NAD^+ levels decline with age. They are also depleted in conditions associated with oxidative stress as occurs with chronic inflamed states such as hypertension, diabetes, and obesity. These comorbidities have high mortality following COVID-19 infection.

Sirtuins are comprised of seven NAD^+-dependent signaling proteins, which regulate metabolic rate and cellular homeostasis. Silent Information Regulator 1 (SIRT1) is the most significant because it downregulates levels of inflammatory cytokines TNF-α, IL-1b, and IL-6. Interestingly, SIRT1 is involved in obesity-associated metabolic diseases, cancer, cellular aging and stress, and inflammatory signaling in response to environmental stress. In its inactive (open) state, it contains a Zn^{2+} module and an NAD^+ binding site. SIRT1 is activated when it binds to zinc and causing a structural change whereby SIRT1 is activated (closed). Zinc and NAD^+ are required for optimal function of SIRT1. This suggests that nutritional support with NAD^+ and SIRT1 activators could minimize disease severity if administered prophylactically and or therapeutically.[124]

Specialized Pro-Resolving Mediators (SPMs)

Bioactive lipids (BALs) inactivate SARS-CoV-2. Therefore, they may confer benefit in the prevention and treatment of COVID-19. It is understood that macrophages and T cells (including NK cells, cytotoxic killer cells and other immune cells) release arachidonic acid (AA) and other BALs, especially in lungs to inactivate various microbes. Pro-inflammatory metabolites prostaglandin E2 (PGE2), leukotrienes (LTs), and anti-inflammatory lipoxin A4 (LXA4) derived from arachidonic acid facilitate the development of pro-inflammatory M1 macrophages. Resolvins (AKA specialized pro-resolving mediators, or SPMs), protectins, and maresins derived from eicosapentaenoic acid (EPA) and docosahexaenoic acid (DHA) generate anti-inflammatory M2 macrophages. These BALs inhibit interleukin-6 (IL-6) and tumor necrosis factor-α (TNF-α) synthesis. Of note, BALs influence cell membrane fluidity and thus, regulate ACE-2. BALs therefore, may support the management of COVID-19 and other enveloped viral infections.[125]

Quercetin

We have been using the flavonoid quercetin as a mast cell modulator for post-COVID and many other conditions in which pro-inflammatory histamine levels are driven up. Quercetin also acts as a zinc ionophore, which helps transport zinc safely across lipid membranes. Quercetin has also been shown in the lab to block the activity of an enzyme critical for coronavirus replication.[126]

Resveratrol

Resveratrol is a potent anti-inflammatory supplement via many mechanisms. Resveratrol downregulates IL-6, TNFα, and promotes sirtuins, thus supporting metabolic and blood sugar balance. Resveratrol has been studied in SARS-CoV-1, and it was shown that resveratrol protects lung soft tissue against the effects of cigarette smoke via upregulation of the Nrf2 gene (nuclear factor erythroid factor 2 – related factor 2) to promote the master antioxidant, glutathione (GSH).[127]

NAC

Glutathione (GSH) and *N*-acetylcysteine (NAC) are the primary antioxidant support in a COVID-19 infection. GSH plays a key role in the regulation of oxidant and antioxidant homeostasis in the lung. The level of GSH in the lung epithelial lining fluid strongly correlates with the extent of lung inflammation present. GSH is also essential for the innate and adaptive branches of the immune system, which includes T-lymphocyte proliferation, phagocytic activity of polymorphonuclear neutrophils (PMN), and dendritic cell (DC) functions. DC's function as the professional antigen presenting cell (APC) for the adaptive immune system. Oral NAC is cheap, shelf stable, and readily absorbed through the gut. It is converted to cysteine in the liver via first pass metabolism. The majority of cysteine is secondarily incorporated into GSH and released into systemic circulation. Cysteine recycling is the rate-limiting factor in GSH synthesis.[128]

Repurposed Drugs/Pharmacology

"Soft pharma" cocktails such as LDN, resveratrol, hyperbaric oxygen, NAC, NAD+, anti-histamines or mast cell stabilizers, zinc, active vitamin D metabolites (calcifediol +/- calcitriol, especially in high risk patients with early active infection), other vitamins, and "hard pharma" immune modulators or other interventions are necessary to combat an ever changing foe.

Microbiome Restoration

Indeed, there is a complex relationship between the microbiota of the lung and GI tract. There is bidirectional influence with the immune system. Acute viral infections drive dysregulation of the gut microbiome, which has been shown to be a source of systemic inflammation. Intestinal metabolism of dietary fiber causes an increase in short chain fatty acids (SCFAs), specifically propionate, which has been shown to enhance the maturation of macrophages and DC's seeding the lungs. These DCs maintain an increased ability for phagocytosis and overall reduced Th2-mediated inflammation. There is a hypothesis that chronic lung diseases are being driven by lung microbial dysbiosis.[129] More and more, the current body of viral research is showing that a more diverse and balanced the gut microbiome leads to a homeostatic and resilient system, which is better able to withstand pathogenic infections and suppress reactivation of latent viral infections.

Suppressing the Reactivation of Herpes viruses During COVID

An important review article by Dr. Jonathan Kerr discussing EBV reactivation and therapeutic inhibitors summarizes the mechanisms whereby reactivation is prevented by efficacious cellular immunity. However, under situations of physical or psychological stress and weakening of cellular immunity, EBV reactivates via the activation of a lytic (cell-killing) phase. Reactivation occurs in populations with a variety of different cancers, autoimmune diseases, post-viral infections, or diagnoses of chronic fatigue syndrome/myalgic encephalitis (CFS/ME) and under other circumstances such as being an inpatient in an intensive care unit or other acute stressor. Many clinicians do not understand that chronic EBV reactivation is a real condition in people without known immunodeficiency, so it is not often tested in these patients. A summary of licensed pharmaceuticals for treatment of other herpes viruses, licensed or experimental drugs for various other indications, compounds at an early stage of drug development and nutritional constituents such as vitamins and dietary supplements are reviewed. It makes sense that these supplements, which are effective at preventing EBV reactivation, now known to be a factor in patients developing long-COVID symptoms, would be therapeutic adjunctive agents for immune system support.[130]

Traditional anti-herpes drugs including acyclovir inhibit EBV reactivation, while other drugs with the same overall inhibition include the anti-retroviral agent zidovudine and the antihistamine cimetidine. Other experimental treatments are introduced for future consideration. Of note, vitamins C, D, A (retinoic acid) especially are discussed. Vitamin C inhibits EBV activation in human cancer cells (such as EBV+ Burkitt lymphoma cells). Vitamin D is known to directly inhibit enveloped viruses and helps upregulate AMPs LL-37 and human beta-defensin. LL-37 may in turn be able to disrupt the viral envelope. Vitamin A supports the inhibition of the EBV lytic cycle and irreversibly inhibits EBV-transformed lymphocytes (pre-cancerous).

Specific dietary constituents and prescription-grade supplements of note include the following:

- Resveratrol: inhibits EBV lytic cycle via effects on many molecular targets.
- Luteolin: inhibits gene expression of EBV early in lytic cycle, reduces genomic instability and suppresses EBV's ability to promote tumor formation.
- Apigenin: inhibition of immediate-early proteins which are required to enter the lytic phase of infection,
- Astragalus: inhibition of multiple proteins including EA-D antigen during the EBV lytic cycle.
- Epigallocatechin-3-gallate (a green-tea polyphenol): inhibition of EBV-induced B lymphocyte transformation.
- Sulforaphane (found in cruciferous vegetables such as broccoli, Brussels sprouts, and cabbage): inhibition of Rta, a protein which triggers the expression of a panel of early EBV lytic proteins.
- Curcumin: enhanced programmed-cell death-mediated inhibition of EBV transformed lymphoblastoid cell line.

Most importantly there is the need to discuss stress mitigation and an unprocessed, anti-inflammatory diet.[131] These lifestyle modifications are paramount, yet tough to discuss in a primary care setting. Speaking from an American perspective, more and more we have greater stressors placed upon families struggling financially to make ends meet. So often we have the choice between either a two-income household, or a stay-at-home parent due to rising costs of childcare. Slow down and stop glorifying the religion of busyness. We Americans can take a lesson from our counterparts in Europe and many other places, where it is in fact mandated to take breaks. This is much more difficult when we do not even have guaranteed maternity leave (up to 52 weeks in England vs zero in the United States), but I digress. Families are spending less time making home-cooked meals a priority. We have food deserts, places without access to fresh fruits and vegetables. Our soil itself is less nutrient-dense. Much of our population has no land to grow food and lost knowledge of how to do so otherwise. We have our youth unable to cook.

In short, the answer is to remember our past. Reclaim our family traditions. Return to simple home-cooked meals. Invest in local shares of fruits and veggies from local farms or plant family or community gardens. There are now ways to grow small amounts of herbs and fresh produce indoors. Reclaim your traditions of your familial heritages and embrace the different traditions in homes with different cultures. Record and treasure the stories of your elders, including the wisdom of using herbal remedies. Use traditional methods of food preparation, including fermentation, sprouting, and soaking, which enrich the gut microbiome and our immune systems. When we remember our collective ancient wisdom, and open our eyes, we conclude the need to use all at our disposal for treating the next pandemic illness. We must embrace the marriage between natural medicine (soft pharma) and hard pharma (novel therapeutics and the repurposing of old drugs). The countries that enrich the health of their populations utilizing these tenants will ultimately thrive in the face of COVID or another viral foe.

FOUR

LDN and Longevity

Yusuf M. (JP) Saleeby, MD

Since our earliest ancestors first walked upright and gained the capacity to think and dream of the future, our species has yearned for a longer life. Some have even sought substances, whether real or imagined, to extend lifespans. Chinese emperor Qin Shi Huang, in the third century BCE, was convinced by his court's scientists to consume cinnabar (mercury sulfide) in efforts to achieve immortality.[132] Obviously, this elixir did more to shorten his life than extend it. Sixteenth-century Spanish explorer Juan Ponce de Leon was so caught up in the longing for longevity that he searched the New World for the fountain of youth. Today, contemporary writers such as Dave Asprey, author of the book *Super Human*, express the desire to live to 180.[133]

Whether you believe aging is a disease or just a part of life, the end result is the same. There are some people who do all the "right things" yet die earlier deaths than predicted given their lifestyle. Then there are folks who seem to do it all wrong yet live well beyond the average lifespan, for example the late Jeanne Calment who passed away in 1997 at the age of 122 years, despite daily enjoying a single Dunhill cigarette and a glass of port wine.[134]

Aging can be loosely defined as a complex biological process to which the body—its organs, cells, and even molecules—is subject. The process is a progressive, inescapable, and eventual decline in function of the body and its systems' ability to act on both internal and external stressors. Aging can further be defined as a gradual functional decline across all systems, a continuum that persists from optimal health to dysfunction to failure and ultimately death as the endpoint.[135] [136]

Theories of Aging

There is no universally held or accepted theory of aging. Aging principles are in reality a constellation of theories with each contributing in its own way. Among the more popular are the disengagement theory, activity theory, neuroendocrine theory, free radical theory, membrane theory, decline theory, and the cross-linking theory. One should also add in the genetic age limits and the immune system's impact on aging.[137] [138]

While presently no consensus agreement yet exists to form a comprehensive unifying theory of aging, the ones discussed here may all contribute. To what degree remains to be seen. Some theories and hypotheses we consider and weigh in heavily today may one day carry less significance or be invalidated.

Programmed Theories of Aging

Programmed longevity theories consider aging the result of genes that control senescence (cell slowing down and dysfunction) switching on and off; when that happens, age-associated deficits occur. According to the endocrine theory, our biological clock is determined by hormones that control the pace of aging, while the immunological theory posits that our immune systems seem to be pre-programmed to decline over time, leading our body and systems to become much more susceptible to infectious diseases. This vulnerability eventually leads to decline, aging and death.

A more focused programmed theory involving neuroendocrine was first proposed in 1992 by Drs. Ward Dean and Vladimir Dilman in a theory referred to as the neuroendocrine theory of aging. Their theory places the emphasis on a small structure in our brains called the hypothalamus. The hypothalamus is responsible for a complex network of biological chemicals such as hormones and neurotransmitters that can impact the aging process. Once corrupted, the effect by this gland is lessened, and there is a reduction in the release of hormones, resulting in aging.[139]

Damage Theories of Aging

Another class of aging theories is focused on accumulated damage to the body and its systems. The wear-and-tear theory describes how the vital parts of our cells, organs, and tissues wear out over time and use, much like the parts of a machine, leading to aging and death. The rate-of-living theory supports the idea that the greater an organism's basal rate of metabolism, oxygen consumption, heart rate, etc., the shorter the life expectancy. The cross-linking theory states that the accumulation of cross-linked proteins and DNA via glycosylation, for example, gum up the inner workings and slow the cellular process down, resulting in aging and eventual death.

The combination of simple sugars with oxygen (analogous to iron and oxygen yielding rust) is a process called glycosylation. The free radical theory proposed by Dr. Denham Harman at the University of Nebraska in 1956 purports that aging happens with the destruction of healthy molecules by oxidation and free electrons' destructive powers. We know that poor diet, unhealthy lifestyles, use of tobacco and excessive alcohol, along with environmental radiation and other factors accelerates free radical production and its negative effects.[140] Overproduction of free radicals by poor life choices can lead to premature aging. The neutralization of free radicals has, by contrast, a beneficial effect.

Many of these theories can be distilled down to a common issue, let us say, with the mitochondria. The mitochondria of each cell in every organ are the powerhouses producing adenosine triphosphate (ATP) for energy cycles within the body. Life and longevity depend on proper mitochondrial function. Whether you subscribe to wear-and-tear, glycosylation, or free radical theory, they can all perform a negative role in mitochondrial function. Supporting the mitochondria with antioxidants and nutrition can reduce the untoward effects on performance. Functional medicine doctors advise the benefits of coenzyme Q10, B-complex vitamins, NADH/NAD+, L-carnitine, N-acetyl cysteine, glutathione, and other antioxidants to protect and support the mitochondria.[141]

Yet another theory involves the membranes of our cells. Again, the previously mentioned theories can have an effect on membranes.

The membrane theory of aging focuses on the ability of the cells to transfer chemicals, heat, and electrical impulses across the cellular membrane. If impaired, the cells will slow down. Their inability to exchange nutrients for waste products and therefore accumulate toxins is the basis for this theory. Eventually the cell succumbs and dies, while aging along the way. This theory was put forth by Dr. Imre Zsolnai-Nagy an experimental gerontologist from Hungary in 1994.[142]

Finally, one cannot ignore the psychological aspects of aging with theories that focus on psychosocial aging and what can be called the activity theory, which evaluates the role and importance of ongoing social activity. This has been a serious problem in premature aging during the recent COVID-19 lockdowns of 2020 and 2021.

In the early 1900s, a researcher put forth the hypothesis that in a given environment with higher organisms, cell division would be continual and possess immortality. So, the goal was to provide an optimal environment to achieve a long-lasting life. This soon-to-be-challenged theory was put forth by Dr. Alexis Carrel, a French surgeon and Nobel Prize-winner in Physiology & Medicine in 1912, whose achievements in medicine include vascular suturing techniques and development of the first perfusion pumps that opened the world of medicine to transplantation. However, his theory was later invalidated by Dr. Leonard Hayflick. In the 1960s, Dr. Hayflick disproved the theory of an immortal cell in an optimal culture by coming up with what we refer to today as the "Hayflick Limit." This limit is the number of times a cell can divide before it becomes idle and thus eventually dies. This number of limited cell divisions equated to a lifespan of about 115 years.[143] Today, some researchers are convinced this limit can be overcome.

Today, we have a way of looking at repair and restoration of telomeres (little segments of DNA at the end of each chromosome), with telomerase and agents including resveratrol and *Astragalus membranaceus*. It appears that with every cell division/replication, a tiny portion of the telomere is sacrificed. Eventually, the enzymes responsible for DNA replication have nothing left to grab hold of and the process stops. When one looks at cancer cells it appears they are immortal and can defy the Hayflick limit by dividing indefinitely. Cancer cells seem to learn how to overcome this limit by not losing DNA endpieces on chromosomes during each cell division. Discovered on Christmas Day in 1984 by Drs. Carol Greider and Elizabeth Blackburn, telomerase is an enzyme consisting of RNA and some proteins that can extend and repair the telomere. They shared the 2009 Nobel Prize in Medicine with Dr. Jack Szostak for this discovery.[144]

~

Human longevity is limited by many factors. To understand and counteract those life-shortening agents of death, we must define them and treat them alongside aging as an umbrella disease. As clinicians we think of the leading killers that shorten our lifespan as: heart disease, cancer, unintentional injuries, chronic lower respiratory disease, stroke and cerebrovascular disease, Alzheimer's disease and other dementias, diabetes, and influenza or other infectious diseases.

There has been much debate as to the upper limit of human longevity, such as 120 to 150 years of age. But our approach to longevity should be more than just a numbers game, and accompanied by the goal of sustaining a good quality of life (morbidity reduction). How many of us really want to live to 130, but spend the last decade or two in a nursing home? Not many, I would imagine.

Before employing "fountain of youth" interventions to extend longevity, attention should be paid to the basics, i.e., maintaining the body "temple" with proper nutrition, exercise, relaxation, sleep, proper work-life balance, avoidance of environmental toxins, and proper personalized preventive medicine and healthcare. Once comfortable with this, we can then discuss and embrace some rather astounding medical and scientific interventions that can prolong life and lower incidence of chronic disease. Another way to look at longevity is not avoiding what can take us out of play, but what one can do proactively to enhance ourselves at a cellular level to cheat an early death. This can include the use of hormones and peptides and other agents to keep our cells youthful, elongate our telomeres, and such. Whether they are ultimately effective remains to be seen.

This book, as well as both volumes of *The LDN Book*, details the benefits of low dose naltrexone (LDN) in treating a variety of conditions. Some of these conditions can certainly shorten life expectancy. Others are nuisance disorders. The following sections are not intended to repeat, but rather to reemphasize what has already been published.

LDN and Inflammation

We know that prolonged and chronic inflammation can lead to a rise in cardiovascular conditions and insults to the endothelium and glycocalyx of our vessel walls. Researchers have delineated inflammation as often responsible for autoimmune disorders. Researchers have shown that inflammation can lead to a variety of cancers. If we address inflammation and have the ability to reduce "bad inflammation" then it is logical to conclude that we are knocking out one mechanism that can shorten life span via several causes. When I refer to inflammation as ''bad inflammation,'' I am purporting that a limited amount of inflammation is a necessary part of our body's immune system function. Short-term (acute) inflammation is a part of the healing process and a protective mechanism.[145] However, as we are all aware, protracted and extended (chronic) inflammation can be dangerous to our health and wellbeing.

The four classical, overt signs of inflammation that a clinician can use in a diagnostic workup of an injury or infection are rubor (redness), calor (heat), tumor (swelling), and dolor (pain). However, what may be more difficult to ascertain is inflammation that is less observable during a physical exam. Laboratory analysis with serology biomarkers is one way to determine if inflammation exists and to what degree. This may be helpful to a clinician in determining an underlying problem or condition.

The inflammation process is activated and amplified by a series of intracellular and extracellular factors. They are organized and tightly coordinated in the process. The innate immune system has been programmed through evolution to respond rapidly to any new infection or injury, but it is the sustained process that can be detrimental. Macrophages, natural killer cells, CD8 + T-lymphocytes, and neutrophils, along with cytokines, coordinate the efforts. From a localized inflammatory response, it can segue into a more systemic inflammatory response syndrome involving the adaptive immune response mediators such as CD4 + T-lymphocytes and their assorted cytokines and chemokines. Examples of chronic inflammatory diseases that cause morbidity and shave years off your life include: rheumatoid arthritis, psoriasis, and inflammatory bowel disease (IBD) such as Crohn's disease and ulcerative colitis, to name only a very few.

This book and previous books discuss the TLR4 mechanism of action of LDN. For a better understanding of toll-like receptors and their interaction with pathogen-associated molecular patterns (PAMPs) and the sterile damage-associated molecular patterns (DAMPs) let us discuss these principles for clarity.[146]

The importance of leukocyte trafficking in inflammation has led to some therapeutic breakthroughs, but there remain some pathologies that defy conventional interventions. If we take PAMPs and DAMPs, we can then see how they bind to specific receptors (pattern recognition receptors, or PRRs) to activate inflammation, which mobilize and recruit leukocytes for proinflammatory purposes. When the acute inflammatory process is not turned off properly to allow for reparative cellular processes, chronic inflammation sets in. Harmful prolonged inflammation via inappropriate leukocyte activation drives many chronic diseases. This persists when the program switch or reverse transmigration of DAMPs and PAMPs fail. In this environment, natural killer T-cells are allowed to continue with an inflammatory milieu we see as a non-desirable immunostimulatory condition. Further insult can be compounded with LAMPS (lifestyle-associated molecular patterns). Toll-like receptors (TLR) are involved in this process. Inhibition of TLR4 is a key factor at suppressing inflammation and thus its damage to mitochondria, cells, tissue, and organs. LDN plays a key role in suppressing TLR4 activity.[147]

Taking a closer look at DAMPs, they are endogenous, low molecular-weight danger molecules that emanate from dying or damaged cells and activate our innate immune system by binding to PRRs. TRLs and inflammasomes are classified as PRRs. In small, localized, and limited amounts these DAMPs are beneficial for our host defense. However, in larger more protracted amounts these DAMPs contribute to pathological inflammatory responses (some may describe as chronic inflammatory response syndrome, or CIRS). Studies have suggested that agents such as heat shock proteins (HSPs) along with S100 proteins and high-mobility group box 1 (HMGB1), all considered DAMPs, participate in the process. These DAMPs along with PAMPs and even LAMPs can all contribute to conditions of inflammatory etiology such as rheumatoid arthritis (RA), systemic lupus erythematosus (SLE), atherosclerosis, Alzheimer's disease, Parkinson's disease, other autoimmune disorders, and cancers. So, these underlying processes contribute to the more superficial conditions we recognize in medicine.

If we look closer at PAMPs and TLR4 when a human subject is attached by gram- negative bacteria with lipopolysaccharide (LPS) molecules on the surface, we witness the following. As part of our innate immune system response activation of circulating macrophages, first the PRR TLR4 (there are 10 types of TLRs identified in humans) is bound by the PAMP LPS on the macrophage membrane with the help of CD14 and LPS monomers through a process involving a glycosylphosphatidylinositol anchor. The now bound TLR4, with the help of MD-2, is able to detect LPS from CD14. This complex of TLR4 + CD14 + MD2 on the cell surface now activates an intracellular process involving Toll-IL-1 Receptors (TIR) within the cell that recruits adaptor proteins. Adaptor proteins such as MY-D88 leads to a cascade of events producing nuclear factor-kappa B (NF-KB), considered the activator of inflammation. NF-KB causes transcription in the nucleus of the cell producing cytokines and chemokines released by the cell into the extracellular space to address the invading gram-negative bacteria (originating LPS). Runaway NF-KB will lead to unwanted effects of high levels of inflammation and autoimmunity. Restraining NF-KB via TLR4 inhibition can dampen down this response and lead to a lower inflammatory response in avoiding a hyperactive immune (autoimmune) response. LDN can intervene in this process to diminish this inflammatory cascade by inhibition of TLR4.

Now for a look at DAMPs. In a similar way DAMPs act as PAMPs. Activation of inflammatory cells due to TLR2 and TLR4 in association with several DAMPs including high mobility group box-1 (HMGB-1), histones, S100 proteins, and heat shock proteins (HSPs) among others will result in a chronic inflammatory pattern. LDN apparently blunts this response. Thus, LDN, by reducing chronic inflammation pathways, is a way of increasing life expectancy by reducing the detrimental effects on longevity seen with chronic inflammation. This can be appreciated in a variety of tissues including brain and cardiac.

In research studies, LDN was associated with reduced plasma concentrations of interleukin (IL)-1β, IL-1Ra, IL-2, IL-4, IL-5, IL-6, IL-10, IL-12p40, IL-12p70, IL-15, IL-17A, IL-27, interferon (IFN)-α, transforming growth factor (TGF)-α, TGF-β, tumor necrosis factor (TNF)-α, and granulocyte-colony stimulating factor (G-CSF). This was elucidated in a 2017 study involving fibromyalgia patients.[148] The reduction in cytokines and inflammation revealed LDN as a key anti-inflammatory agent for use in this and other conditions.

Cell senescence can be induced by inflammation and a hyperactive Th17 process. Sarcopenia and bone loss are factors that can be easily seen and observed as clinically attributed to aging. Senescent cells secrete toxic substances and lead to many disruptions in cell function, organ function, and ultimately vitality and longevity. Senescence-associated secretory phenotypes (SASP) are phenotypes linked with senescent cells. Those cells can release inflammatory cytokines, growth factors, and proteases. SASP likely consist of ectosomes and exosomes with enzymes, microRNA, and other bioactive substances initially immunosuppressive (TGF-β1 and TGF-β3), but then progressing to proinflammatory (IL-1β, IL-6 and IL-8). SASP is a primary cause of senescent cells' detrimental effects on many tissues and organs, including those of muscle and bone mass.

LDN and Cancer Reduction

Cancer in its many forms is the second most fatal medical condition, and often the aggressive treatments for cancer currently offered in the early 21st-century can also have damaging effects and complications that can either lead directly to death or reduce longevity overall. Low dose naltrexone is an agent that can reduce the occurrence of cancers across the board. It can also be used as an adjuvant to many current conventional or complementary and alternative (CAM) therapies for a wide range of cancers.[149] LDN's ability to inhibit tumor growth is by actions on cell signaling and immune modification. LDN's actions on opioid growth factor receptors (OGFr) as an antagonist will inhibit the biological pathways in human cancer cells directed by the OGF-OGFr axis. Early studies show LDN as having promise as an anti-cancer agent.[150] This principle will be discussed in other chapters and has been discussed in previous volumes of *The LDN Book*. Since primary cancers of the genitourinary system, liver, lung, breast, colon, and lymphatics are seen as conditions that impact life expectancy, it can be presumed that by limiting that burden either in mass or occurrence would have a positive impact on longevity. Research in autophagy has enlightened us with regard to the impact of this discovery within our own cells.[151] Autophagy is the process by which the lysosomes clean up and recycle worn out or expired molecules and proteins. This keeps the cells running like well-oiled machines. It also apparently has a part to play in cancer. Clog up the cells with dysfunctional molecules, proteins and organelles, and you are set up for cancer. LDN influences autophagy in a positive way.

LDN and Telomere Length

Human telomeres are composed of 10 to 15 kb of a sequence 5'-TTAGGG-3' DNA that is repeated and a complex of protein that is telomere-associated called shelterin. Shelterin is a protein complex consisting of six telomere-associated proteins.[152] They are referred to as: telomeric repeat-binding factors 1 and 2 (TRF1 and TRF2), TRF1-interacting nuclear factor 2 (TIN2), protection of telomeres (POT1), POT1 and TIN2-interacting protein 1 (TPP1), and TRF2-interacting protein 1 (Rap1). Telomerase is a reverse transcriptase enzyme that maintains the telomere length by adding nucleotides during cell division to the single-stranded DNA (ssDNA). The shelterin complex protects the telomeres from being recognized as a double stranded (ds) break in DNA. There are mechanisms that will repair damaged or broken DNA and this would disrupt the process of telomere lengthening. So, this shelterin complex blocks the initiation and activation of the DNA damage response and repair process. This repair process for dsDNA would defeat the purpose of the mechanism of elongation or maintenance of the length of the telomere. Thus, it is the partnership of both the enzyme and the protein bundle that works the magic.

When you have low telomerase activity and hence the inability to repair and lengthen (or maintain adequate length of the telomere) you have a more progressive and rapid rate of aging or in some cases disease states. Take the example of mutations in genes encoding for telomerase or telomere-binding proteins. These genetic or congenital disorders can in fact cause issues with bone marrow, lung, and skin. Telomerase controls the hematopoietic stem cell differentiation and senescence. These diseases are linked to the presence of shortened telomeres and to defects in stem cells in the bone marrow. Insufficient cell division in these stem cells can lead to anemia. In the case of dyskeratosis congenita, a congenital progressive telomeropathy, there is a mutation in the telomerase non-coding RNA (ncRNA) gene (TERC-gene) that leads to accelerated cellular senescence and premature aging in those with the mutation.[153] The same applies for mutations in the telomerase reverse transcriptase gene (TERT-gene). If there is a mutation in the DKC1-gene (the gene that codes for the telomere-protein complex) one realizes disorders such as aplastic anemias, and pulmonary and liver fibrosis.

Despite all that we know about telomeres and premature aging, senescence of cell telomere biology cannot explain all of human aging. Telomere shortening and attrition does lead to cell senescence and the Hayflick phenomenon, but some of the congenital telomeropathies such as dyskeratosis congenita (DC), which can sometimes be misclassified as Hutchinson-Gilford progeria or Werner's syndrome, as they are a tad dissimilar. Those with DC in general do not appear old nor do they have premature Alzheimer's disease, osteopenia, T2DM, or atherosclerosis. This is likely the case because mutations in TERT and TERC do not have a uniform effect on all tissues.[154] For instance, it may show variations in brain and heart tissues. And for that matter, decreased telomere length over a human's life does not really establish a cause for aging. However, it is known that shortened telomeres are linked to a weak immune system and chronic/degenerative diseases like coronary disease, congestive heart failure, cancers, diabetes, and osteoporosis, all which increase the risk of shortened life expectancy or reduced quality of life at the very least. Many functional and anti-aging medicine doctors still use telomere length testing as a way to measure risks and report a biological age to compare with a patient's chronological age. Obviously, we don't have all the answers and more research is needed.

On the other side of the spectrum, high telomerase activity as seen in cancer cells may lead them to divide indefinitely and thus refer to some cancer cells as immortal. It has been found that telomerase activity is increased in about 80 to 90% of cancers.[155] One must be careful when attempting to maintain or increase the telomere length. Steroid hormones and growth-hormone, while not necessarily implicated in sparking cancer, certainly can perpetuate and contribute to those aberrant cells.

Autophagy and Lifespan

As a human cell ages over time some of its components become damaged or worn out. The damaged components can build up in a cell and cause cellular dysfunction. This bioaccumulation of cellular debris can impact the day-to-day activities of a cell and thus its health and lifespan. To keep cells working optimally in function, structure and how genes perform, a complex process known as autophagy clears our damaged or suboptimal performing cells. Research in the process of autophagy is in its infancy but scientists are looking at ways to enhance this process to increase lifespan. Caution must be exacted as enhancement of autophagy may on the other hand have detrimental effects, so it must be well-controlled.

The word autophagy is derived from the ancient Greek meaning to "eat thyself." We recognize it today as the process our cells have to remove dysfunctional components or unwanted molecules within our cells. This process is highly regulated and results in a recycling of inefficient cellular components and the removal of damaged cellular material. Autophagy can be triggered by outside influences such as fasting, meditation, R&R vacations, and agents such as curcumin, quercetin, resveratrol, peptides, and some hormones. In 1955, the Belgian cytologist and biochemist Dr. Christian de Duve discovered the lysosome (a previously unknown cellular organelle) that defined autophagy. Since then, research has progressed in the targeting of cytoplasmic material for lysosomal degradation in what we now refer to as autophagy. Following its discovery it has been realized that autophagy deficiency is linked to a variety of diseases, cancer being chief among them. This work won Dr. de Duve the Nobel Prize in Physiology or Medicine in 1974.

Low dose naltrexone appears to upregulate a unique gene expression affecting autophagy and apoptosis in cancer cells.[156] This effect is not seen in normal dosing of naltrexone for the purposes of opioid and alcohol addiction. The mechanisms of action are only associated with lower doses of naltrexone. As a matter of fact, one must be very careful with autophagy, as over expression can have the opposite intended effects.

Exosomes (decellularized nanoparticles) and Stem Cells

Exosomes are a very hot topic these days. So hot that the FDA has insisted on renaming them "decellularized nanoparticles." Exosomes can be classified as nanoparticles based on their size. Exosomes can be developed for drug delivery as a novel way to transport small-molecule synthetic drugs to targeted organs, tissues, and cells.[157] [158] This type of technology may limit the cytotoxic effects seen with standard types of chemotherapy in the treatment of cancers. In nature, these nanoparticles are usually packed with proteins, RNA/micro-RNS (miRNA)/small interfering RNA (siRNA) both classified as non-coding RNA (ncRNA), cytokines, growth factors, and lipids, among other things, and are generated, secreted from donor cells to eventually connect with recipient cells. Exosomes are very small (30 to 100ng) particles made up of the membrane or cell wall of most types of cells. The outward budding process occurs when internal vesicles for what is referred to as multivesicular bodies (MVB) are formed. MVBs migrate and fuse with the plasma membrane and these internal vesicles are then jettisoned into intercellular spaces as exosomes. They then can migrate to a recipient cell and deliver their payload to exact different physiological and cell behavior on that recipient cell.

How exosomes or decellularized nanoparticles can help with longevity is obvious.[159] From a cancer perspective they can deliver chemotherapeutic agents to targeted cells with less collateral damage. Fighting cancer can increase the lifespan of a patient burdened with this disease. There may be future ways of delivering DNA via this modality as gene therapy, again conquering some congenital conditions known to shave years off a person's life.

In the laboratory, model studies have shown that mesenchymal stem cells enhance the repair effect with myocardial infarction. In one study exosomes derived from TIMP2-modified human umbilical cord mesenchymal stem cells (hucMSCs) repaired the ischemic heart muscle of lab mice suffering from ischemic injury. In another study in 2019, noted in the *Journal of Oxidative Medicine and Cellular Longevity*, it was determined that exosomes can prevent aging-induced cardiac dysfunction. This can obviously have an impact on aging and impact public health. These are just two examples of how exosome technology may impact humanity and longevity.[160]

The connection between LDN and exosomes is a bit less evident as our exploration into exosomes is in its early stages and once better understood studies of the impact of naltrexone can be explored.

Peptides and Hormones

The 1902 winner of the Nobel Prize in Chemistry, Dr. Emil Fischer, is considered the founding father of peptide chemistry. He is also likely the originator of the term peptide. In the early 20th century, the renowned chemist had a vision foreseeing the day when a protein would be synthesized not just extracted from animal organs. Fischer's vision was correct as scientists in China were able to synthesize insulin in 1965. Insulin was the first synthetic peptide produced. It is now widely used in medicine and it's not an overstatement to say it has saved many lives and reduced morbidity as well. The same year Dr. Fischer was awarded the Nobel Prize, researchers Sir William M. Bayliss and Dr. Ernest Starling discovered secretin. Secretin is a peptide released from the jejunal mucosa when acid from the stomach activates it. This secretin hormone coursed through the bloodstream acting as a messenger that excited the pancreas and releases pancreatic enzymes. For this discovery they were themselves nominated for a Nobel Prize in Physiology.

Following insulin in 1970, there was a new hot topic: research focused on neuropeptides. Enkephalin and the opioid peptides were discovered and since that time biochemists have been able to synthesize peptides by artificial methods. In 1931, Substance P (SP) was discovered and later in 1953, Oxytocin was discovered. Both of these considered as neuropeptides helped push research into peptides further. On the heels of all this interest, Drs. Rita Levi-Montalcini and Stanley Cohen identified a healing peptide they called nerve growth factor (NGF) in 1960. With the ability for biochemists to synthesize peptides by artificial methods for more than 40 years, developments in molecular biology and biochemistry have advanced peptide research at a rapid rate.[161]

While there is too much to discuss about the healing effects of peptides, which have been heavily researched for over three decades, they will briefly be touched upon here. Worth a mention is that optimal hormone balance is essential for proper health and wellness and contributes to longevity. Behind the Iron Curtain much of the research was published in Russian language journals, but with the collapse of the USSR, research continued within Russia and Ukraine. Now that secrecy has been broken and journals translated, Sweden and other European countries are continuing the research of peptides for use in healing and fighting cancer. It is worth mentioning that peptides came late to the Western hemisphere, and once they arrived things got shuttered in early 2021 when the FDA moved to redefine and recategorize natural-occurring and synthesized peptides. This restriction on their synthesis and availability has hampered clinicians from prescribing them. There are outlets in which they can be acquired and providers in the know can offer guidance on their use and doses.

Peptides worth mentioning here are: thymosin alpha-1, thymosin beta-4 (TB500 or thymosin beta-4-frag), and body protection compound (BPC)-157. Thymosin is a peptide found in the thymus gland and while TB500 and TB4-frag are used interchangeably they probably should not. While thymosin beta-4 is a natural compound TB500 is a synthetic version produced in the laboratory. TB-4-frag is a fragment of the larger TB-4 peptide and being only a few amino-acids long appears to have greater function as a healing peptide than the full-length 43-aa peptide. Thymic gland function is decreased as we age out of childhood and by age 40, we do not retain much of the thymus gland. Thymosin alpha-1 and thymosin beta-4 are two peptides that replace what is lost as far as thymic function peptide hormones.[162] This can be useful in the aging patient.

Epithalon and pinealon are pineal peptides, delta sleep-inducing peptide (DSIP), DIHEXA, cerebrolysin, lysine-proline-valine (KPV) a tripeptide known to mitigate inflammation, often used to heal intestinal permeability (leaky gut) are examples of peptides that have a positive effect on the aging process and tissue repair and rejuvenation. Still others include bremelanotide, CJC-1295, ipamorelin (often use in combination with CJC-1295), ibutamoren (MK-677), IGF-1 LR3, RAS, sermorelin (and the modified longer acting analog CJC-1295), AOD-9604, KISSPEPTIN-10, SELANK, SEMAX, LL33 and LL37, to name a few.[163]

When in balance, hormones all along the HPA-axis contribute to wellness, increased performance, and longevity. Those are a balance of DHEA, cortisol, pregnenolone, testosterone, progesterone, and the estrogens for the most part.[164] One can go further to the myriad of metabolites along the way, as testing for them is available. Additionally, a big player in human metabolism are the thyroid hormones. Chief among them is triiodothyronine (T3), but there is some activity seen in thyroxine (T4) (considered a pro-hormone for T3) and diiodothyronine (T2) (a metabolite of T3 lacking an iodine atom). This chapter does not allow for a lengthy discussion on gonadal-hormones, adrenal hormones, or thyroid hormones, but one cannot have a meaningful conversation about longevity without mentioning these hormones. Proper balance of these hormones is essential for good health and longevity and when they are out of balance or lacking appropriate levels, the body ages. Management in appropriate ways to keep in balance and at suitable levels is a critical step to longevity medicine when they are found to be out of equilibrium. Entire books have been written on the value to human health of these hormones. Seeking to keep them in balance in physiologically appropriate levels with replacement or correcting underlying issues that are the root cause for their disequilibrium are necessary to identify.

Select Nutraceuticals: Antioxidants, NAD+, et al

A full discussion of dietary supplements or nutraceuticals would require its own book. One cannot begin to have a detailed dissertation on supplements here related to antiaging or longevity, so we will cover them with broad strokes. Antioxidants in general seem to be protective against major chronic disease-inducing entities that shorten human life expectancy. Antioxidants interfere with the pathology of cardiovascular disease and cancer. Research into agents such as superoxide dismutase (SOD), catalase (CAT), resveratrol (Res), lipoic acids, coenzyme Q10, curcumin, multiple polyphenols and anthocyanins, nicotinamide-adenine dinucleotide (NAD+/NADH) and nicotinamide mononucleotide (NMN) or nicotinamide riboside (NR) has been conducted for many years. Sulforaphane, epigallocatechin gallate (EGCG) and even synthetic antioxidant nanoparticles should be included in any review. Not to be excluded in this brief discussion are vitamin C, vitamin A, α-tocopherol, selenium, glutathione peroxidase, and reductase, melatonin, and the many other micronutrients that support and promote the production of antioxidant and anti-aging agents.[165] While research in lower lifeforms (such as nematodes and fruit flies) has remained equivocal, positive, and negative in some peer-reviewed research papers, the more complex human organism may be a better model for proving antioxidants effective in the aging process, and more recent research published in human studies seems to concur.[166] Naltrexone is an antioxidant worth noting again in this discussion. LDN serves as a synthetic agent yielding antioxidant and anti-aging properties. LDN can be suggested, used singularly or in combination with other agents for a symbiotic effect.

Meditation (Mind-Body/Social Interaction)

Social interaction has been shown in studies to extend life. Humans are social animals and as such, thrive on interaction with others. Healthy socialization, is important and even socializing among other species (pets for example) can add years to our lives. The principles of social distancing we have witnessed during the COVID-19 pandemic as a means of the first pillar of a pandemic response has provided even more evidence of how this can impact our longevity.[167] The term social distancing should be replaced with the term "physical distancing" so as not to confuse and ignore the socialization aspect so important to human mental health. Social distancing can lead to social isolation and loneliness and that correlates with a loss of longevity. Depression can ensue with isolation and loneliness. In fact, there is evidence that beyond repairing the damage of social isolation by reinstating more of the social norms and interactions, adding in agents to reduce depression is helpful. Adding to the list of natural and synthetic antidepressants you cannot leave out LDN. LDN has been shown clinically to help with major depressive disorder (MDD).[168]

Meditation is yet another human activity that lends itself to longevity, though as with dietary supplements we do not have room for lengthy discussion on meditation and other forms of energy medicine in this chapter. Instead, I want only to make mention of meditation as a general contributor of wellness, good health, and how calming the mind affects the hypothalamic-pituitary-adrenal axis (HPA-axis), promoting a much healthier and longer life.

Exercise, Stretching, Aerobic and Resistance

Along with a good diet, exercise plays a crucial role in longevity. Exercise comes in many forms, from basic aerobic activities such as walking, jogging, or running, to bicycling or swimming laps, to more recent variations such as high intensity interval training (HIIT). Then there is functional exercise to support individuals as they advance in years. On the other side of the continuum of exercise is resistance training, which may consist of weight training, cross training, or other programs.[169] Somewhere in between is passive and active stretching and activities such as yoga or Pilates. Most people are advised to find a balance between aerobic and resistance to achieve the best outcome. From an antiaging perspective, it is advised to not overdo exercise since extreme intensity or duration (especially without supervision) can lead to injury that can either temporarily or permanently result in the inability to perform future exercise. Over exercising can result in the production of un-countered oxidative stress or inflammatory loads. Regular moderate exercise has been associated with an increase in life expectancy of several years. For example, 150 minutes of exercise or more each week increased life expectancy by about 7.2 years over those who did not do regular moderate exercise at all, who were inactive or obese according to studies published in 2012 and 2021.[170] [171]

Restorative Sleep

Sleep is one of the prime anti-aging modalities and also the most cost-effective. Not just any sleep, however, but restorative sleep. In healthcare we debate the proper number of hours of sleep required to be healthy. Some say that between seven and nine hours is best, though some people can survive and thrive on less. The literature reports that for most people seven hours is the most restorative and leads to longer life. A study published in 2014 by *Frontiers in Aging Neuroscience* revealed that longevity was associated with regular sleep patterns and the maintenance of slow-wave sleep.[172] In one meta-analysis of 16 sleep studies, it was revealed that too-short and too-long durations of sleep were associated with a higher degree of mortality, so there is a sweet spot, though it may vary from person to person.[173]

Aiding sleep with LDN should be a positive undertaking. LDN and VLDN (very low dose naltrexone) are ways to achieve better sleep as they can modulate sleep by abolishing the cortisol surge in the evenings associated with many disorders hampering REM sleep (one component of the sleep cycle that has restorative properties when in balance) and delaying falling asleep. There are some that find LDN therapy disruptive to sleep and those are the outliers; again, LDN may not be for everyone. About 37% of patients taking LDN will report vivid dreams, which is a common side-effect of LDN therapy. Some may endorse sleep disturbance but with ongoing therapy, dose adjustments, and timing this usually resolves spontaneously.[174]

Breathing

Yoga, yogic breathing, and other breathing techniques such as square or box breathing have been studied with regard to longevity, and how they affect the HPA-axis among other biomarkers to promote life extension and longevity. This was noted in a 2009 study and more recently in a 2017 study, which identified biomarkers associated with aging and the influence of yoga and yogic breathing exercises in conjunction with other lifestyle modifications. The study led by Dr. Tolahunase used the terminology yoga and meditation-based lifestyle intervention (YMLI) on cellular aging in a healthy adult cohort.[175] During a 12-week prospective, open-label study, 96 healthy individuals were enrolled to receive YMLI. Cardinal biomarkers of cellular aging such as DNA damage marker 8-hydroxy-2'-deoxyguanosine (8-OH2dG), oxidative stress markers reactive oxygen species (ROS), and total antioxidant capacity (TAC), and telomere attrition markers, telomere length and telomerase activity were measured. Other endpoint markers such as cortisol, β-endorphin, IL-6, BDNF, and sirtuin-1 were also evaluated. After 12 weeks of YMLI, there were significant improvements in both the cardinal biomarkers of cellular aging and the metabolic biomarkers influencing cellular aging compared to baseline values. The levels of 8-OH2dG, ROS, cortisol, and IL-6 were significantly lower and mean levels of TAC, telomerase activity, β-endorphin, BDNF, and sirtuin-1 were significantly increased, all statistically significant. Therefore, YMLI significantly reduced the rate of cellular aging, and this would impact longevity.[176]

Caloric Restrictions: SIR-2 gene, FOXO3 gene, CETP gene, MOD-1 gene

Many animal and human studies over the years have shown a positive relationship between caloric restriction (CR) and longevity. Caloric restrictions can also include intermittent fasting, but one does not have to fast to achieve CR. Decades of research on a variety of animal models from snails to rodents to humans show if calories are restricted, the onset of age-related disorders is limited and in some cases lifespan extended. A growing body of evidence has shown that CR can reduce risk factors and pathophysiology of diabetes (T2DM), cardiovascular disease, cancer, and neurological disorders that all chip away at our life expectancy. Mechanisms of action that drive CR-induced longevity include those involving energy metabolism, oxidative load, and inflammation. CR also affects glucose homeostasis and the neuroendocrine system in ways to support a longer lifespan. In one study published in 2018 in the journal *Communications Biology*, CR accelerated gray matter atrophy in the animal model (mouse lemurs).[177] This one study shows a potential negative impact that CR has on brain integrity and warrants further study. That study may be one of the few outliers.

Genetics impact on longevity include some genes by cryptic names such as silent information regulator gene (SIR2), decay accelerating factor (Daf-2), Pit-1, AAK-1, CLK-1 and P66Shc, and several others discussed here. SIR2 is found in organisms from yeasts to humans and variants in this gene and extra copies of this gene yield an increase in longevity. Researchers are looking into how these genes can be expressed (epigenetically) in a beneficial way for human longevity. Research findings suggested that aging in mother cells was caused by some form of ribosomal DNA (rDNA) instability that was mitigated by the SIR proteins and enzymes encoded by SIR2 after a mutation in the SIR4 gene affected it. When researchers added extra copies of SIR2 genes to organisms, it increased life expectancy (in yeast it was extended by 30% and in roundworms by as much as 50%).[178] Will this work in humans? Well, to increase the expression of SIR2 gene CR seems to be one mechanism. CR and Resveratrol activate SIR2 and lead to longevity in higher organisms. There is a second pathway involving NAD/NADH ratios that influence SIR2 activity. In mammals, the version of SIR2 gene is known as SIRT1 and it results in the production of SIRT1 enzymes much like the SIR enzymes in lower forms of life. Manipulating these genes will likely have an impact on human longevity as it is seen in other forms of organisms. Apparently, SIRT1 has a regulatory activity on other cellular proteins such as FoxO, Ku70 and p53. Research into the four forkhead box (FoxO) subtypes in mammals found that FoxO3 regulates cellular hemostasis in stem cells and cell cycle arrest, apoptosis and cell repair. The key to longevity may be the manipulation of FoxO3 by therapeutic agents. Another gene known as CETP having to do with cholesterol transfer protein, affects HDL-cholesterol. Defects in this gene can cause hyperalphalipoproteinemia 1 (HALP1) and have an effect on the cardiovascular system as it relates to longevity. When studying a particular region (a non-blue zone region) in China, researchers studied a population of Han Chinese from Yunnan province for single nucleotide polymorphisms (SNPs) of the CETP gene and at least in this population mutations or variants of this gene did not seem to have an impact on aging. These findings emphasize the point that further study is needed.[179] [180]

Mutations that decrease the activity of DAF-2 can lead to longevity in some lower animal forms. It also involves the DAF-16 gene and IIS activity leading to effects on cellular stress response (heat-shock proteins, superoxide dismutase, and catalase), metabolism, and autophagy. Manipulation of DAF-2 and DAF-16 and their effects on FoxO transcription plays a role along with a class 1 ARF GAP domain (AGD-1) gene in aging. One mechanism whereby CR works on a cellular level is described as TOR signaling, where a mammalian mechanistic target of rapamycin (mTOR) and a serine/threonine kinase regulates cell growth, proliferation, motility, and survival in the aging process. TOR signaling ultimately impacts autophagy and transcription. By reducing TOR activity by nutrient- or energy-lacking conditions such as caloric restrictions, it was hypothesized that this process was involved in increasing the lifespan of *C. elegans* in a DAF-16-dependent manner. The same rules apply in higher life forms (mTOR). One can postulate that naltrexone even in lower doses may have an effect on caloric intake (reduction in food addiction and overeating) to manifest in similar fashion. More research needs to be undertaken.[181]

New Paradigm

For integrative and functional medicine practitioners, aging is treated as a disease to prevent. Conventional mainstream medicine today is focused on the mindset of treating the diseases associated with aging as they present. There is a lack of focus or attention directed to a holistic approach on prevention. Within mainstream medicine, a lot of lip service is given to prevention, but in actuality that paradigm is well entrenched in sick care and not wellness or genuine prevention. The sick care paradigm is a multi-billion dollar a year industry entrenched deeply in the medical-industrial complex where profits trump science and prevention. Little money is to be made in the long term by these huge systems of healthcare if we keep the populace well and free of disease. For this reason, one must look to another paradigm that is embraced by practitioners of integrative, anti-aging, and functional medicine. Within this wellness-based (well-care) system there is a mindset of early interventions to lower or eliminate the risk of chronic illness setting in. The chief concern is with interventional protocols to promote health and wellness.

Low dose naltrexone is one of many tools to assist with morbidity compression and vitality expansion. LDN as it is discussed in this book as well as the past two volumes has properties that help with autoimmune disease, cancer, immune enhancement, and some chronic illnesses that can shorten life and reduce vitality. LDN (by reducing the effects of the major killers and life-shortening issues we face) may play a crucial role in our longevity.

FIVE

An Integrative Approach to Mixed Connective Tissue Disease

Deanna Windham, DO

Mixed connective tissue disease (MCTD) is a complicated, poorly understood, and often misdiagnosed disease process. Diagnosis of MCTD is partially one of exclusion and is easy to miss. Treatment options are limited and focus solely on symptom management. Together, these aspects make MCTD difficult for both practitioners, who can feel useless in helping their patients to improve their lives, and patients, who seek out doctor after doctor looking for a diagnosis or a treatment plan that offers some hope.

In this chapter, we will discuss the nuances of mixed connective tissue disease, what research tells us about its pathological basis, and how to nail the diagnosis every time. But more importantly, for our sanity as clinicians and for the good of our patients, we will delve into the science behind effective treatment methods and highlight the benefits of treatment with low dose naltrexone.

Diagnosis of MCTD

For many years, it wasn't clear if MCTD was an independent disease process or if the symptoms recognized as MCTD were in fact a manifestation of a combination of other autoimmune diseases such as lupus, scleroderma, or polymyositis. However, research over the last few years has elucidated a distinct pathological process although the diagnostic process is still complicated due to its overlapping features with other autoimmune diseases. So first, let's discuss how to diagnose MCTD correctly with three easy guidelines:

Diagnostic Guideline One: Maintain a high level of suspicion. Most autoimmune patients have symptoms from multiple systems, see multiple doctors, and suffer needlessly for years before they get a correct diagnosis. Begin suspecting autoimmune disease if your patients experience brain fog (in any/all of its many forms), fatigue despite getting enough sleep or sleep disturbance they haven't been able to overcome, post-exertional fatigue (not just for chronic fatigue syndrome), symptoms of hormone imbalance, chronic pain of any type, chronic gastrointestinal concerns of any type, sensitivity to chemicals or smells, early response to medications that later fail, any psychiatric conditions that are difficult to treat or recalcitrant to treatment, any "weird" or "crazy" symptoms that don't seem to make sense. Family history of autoimmune disease should be considered as well, though lack of family history does not exclude the diagnosis. None of these are specific to autoimmune disease, but all of them, especially if two or more are seen together in the same person, are red flags.

More specifically, MCTD can have many presentations due to its systemic impact. And, like most autoimmune diseases, it can be difficult to detect. However, research has given us common presentations and system-specific signs and symptoms that should alert practitioners to the possibility of MCTD. These serious conditions, which are outcomes of MCTD, also highlight the need for a comprehensive approach to treatment. Mixed connective tissue disease system-specific signs and symptoms:[182]

- Most common presentations include: arthralgia, myalgia, malaise, and low-grade fever.
- Dermatology: Raynaud's, hand edema, telangiectasia, erythema nodosum, alopecia, vasculitis of digits, acrosclerosis, calcinosis, discoid plaques, and malar rash.
- Joint: deformities similar to rheumatoid arthritis or psoriatic arthritis.
- Muscle: inflammatory myopathy with myalgia.
- Lung: 73% of patients have lung disease with dyspnea, pleural effusion, pulmonary hypertension, interstitial lung disease, vasculitis, thrombus, chronic or recurrent infection, or COPD.

- Heart: pericarditis in 40% of MCTD patients in their lifetimes, pericardial effusion, mitral valve prolapse, myocarditis, cardiomegaly, accelerated atherosclerosis.
- Kidney: 15-25% of patients have renal disease that most commonly presents as membranous nephropathy although usually asymptomatic, risk of hypertension and rare hemodialysis result.
- Gastroenterology: GERD or reflux, esophageal hypomotility requiring dilation, pancreatitis, mega colon, autoimmune hepatitis, duodenal bleed, portal hypertension.
- Neurology: brain fog and brain fatigue are common, trigeminal neuralgia, chronic or recurrent headaches, nuchal rigidity, sensorineural hearing loss, aseptic meningitis, even psychosis.

Diagnostic Guideline Two: While there are several diagnostic criteria for MCTD, let's simplify our understanding to make it easier to find. Anti-U1 ribonucleoprotein (RNP) complex is an intramuscular protein that converts pre-mRNA to mature RNA. Anti-U1-RNP antibody reactive T lymphocytes circulating in peripheral blood is the hallmark of MCTD. At a basic level, MCTD is defined by the presence of anti-U1-RNP complex in the presence of one, both, or a combination of the following:

- Features of at least two connective tissue diseases: lupus, RA, polymyositis, dermatomyositis, systemic sclerosis. If none of these disease processes have been diagnosed, the diagnostic process can be simplified to identifying someone with chronic joint pain, especially when accompanied by morning stiffness or joint swelling; chronic muscle aches or pains; chronic characteristic skin lesions; chronic spinal pain or headaches; and, often, other general signs and symptoms of autoimmune disease.
- Three or more of the following: hand edema, synovitis, myositis, Raynaud's, or atherosclerosis. As you can see, the first three of these—joint pain, muscle pain and swelling—are all symptoms from the first list of criteria with the added recognition that vascular issues such as Raynaud's and atherosclerotic disease may also be present.

Diagnostic Guideline Three: Breaking these criteria down to their simplest form, if a patient has two or more of the aforementioned symptoms, test them for anti-U1 RNP. All major labs do this test both individually and as part of the ANA and other autoimmune profiles. If the result is positive, you are working with mixed connective tissue disease.

However, if we want to understand mixed connective tissue disease to help us treat it more effectively, then we must take into account the genesis of the disease. MCTD, like all autoimmune diseases, is an epigenetic disease with triggers. Let's break that down into its component parts because these must be understood to truly get a grasp on mixed connective tissue disease.

What Is Meant by "Epigenetic Disease"

Epigenetics is, put simply, the science of how one's DNA changes its expression based on various exposures. I call these exposures triggers because they trigger your body to develop autoimmune disease. We have all seen pictures of the double helix of a DNA strand. However, our DNA is actually folded up into a mass that looks like a cloud and is hard to recognize. It is partially in the folding that the key to epigenetics can be found. By folding in different ways, different parts of the genetic code come into contact with one another and copying of the material in the code produces varying results. Depending on which parts are folded together while being copied, there would be a different message than if the strand were stretched out fully.

Other ways that epigenetic changes are triggered include methylation of the DNA strand which effectively "turns on" or "turns off" certain parts of the genetic code, as well as the recognized processes of apoptosis modification and molecular mimicry that create epigenetic changes leading to MCTD.[183] Although I am oversimplifying these concepts for the sake of brevity, the point is that there are well-researched and well-understood ways by which our human DNA makes changes during our lifetimes in response to certain known triggers.

MCTD is an epigenetic disease with known risk alleles and

protective alleles.[ii] That means that the epigenetic factors that make one more or less susceptible to MCTD have been, at least partially, identified. The genetics of MCTD are associated with HLD-DR4 and DR2 positive genetics, indicative of T cell receptor and HLA molecule involvement.[184] There has been further research to identify the epigenetic changes that lead to MCTD, of which there are many.[185] In addition, miRNA (microRNA) molecules have been shown in research to epigenetically increase the risk of developing MCTD.[186]

Next, with full understanding that the epigenetic factor of MCTD has been established, let's explore the triggers that lead to these epigenetic changes because it is here that we are able to impact the disease process. Identifying triggers also means identifying individualized treatment targets that we can use to help ourselves or our patients heal.

The only triggers that are recognized by the mainstream medical approach to increase the risk of developing MCTD are: certain drugs, toxins, chemicals including vinyl chloride and silica, and UV radiation (all of which fall under the one category of environmental toxins, which is one of 12 categories of triggering factors). However, while some of these triggers may be addressed in the literature, a complete evaluation of each patient's triggers that precipitated their development of autoimmune disease need to be addressed if we are to have long-lasting positive impact in the disease process.

MCTD is rare enough that there hasn't been much research in the field of treatment. What research has been published is sparse and focuses on diagnosis and treatment with the mainstream approach of steroids, pain medications, DMARDS, and immunosuppressing drugs. This approach focuses solely on symptom relief. Triggers or root causes of disease are not addressed or treated in this purely Western medicine approach. Anyone who has worked with autoimmune disease knows the abysmal impact this approach has on overall quality of life.

While there is no significant research on the integrative medical

ii   Alleles are defined as one of two or more alternative forms of a gene that arise by mutation and are found at the same place on a [DNA] chromosome.

approach through identifying and treating triggers, practitioners who treat this way have much higher success rates in the form of improved quality of life, slowing or reversing the disease process, and decreased risk of development of other diseases or negative outcomes as a result of MCTD.

The Triggers

The triggers that turn on the epigenetic risk for autoimmune disease have been identified in research and occur in four broad categories:

1. Body factors
    1. Microbiome: all the bacteria on and in the human body, especially in the gut
    2. Nutritional deficiencies
    3. Endocrine (hormone) imbalance
2. Environmental factors
    1. Pathogens (viruses, bacteria, parasites and other infectious agents)
    2. Chemical and environmental toxicity
    3. Diet
3. Lifestyle factors
    1. Sleep disturbance or deprivation
    2. Movement / exercise
    3. Autonomic nervous system imbalance
4. Mind factors
    1. Stress / Emotions
    2. Beliefs
    3. Social Circumstances

In this section, we will discuss each trigger separately, as well as how LDN works to impact each particular trigger, starting with the microbiome because this is one of the potentially most significant triggering factors. All or most autoimmune diseases in which the microbiome has been researched have found that imbalances in the gut microbiome, termed dysbiosis, are a significant epigenetic trigger. There is good reason for this.

Body Factor 1: The Microbiome

Many people have heard of the microbiome but don't understand its significance. There are trillions of bacteria in your gut. In fact, bacteria cells in our bodies outnumber our human cells by more than 10 to 1. The bacteria in our gut work hard on our behalf to keep us alive and healthy. The microbiome:

- Trains your immune system.
- Is your first line of defense against the outside world (other invading microorganisms).
- Helps you digest your food and synthesize nutrients from it.
- Helps you to inhibit uptake of and eliminate toxins.
- Aids in detoxification of poisons, drugs, and toxins.
- Contributes to your human genetic expression.

In addition, your microbiome has connections throughout the body that assure its optimum functioning:

Gut ↔ Hormones
- Many hormones are produced, recycled, or eliminated by the gut microbiome.
- Hormones have documented effects on the microbiome (bidirectional impact).
- Male/female variance in the microbiota is one contributory factor of the difference in autoimmune susceptibility.

Gut ↔ Brain
- More than 80% of neurotransmitters (chemical messengers in the brain) are produced in the gut.
- The microbiome produces cytokines (chemical messengers) that impact your brain health.
- Unhealthy microbiota secrete metabolites that alter the blood brain barrier, allowing toxins and other substances access to the brain.

Gut ↔ Immune
- 80% of your immune system is located in your gut.
- Immune responses are often initiated in the gut.
- Many immune diseases are triggered and maintained by microbiome dysfunction or dysbiosis.

- Damage to the lining of the gastrointestinal tract (ubiquitous in autoimmune disease) leads to broken tight junctions between the enterocytes (cells that line the gut) which in turn creates the condition for autoimmune disease in the form of abnormal immune responses and induction of inflammatory cytokine cascades.

Human bodies have 350 times more microbial genes than human genes according to the National Institute of Health (NIH).[187] Bacteria can exchange genes to change, function, or adapt to the environment. Bacterial genetics change much faster than human genetics, giving us an advantage in a changing world. In 2015, researchers at the University of Cambridge determined that humans have 128 microbial genes in our genetic code as a result of horizontal transmission.[188] Amazingly, research has shown that, therefore, changes to the structure of our microbiome changes our human genetic expression. This means that changes to the microbiome are a strong epigenetic factor contributing to disease activation or deactivation. The impact of the microbiome is in no disease process so clear as it is in autoimmune disease and recently has been shown to be impactful in MCTD, specifically.[189]

How LDN helps the microbiome

As can be seen from the extensive research gathered by the LDN Research Trust, LDN has been shown in many studies to have positive benefits in immune diseases that center on the GI system, such as Crohn's disease, ulcerative colitis, inflammatory bowel disease, and irritable bowel syndrome. Research has shown improvements in both symptoms and pathology. LDN decreases the damaging inflammatory cytokines produced in the gut and alters the pathological cellular balance of autoimmune disease. It also supports the immune system to improve the balance of the microbiome and decreases cravings for foods that are harmful to the microbiome.

Body Factor 2: Nutritional Deficiencies

With all nutritional deficiencies, as with everything else, there is an art to correct diagnosis and optimal treatment to ideal, not just "normal," ranges. Deficiencies are rampant in our society due to the abysmal quality of a Standard American Diet (SAD, pun intended) which is high in sugar, carbohydrates, and saturated fats but low in vitamins, minerals, enzymes, probiotics, prebiotics, fiber, antioxidants, and thousands of trace phytonutrients that help our bodies sustain healthy cellular activity. Likely, there are dozens or even hundreds of as-yet-undiscovered nutrients that are important to human health and disease management. Only a few have been researched.

The most widely researched and widely accepted nutritional deficiency associated with increased risk of developing or worsening MCTD is vitamin D deficiency. Vitamin D deficiency has been shown to epigenetically alter the gene expression by histone modification and methylation.[190] In addition, having ideal levels stabilized several aspects of disease including inflammation, immune system function and stabilization, and improves immune tolerance to self.

About 75% of people with MCTD have iron deficiency anemia, likely from loss through the damaged intestinal tract. It is important to test levels and treat appropriately as high iron levels are dangerous and inflammatory.

Vitamin C deficiency is common in connective tissue diseases in general. This is easily understood if you know that collagen, part of the glue that holds our connective tissue together, requires vitamin C and other nutrients for its production. Both vitamin C and vitamin D have anti-inflammatory effects and are protective for the cardiovascular system. Both vitamins are also protective against the epigenetic changes that lead to autoimmune disease manifestation.

How LDN helps in the case of nutritional deficiencies

LDN changes the appetite, making it easier to stick with a diet that has higher nutritional value. Research in mice and humans has shown that LDN has a positive benefit on dietary choices, decreases appetite and improves the ability to make healthier food choices.[191] Perturbed mitochondrial function in the enterocyte is believed to be an activating factor in inflammatory changes associated with increased intestinal permeability and chronic disease states of many types. Research published this year showed that LDN improved the mitochondrial function of cells and improved oxidative phosphorylation, i.e., improved energy production.[192]

Body Factor 3: The Endocrine (Hormone) System

The entire endocrine system—including the thyroid, the sex hormones (male and female hormones) and the HPA axis (Hypothalamus, Pituitary and Adrenal glands)—impacts the development and progression of autoimmune disease.

Sex hormones directly affect immune mechanisms, including the homing of lymphocytes, the expression of adhesion molecules, the balance between Th1 and Th2 responses, the transcription and translation of cytokine genes, antigen presentation and costimulation, and T cell receptor signaling.[193] Estrogen dominance specifically and lower than ideal hormone levels in general have been shown to increase the risk of immune diseases including autoimmune disease, cancer, and chronic infections. Hormone differences between men and women have also been implicated in the increased risk of autoimmune disease for females that has been noted in the research.[194] Balancing and optimizing hormones with bio-identical forms of hormones has been shown to have strong impacts in some patients.

HPA axis dysregulation is known to have negative impact in patients with autoimmune connective tissue diseases by several mechanisms of action. Healthy HPA axis function is part of what maintains a healthy cytokine balance, and dysregulation of the HPA axis is like removing the brakes from a car that is going downhill. The HPA axis is known to modulate inflammatory processes in the body, such as autoimmunity, through the glucocorticoid pathway, and imbalance in this is a known contributor to connective tissue diseases.[195] Testing and treatment of this axis can be both complicated and simple. There are specialty labs but one must be savvy and knowledgeable because a lot of testing is neither helpful nor accurate.

Most people with chronic fatigue, which is typical of patients with MCTD, have their TSH tested to determine if their thyroid is low. However, other measurements of thyroid function, such as Free T3 (the active form of thyroid and arguably the most important test), Free T4, Reverse T3, and autoimmune markers for thyroid disease are rarely checked. But patients with autoimmune disease often have what has been termed subclinical hypothyroidism, which means that their thyroid numbers are in the normal but not ideal range, and they are symptomatic of hypothyroidism. In those cases, treating the thyroid with both T3 and T4 can be life-changing for patients.

How LDN is helpful for the endocrine system

LDN has been in use for over a decade to balance hormones and has been shown to help in PMS, fertility, premenstrual dysmorphic disorder (PMDD), postmenopausal symptoms and more, all of which are symptoms of hormone imbalance. LDN is known to help balance stress hormones as well. LDN has a balancing effect on the HPA axis and all the body's hormones. By improving endorphins, which are key signaling and controlling molecules, LDN helps to control and direct improved balance in the endocrine system.

Environmental Factor 1: Pathogens (Chronic or Latent Infections)

Chronic infections are among the top three triggers for autoimmune disease, the most common and virulent of which are mold and chronic Lyme disease. Other known latent infectious triggers for autoimmune disease include: (methicillin-resistant staph aureus (MRSA), herpes simplex virus (HSV); cytomegalovirus (CMV); Epstein-Barr virus (EBV); candida and other overgrowth issues in the microbiome; human herpes virus (HHV); retroviruses, COVID-19, flu viruses, and many others.

There are several recognized mechanisms by which latent infections lead to activation of autoimmune disease: molecular mimicry, bystander effect, and epitope spreading model. When the body is fighting infection, cytokines that regulate sleep, as well as the HPA axis, undergo changes that may stimulate the development of autoimmune disease.

Because chronic infections are such a large contributor to the epigenetic activation of autoimmune disease, this category of trigger must be evaluated with testing. Testing is imperative to healing, especially when there are signs or symptoms of chronic infection such as "sick behaviors," intermittent fevers, swollen lymph nodes, or recurrent infections of any type.

Other signs that this trigger needs to be evaluated is exposure, including if patients have spent time in a home with known mold or water damage; if they've spent a lot of time in nature or live in a rural area; or if they've had a root canal, as infections can lurk under the now-dead tooth and can only be detected by a dentist trained in appropriate diagnostic and treatment methods.

Lastly, there is a test that can be used as a screening tool for chronic Lyme infections called CD57 (also called HNK-1). I often use this test if patient symptoms aren't clear because follow up testing is often only partially or not at all covered by insurance. You can look up the history of this test online for further information. While it was tested for chronic Lyme, I have found some patients with other chronic infections that were detected due to a low result on the CD57 test.

LDN and infection

LDN has been shown in research to have a positive benefit in many types of infections including HIV, herpes, hepatitis, EBV, yeast, chronic Lyme, chronic mold, and more. Patients with chronic infections of many types respond well to LDN with fewer, less frequent, and less severe infections as well as improved response to therapy. LDN's positive benefits are in part due to its immunomodulatory effects on T cells, monocytes, and macrophages. Additionally, LDN decreases the inflammatory cytokines associated with and TLR response to chronic infections.

Environmental Factor 2: Chemical and Environmental Toxins

Environmental toxicity is one of the well-known and -investigated triggers for autoimmune disease. However, only a couple of toxic exposures are known and have been evaluated for most disease processes, MCTD included. Others are overlooked and ignored. But the impact of environmental toxicity has been established and we know that it leads directly to epigenetic change that "turns on" the risk of autoimmune disease. While there are only two toxins (silica and vinyl chloride) that are known and accepted to be causative in creating the epigenetic risk associated with MCTD, there are likely many more that are untested.

According to the Worldometer, over 10 billion tons of chemical toxins are released into the environment every year, and of those, over 2 billion are known or suspected carcinogens.[196] The Environmental Working Group states that we are currently exposed to over 85,000 chemical toxins on a regular basis.[197] And the CDC has found more than 400 toxic metabolites (breakdown products of toxins that have gotten into the body) in the samples of 100% of people tested.[198]

Some of the known or theorized mechanisms of actions by which environmental toxins trigger autoimmune disease are through mimicry, endocrine disruption, blocking the uptake of nutrients, or activation or inactivation of epigenetic changes through oxidative damage.[199] [200] [201] [202]

How LDN can help with environmental toxicity

LDN improves the body's ability to eliminate and manage toxic exposure in several ways. It improves glutathione levels, thereby aiding detoxification. It decreases oxidative damage caused by toxic exposure, making it easier for your body to clear the toxins. It decreases the autoreactive T cells and inflammatory cytokines that are a hallmark of environmental toxicity. It helps to repair the damage to the epithelial cells of the gut and BBB that is caused by toxins. And lastly, LDN helps to repair the toxin-induced DNA methylation that leads to epigenetic change.

Environmental Factor 3: Diet

Many people have successfully treated or improved their disease process by changing from a SAD diet to any of the multiple diets often recommended for people with autoimmune disease. While not a comprehensive list by far, you can look up: The AutoImmune Protocol diet (AIP); microbiome diets, my personal favorite; the Carbohydrate Specific Diet (CSD); Mediterranean diets; ketogenic and paleo diets; and many more. All significantly improve nutritional status and improvements to diet are almost universally helpful.

Food sensitivities are common in people with autoimmune disease. Food sensitivities are not the same as food allergies. A food allergy is mediated by the IgE immune response and is usually immediate and happens every time you eat a certain food. A food sensitivity is mediated by the IgG immune response but is slower, taking 24-72 hours to present itself, doesn't involve a consistent response that can be tracked, and is often marked by atypical symptoms. Food sensitivities are often a result of damage to the enterocytes in the intestinal tract causing increased intestinal permeability, and can be tested for, treated, and resolved.

Sensitivity to grains, however, is not a food sensitivity that can be mediated. Grain intake has been linked to higher risk of autoimmune diseases, cancer, and neurodegenerative disorders. This is partially because gluten, casein, and other foods can produce exorphins in susceptible individuals.[iii] Some research has indicated that exorphins are the cause of side effects from food allergies or sensitivities while also stimulating cravings for the allergenic food.[203] Chronic grain and gluten intake has also been shown to lead to dysbiosis and directly to molecular mimicry, both of which result in the induction of autoimmune disease.[204]

The research indicating the many problems with a diet that contains grains is mounting and there are hundreds of studies and entire books written on the subject. Eating grains in your diet regularly is known to:

- Increase inflammatory cytokines
- Disrupt the HPA axis
- Significantly impair and have an inhibitory effect on an individual's immune system
- Stimulate tumor cell growth
- Inhibit the healing functions of the body
- Produce vulnerability to infection
- Damage the lining to the intestinal tract leading to increased intestinal permeability, aka, leaky gut syndrome.

Therefore, any dietary recommendations for MCTD need to include the elimination of all grains and dairy. This step is tough for most people, but it's worth the inconvenience. Some of my other

---

iii   Exorphins are opioid peptides made by the human body in response to the intake of certain foods, which is to say that they are morphine-like compounds derived from the incomplete digestive breakdown of grains and dairy products.

favorite recommendations that have high benefit in research and/or patient response are:

- Eliminate white sugar, artificial sweeteners, high fructose corn syrup, gluten, dairy, corn, and sodas.
- Avoid additives, preservatives, chemicals, hormones, genetically modified organisms (GMOs), herbicides, pesticides, hormones, and antibiotics. The most common genetically modified foods are corn and soy.
- Eat only organic, free-range, hormone-free, antibiotic-free foods as much as possible.
- Decrease grain intake to 1-2 servings daily if a grain-free diet is too challenging to start. All grains should be organic and gluten-free. Non-organic grains are sprayed with pesticides just before harvesting, which are known to kill your microbiome.
- Eat more healthy fats: real butter, olives and olive oil, nuts and nut butters, eggs, fatty fish, avocados, seeds, sesame and coconut oil, ghee, almond milk, coconuts, cheese except blue cheeses.
- Eat the healthiest vegetables: leafy greens, lettuces, collards, kale, chard, cabbage, mushrooms, broccoli, cauliflower, watercress, garlic, leek, fennel, spinach, onions, Brussels sprouts, alfalfa sprouts, artichoke, bok choy, radishes, shallots, scallions, ginger, jicama, parsley, turnips, asparagus, carrots, and okra.
- Eat the best fruits: tomatoes, avocados, bell peppers, cucumbers, zucchini, pumpkins, squash, eggplants, lemons, and limes.
- Eat more fermented foods. Among the most common are yogurt, kefir, kimchee, sauerkraut, pickled fruits and vegetables, fermented meat /fish/eggs, and kombucha.
- Eat prebiotic foods to feed a healthy microbiome: acacia gum, raw chicory root, artichokes, dandelion greens, garlic, leeks, onions, asparagus, and inulin contained in foods or supplements.
- Season your food with: mustard, horse radish, tamponade, salsa, cinnamon, garlic or onion powder, and turmeric.

How LDN helps with diet

LDN improves the microbiome, thereby changing the appetite and improving the ability to make healthier food choices. LDN decreases the appetite and cravings for carbs, sweets, and other unhealthy foods. LDN improves brain function, energy production, and elimination of toxins, all of which make it easier to tackle new tasks such as dietary changes. LDN improves sleep, which decreases cravings for carbs and sweets, especially late-night cravings.

Lifestyle Factor 1: Sleep Deprivation or Disturbance

When you sleep deeply:

- Your immune system is most active and most capable of dealing with immune imbalances.
- Your brain and heart get the most rest.
- Your body repairs and regenerates.
- Your brain processes and makes sense of the day's events.
- The nutrients you have given your body throughout the day are utilized for repair and regeneration.

Humans need sleep, and deep sleep, in order to be healthy of body and mind. There is a well-known link between the development of autoimmune disease and sleep deprivation. Many studies have demonstrated this link including a study published in 2021 showing that people with autoimmune disease had a significantly higher rate of symptomatic insomnia and restless legs syndrome (RLS).[205] Chronic poor sleep is a trigger for the epigenetic change that leads to the expression of autoimmune disease.[206]

Sleep deprivation comes in many forms that are often unrecognized or unappreciated: insomnia, parasomnia (waking multiple times during the night), general restlessness, chronic itching (only when trying to sleep), restless legs syndrome, racing mind with or without insomnia, chronic pain induced, hormonal, exogenous factors (animals, snoring spouse, light sleeper who wakes to everything, etc), undetected sleep apnea or sleep hypopnea (which is more commonly missed), and many others. It is important to ask the patient if they are "sleeping well," meaning that they fall asleep within 30 minutes of going to bed, sleep through the night without waking more than once, and wake up feeling rested. A "no" answer to that question warrants investigation.

Obviously, each of the listed (and many unlisted) causes for chronic insomnia need to be evaluated and treated with unique and individual care. One aspect of sleep deprivation that is often missed is sleep hypopnea. This is a condition in which the patient's throat narrows but doesn't close and creates decreased air flow which leads to lowered oxygen levels, which in turn cause the brain to wake to a lighter level of sleep in order to stimulate the body to take a deep breath, after which they try to go back to sleep and the cycle starts again. This effectively keeps people out of deep sleep and 90% of people don't think they have it when queried (from my unpublished experience with thousands of patients).

The symptoms that should raise suspicion of sleep hypopnea or sleep apnea are three or more of the following:

- Waking more than once a night (even to urinate)
- Snoring, especially but not necessarily loudly
- More than two medications required for blood pressure control
- High morning blood pressure (ask patient to check)
- New onset of heart problems
- Memory problems or brain fog
- Chronic pain or fatigue
- Heart arrhythmia
- Insomnia
- New onset of psychiatric problems (depression, anxiety)
- Obesity (least important)

Remember, you can't treat autoimmune disease without treating sleep. Find and treat the problem because even if this is not a patient's primary trigger, they are not going to heal without addressing it.

How LDN helps with sleep

Research has shown that many disease processes, including autoimmune disease, result in cytokine production that disrupts sleep. LDN has a balancing effect on those cytokines that disrupt sleep. LDN decreases or eliminates the cortisol surge that can happen at night as a result of chronic stress or adrenal fatigue, thereby improving sleep. LDN improves hormone balance, which can aid sleep. While up to 20% of people experience sleep disturbance when starting LDN, most people sleep better and deeper and wake up feeling more refreshed with less daytime fatigue on LDN.

Lifestyle Factor 2: Movement, Exercise, Chronic Pain
Chronic pain of all types is a common symptom of autoimmune disease as well as a trigger for it. Chronic pain depletes the body's endorphin supplies, which is one of the factors in the immune dysregulation that becomes autoimmune disease. And the opioid medications that are used to treat chronic pain in a Western medicine approach further deplete endorphin levels, making pain worse and creates a vicious cycle of increasing pain with decreasing endorphins and worsening immune function.

Movement is a necessary part of a balanced and therefore healthy life. Research since the 1990s has indicated that exercise improves inflammatory markers in the blood and improves quality of life in patients with autoimmune disease, including rheumatic diseases. Pain levels actually decrease with exercise, even if the muscles and joints are affected by the disease process.

But there is a big caveat on exercise with regard to autoimmune disease. Because research has also shown that while moderate regular exercise improves immune function, chronic intense exercise is actually deleterious to immune function.[207] And in autoimmune disease, even minimal exercise can be the equivalent of intense exertion to cells that have poor blood flow, increased cytokine count, and decreased energy production. Post-exertional fatigue and chronic fatigue are common in MCTD and must be treated individually. But whatever the method, this aspect of treatment needs to be addressed.

How LDN helps with chronic pain
LDN treats this aspect of the disease directly by increasing endorphin levels (simplistically stated). LDN has been shown to decrease pain levels and can help patients to wean off of opioid medications, decrease or stabilize dosage requirements, and transition to non-opioid alternatives. Research into LDN and chronic pain has shown it to be useful in multiple types of pain including autoimmune diseases. Decreasing chronic pain improves not just quality of life,

but people's ability to move, exercise, and stretch, which further decreases their pain. In recent research, physical performance improved in 24% of ME/CFS patients treated with LDN.

Lifestyle Factor 3: Autonomic Nervous System Imbalance
In short, the autonomic nervous system (ANS) is the sympathetic nervous system, aka fight or flight, while the parasympathetic nervous system's motto is rest and digest. You can think of the former as the "automatic" nervous system because it takes care of everything you don't think about: digestion, heartbeat, blinking eyes, breathing, etc. Chronic stress, chronic illness, chronic anxiety, all lead to over-activation of the sympathetic nervous system which creates a positive feedback loop that is hard to break. While ANS imbalance is not well researched as far as a trigger for autoimmune disease, it is a commonly treated and often valuable tool in the treatment of MCTD. There have been times when I couldn't proceed with patient treatment plans until I balanced the ANS. This can sometimes be the key.

Factors that may indicate one has an ANS imbalance include: chronic stress/anxiety/depression, brain fog, memory concerns or changes, difficulty concentrating, difficulty controlling emotions/thoughts/feelings, tachycardia (fast heart rate) or bradycardia (slow heart rate), and symptoms or diagnosis of irritable bowel syndrome (IBS).

How LDN helps the autonomic nervous system
Many chronic disease states are marked by sympathetic nervous system over-activation and parasympathetic nervous system under-activation. LDN has been shown to improve ANS dysregulation in CRPS. Research published in Jan 2021 showed that LDN improved SIBO and leaky gut symptoms associated with dysautonomia. Improving endorphin production improves balance of ANS.

Mind Factor 1: Stress
There are many stories of autoimmune disease manifesting after or during a stressful life event. It is understood from decades of research that chronic stress leads to epigenetic changes to our DNA through methylation and HPA axis imbalance. Chronic exposure to stress in

animal studies has shown an activation of the miRNA regions in the genetic code which in turn leads to autoimmune disease.[208]

How LDN helps with stress

LDN improves endorphin production. Endorphins are your "feel good" hormones and have been shown to help with depression, anxiety, sleep, bipolar disorder, hormone imbalance, and ANS balance, all of which improve management of chronic stress. LDN enhances the function of other supplements and lifestyle factors to manage stress. If you can think more clearly, you can meditate easier and treat stress more effectively.

Mind Factor 2: Beliefs and Thoughts

There is a long history of associations between autoimmune disease and depression with or without anxiety. Mounting research is also linking autoimmune disease with increased risk of psychotic diseases. It is now understood that many psychiatric disease processes are in fact autoimmune in nature and the scientific knowledge in this field is steadily growing.

Our thoughts and beliefs have long been understood to have impacts on our body's health or disease expression. New research is indicating that medical treatments that include a mind/body approach alter epigenetic expression away from disease, decreases inflammatory cytokine production and other markers of inflammation and improve immune function in autoimmune, cancer, and HIV patients. Mind-body medicine approaches have also been shown to improve chronic pain, psychiatric functioning, sleep quality and disturbances, overall mental health, perceived control, and quality of life in autoimmune patients. And amazingly, some research has shown that a mind-body medicine approach actually increases the length of telomeres, which is a strong indication of anti-aging benefit.[209]

LDN and beliefs

LDN helps you to help your mind and your body. By balancing the autonomic nervous system, decreasing inflammatory cytokines, decreasing pain, balancing hormones, improving your ability to deal with chronic infections, improving brain health, improving sleep, decreasing cortisol and chronic stress hormones, stimulating and improving detoxification of toxic compounds, and increasing neurogenesis, you are empowered to make the changes to your thinking that will most benefit you and your health.

Mind Factor 3: Social Circumstances

While not, strictly speaking, an aspect of the mind, I mention social circumstances here because they should be one of the factors on the mind of the practitioner, as some can be triggers for autoimmune disease. People who are in chronically stressful social circumstances, unhealthy or discordant relationships at work or home, or jobs that are draining and out-of-sync with their life goals are more likely to develop autoimmune disease.

There is also a social aspect that must be considered in the patient's ability to follow through on a treatment plan based on their family support or lack thereof, as well as available monetary or time resources. Any treatment plan must include consideration of these factors.

A Mixed Connective Tissue Disease Treatment Plan

All patients have a combination of the triggers that have led to the epigenetic shift that created MCTD in their body. Each person is unique and must be evaluated on an individual basis. But with all these factors to consider, it can be overwhelming, though the patient (or yourself, if you are the patient), will usually give you an idea of where to start your search for triggers.

If symptoms presented themselves soon after a dental procedure, look for chronic infections or toxins (especially mercury if amalgam fillings were involved).

If patients blame breast implants or feel their health changed after a surgical procedure, look for toxicity issues, pathogens, nutrient deficiencies, or endocrine imbalance.

If symptoms began or worsened around pregnancy, miscarriage, puberty, or menopause, look at the endocrine system.

If the patient has chronic GI complaints, evaluate the microbiome and gut in depth, consider food sensitivity testing, look closely at diet, and consider chronic overgrowth in the microbiome. Since the gut has so many connections with the rest of the body, you should also consider evaluation of toxic burden and chronic infection if symptoms persist. It is imperative in any comprehensive treatment of MCTD to consider, and often to test, the microbiome. There are specialty labs that can test for imbalances, dysbiosis, chronic overgrowth, digestive or metabolic abnormalities, digestive enzyme production, and GI-specific inflammation. The information from the results of this type of testing are often invaluable.

Likewise, if the patient has a poor diet, assess their nutritional status, look for nutrient deficiencies, and consider gluten intolerance and yeast overgrowth as well as chronic infections.

If symptoms began after exposure to mold, outdoor activities or infection, look for chronic or latent infections.

If stressful life events seemed to precipitate MCTD, look for adrenal fatigue, endocrine imbalance, sleep problems, and ANS imbalance.

Getting started with treatment is easier than you think. Start with lifestyle because these triggers are easier to identify and address. You must have something in your daily arsenal to easily address each of these issues in order to have positive impact in MCTD treatment:

- Start your treatment plan with LDN, which has been shown to be effective in patient case studies specifically in MCTD, and generally the triggers that lead to the development of MCTD are known to be treated with LDN. Given the low side effect profile and the great chance of benefit, there is very little reason not to start LDN right away, even while testing and other treatments are being explored.
- Always ask how patients are sleeping as this is so important for healing. Take a home sleep test or become familiar with them and have a go-to company for ordering them if you are a practitioner. Remember to treat sleep you sometimes have to treat hormone imbalances, adrenal fatigue, subclinical hypothyroid, microbiome dysbiosis, autonomic nervous system imbalance, chronic infection, stress, or even talk to the patient about their life (social) circumstances and determine if they need help or referral in this area.

- Diet is shown to be helpful most of the time and needs to be addressed. Start with eliminating grains and clean up the diet as indicated earlier in this chapter. Review and become familiar with different autoimmune diets because no two people are alike and we need to tailor treatment to many patient factors.
- Movement is important and exercise routines should be individually tailored. I've had chronic pain patients who started out by walking down the hall three times a day, then to the mailbox, then to the end of the street, and slowly regained mobility and decreased pain on a graduated program. Once patients can begin to move better, add in aspects of interval training since this is so much more effective than other forms of exercise. You can do this even with walking by adding in 5-30 second intervals of intense (for you) walking followed by 60-90 seconds of rest or slow walking for a total of 10-20 minutes or as tolerated. Interval training provides the same benefits of other cardiovascular work outs in a much shorter period of time. There are many apps for your phone that can help you institute this in your life in about 10 minutes a day.
- Stress reduction needs to be directed and adjusted based on impact. There are some common apps, books, online courses, meditations, positive affirmations, and handouts that I recommend for patients to help them deal with stress.
- Add in a mind/body aspect of your care.
- Get the help of an integrative or functional medicine practitioner to help guide you through your exploration of your triggers. If you are a practitioner, make sure that you have ways of evaluating all the triggers or become familiar with some. Since your triggers "turn on" your epigenetic risk for disease, there is at least a potential that your epigenetic factors could be "turned off" or "turned down" by treating and eliminating those triggers.

Throughout this chapter, I have written for practitioners and patients alike, shifting between addressing the two. I hope that the thinking and processes outlined here are helpful to both. Many people have treated themselves with an approach that takes into account some of these triggers described here. When they employ a systematic approach to evaluation and treatment, most people find that they have better quality of life than they thought possible. I hope this is true for you as well.

SIX

LDN and Mold Illness

The Updated Protocol for the Rapid Treatment of CIRS

KENT HOLTORF, MD

This chapter is dedicated to detailing new, evidence-based treatments for mold illness and explaining how to diagnose and treat mold-related illness and chronic inflammatory response syndrome (CIRS) most effectively. The chapter will review the groundbreaking work and current standard of care for the treatment of CIRS and the current standard Shoemaker protocol for CIRS (CSSPC) and demonstrate how LDN and peptides can augment and replace many aspects of this protocol to achieve faster recovery and superior efficacy. This chapter will also cover the symptoms and consistent pathophysiology associated with mold illness, illustrating the multisystem pathophysiology seen with mold patients, emphasizing the diagnosis and treatment of immune dysfunction, a hallmark of CIRS. In addition, this section will review the literature on effective methods of mold remediation and explain the use of LDN and peptides to treat mold illness, as well as the correlation between the degree of immune dysfunction, specifically the severity of T cell exhaustion, immunosenescence, and the Th1/Treg to Th2/Th17 shift and the severity of this multisystem condition, CIRS.

Introduction

Mold is a much more common household toxin than most people realize. According to the World Health Organization (WHO), it builds up in homes and other buildings due to water damage and persistent indoor dampness, affecting between 9% and 70% percent of indoor environments worldwide.[210] [211] [212] Not only found in basements, mold can permeate walls, floors, and ceilings, often going undetected until the health problems it causes become more than the body's immune system can cope with. While some types of mold are detectable by their color, fuzzy appearance, and/or musty odor, other types of mold can be invisible. As a result, people can be exposed to mold inhalation through skin contact and, in some cases, ingestion.

Inhalation is the most common mechanism of exposure in indoor environments. Harmful mold in homes continuously releases spores and mycotoxins as airborne inhalants, especially in the presence of electric and magnetic fields (EMFs).[213] [214] [215] It has been reported that 25 percent of people cannot detoxify from mold on their own once they are exposed, making them exceptionally susceptible to mold-triggering chronic fatigue and other serious diseases. Additionally, most individuals suffering from mold-related illness have additional conditions, such as chronic Lyme disease or even significant physiologic stress, that make them more sensitive to the potentially toxic effects of mold due to their preexisting immune dysfunction. Subsequently, the synergistic poisonous effect blamed on toxic mold exposure, chronic Lyme disease, which includes all other coinfections, and reactivating infections secondary to immune dysfunction, or stress, is actually due to the combination of the entities. Often, when one of these immunotoxic effects is eliminated, the patient no longer gets sick from the mold exposure or vice versa.

Another little-known fact about mold is that many of the mycotoxins produced are more harmful to the human body than any other human-made toxins except for certain radioactive elements. They are also fat-soluble, enabling them to accumulate in the body's fat cells, cell walls, and tissues while suppressing the immune system. Because they are fat-soluble, mycotoxins in the body are difficult to eliminate on one's own. Additionally, EMFs will stimulate mold growth, but EMFs can also stimulate mold and fungi to secrete thousands of times more mycotoxins than they usually would.[216] [217] [218]

Current Method of Diagnosis of Mold Illness

Mold illness is also known as mold sickness or toxicity, biotoxin illness, immunologic disease, water-damaged building (WDB) sickness, and environmentally acquired illness. Regardless of how it is termed, it is rarely considered by most conventionally trained physicians as a primary cause or related source of their patients' presenting symptoms. Most physicians do not even recognize mold illness, either because they are unaware of the various ways it can present in the body or are not up-to-date on the science documenting the significant health risks that molds, mycotoxins, and other related contaminants pose. Therefore, it is impossible to accurately estimate how many people suffer from mold illness, though the figure is likely to be in the millions of patients worldwide.

Additionally, the multiple severe symptoms triggered by mold illness are often mistaken by physicians as allergic reactions, blamed on emotional stress, or explained away as being psychosomatic, especially if the patient is female. This results in time being lost as physicians seek to identify potential allergens when in fact, mold illness can induce mast cell activation and an allergic reaction. Most of the time, it is a chronic inflammatory condition and a subset within the broader category of CIRS.

One leading CIRS and mold illness expert is Ritchie Shoemaker, MD. On his website, he defines CIRS as "an acute and chronic, systemic inflammatory response syndrome acquired following exposure to the interior environment of a water-damaged building with resident toxigenic organisms, including, but not limited to fungi, bacteria, actinomycetes, and mycobacteria, as well as inflammagens, such as endotoxins, beta-glucans, hemolysins, proteinases, mannans and possibly spirocyclic drimanes; as well as volatile organic compounds."[219] Shoemaker also coined the term "CIRS-WDB (CIRS-water-damaged building)" and recommends a symptom cluster analysis and a triple-tiered diagnosis system to distinguish mold illness/CIRS-WDB from other illnesses accurately.

Symptom Cluster Analysis

While mold illness/CIRS symptoms can initially present in random sequences, Shoemaker's analysis of patients suffering from these

conditions revealed thirteen distinct symptom clusters associated with mold illness/CIRS-WDB.[220]
The unique clusters of symptoms are:

1. Abdominal pain, diarrhea, numbness
2. Shortness of breath, congested sinuses
3. Impaired memory, difficulty recalling words
4. Heightened skin sensitivity, sensations of tingling, "pin and needles."
5. Watery eyes, metallic taste, disorientation
6. Weakness, body aches, headache, sensitivity to light, trouble grasping new concepts
7. Night sweats, blurred vision, mood swings, red or bloodshot eyes, "ice pick" pain
8. Morning stiffness, joint pain, muscle cramps
9. Severe, persistent fatigue
10. Difficulty concentrating
11. Static shocks, dizziness
12. Persistent cough, extreme thirst, confusion
13. Frequent urination, fluctuating body temperature.

CIRS patients suffer from many more multi-system symptoms than listed above in the current standard Shoemaker protocol (CSSPC), so I have not found the symptom clusters very helpful. Given that the above symptoms in each of these clusters are common in other health conditions and, in my opinion, that this cluster mix misses many symptoms suffered by those stricken with CIRS, it doesn't seem very helpful in the diagnosis of mold illness/CIRS nor does it seem to help differentiate CIRS patients from many other multi-system fatiguing conditions. Therefore, I would add the additional symptoms, including but not limited to sleep disorders, palpitations, depression, appetite loss, dyspepsia, epigastric pain, gastrointestinal dysfunction, tinnitus, various neurologic symptoms, weight gain, leptin and insulin resistance, PCOS, chronic cough, rhinorrhea, rhinosinusitis, post-exertional fatigue, low libido, brittle nails, feeling overwhelmed, stress, and anxiety.

According to CSSPC, the most common misdiagnoses are allergies, anxiety, depression, attention deficit hyperactivity disorder

(ADD/ADHD), chronic fatigue syndrome (CFS), fibromyalgia (FM), irritable bowel disorder (IBS), post-traumatic stress disorder (PTSD), and somatic symptom disorder (somatization). Still, these diagnoses are not mutually exclusive, and CFS, FM, IBS, and PTSD share the same pathophysiology and will often have the same symptoms and biomarkers used to diagnose CIRS. It comes down to the fact that it doesn't matter what you call it; the goal is to fix it and end the patient's suffering. Shoemaker notes that adult patients experiencing symptoms in eight or more clusters (six in children) almost certainly (greater than 95 percent likelihood) are affected with mold illness/CIR-WDB.[221]

As just mentioned, while the syndrome of CIRS appears to be a unique entity with a unique set of symptoms, it shares a common multi-system underlying pathophysiology seen with chronic infections, including Lyme and associated infections, chronic fatigue syndrome (CFS), fibromyalgia, MCAS, PTSD, mast cell activation syndrome (MCAS), autoimmunity, neurodegenerative diseases, and chronic age-related diseases. Thus, CIRS will respond to new innovative immune-modulating and other therapies that have been developed for the above conditions with a few caveats unique to CIRS. As these newly developed therapies have resulted in the ability to see benefits in chronic Lyme patients in months rather than following the standard "enlightened" therapy of antibiotics for extended periods, often years, the Updated Protocol for the Rapid Treatment of CIRS (UPRTOC), which doctors often refer to as the Holtorf Updated Protocol for the Rapid Treatment of CIRS (HUPRTOC), can result in rapid improvement in CIRS patients instead of the usual time frame of years that it typically takes to see progress with the current protocol used for CIRS by doctors trained in this condition.

A greater understanding of the pathophysiology of CIRS, combined with new therapies directed at modification and normalization of the dysfunctional systems, improvement, and resolution of CIRS, can be achieved much quicker than following the current stepwise CIRS protocol that, while revolutionary and groundbreaking, fails to address numerous vital aspects of the dysfunctions seen with this condition.

Testing For Mold Illness/CIRS

The triple-tiered system of diagnosis Shoemaker developed to diagnose mold illness/CIRS consists of a combination of visual, genetic, and biomarker tests, along with analysis of MRI brain scans using NeuroQuant®, an FDA-approved software program, and, most recently, a transcriptomics test. A brief description of each of Shoemaker's recommended tests follows.

Visual Contrast Sensitivity (VCS) Testing

Research shows that mold and other biotoxins, in addition to causing CIRS, also negatively impact nerves, resulting in various nerve dysfunctions and subsequent neurological symptoms. For example, a common nerve dysfunction in mold illness/CIRS patients is impaired visual contrast sensitivity (VCS), characterized by a diminished ability to detect visual patterns. Shoemaker posits that diminished VCS is caused by reduced red blood cell flow velocity into the eye structures that transmit visual information to the brain via the optic nerve.

VCS testing involves showing patients images designed to evaluate their ability to detect visual patterns. Patients affected with mold illness/CIRS typically score low on VCS tests. VCS testing has been stated to accurately determine mold illness/CIRS in 92 percent of cases, with an estimated eight percent of cases resulting in false-negative readings.[222] VCS testing is performed at the initial patient visit and then repeated at follow-up consultations to evaluate the patient's response to treatment. Loss of VCS is not, however, exclusive to CIRS patients.

Genetic Testing: Human Leukocyte Antigen (HLA) Test

The specific gene test used to determine a person's genetic susceptibility to mold illness/CIRS is the human leukocyte antigen (HLA) test. In the body, the HLA system is comprised of genes in chromosome 6. These genes encode cell-surface proteins that play an essential role in the immune system, helping to recognize foreign cells in the body. Therefore, patients in the HLA type category are more likely than other patients to develop CIRS when exposed to mold and other biotoxins.

After reviewing international gene registries matched by case-controlled studies, Shoemaker reported that approximately 25 percent of the population is "mold susceptible" because of their HLA haplotype, making them more susceptible to developing persistent mold illness/CIRS when exposed to mold and related biotoxins.[223] With that said, many patients with CIRS do not have a genetic predisposition, so this test cannot rule out someone from having CIRS or be used to diagnose CIRS.

NeuroQuant® Analysis of MRI Tests
NeuroQuant® is an FDA-approved software program used to detect evidence of brain injury. Most patients with mild to moderate traumatic brain injury (TBI) have normal MRI scans. NeuroQuant® can analyze a properly run MRI of the brain and assess volumes of fifteen different brain areas. These data are then compared to MRI data from normal control subjects to determine possible structural brain damage and brain volume atrophy. NeuroQuant® can detect brain atrophy in specific brain structures, which may be linked to specific biotoxins, but is not specific for CIRS.

Shoemaker Protocol Biomarker Tests
The biomarker tests recommended by Shoemaker to screen for or rule-in mold illness/CIRS are transforming growth factor beta-1 (TGF beta-1), C4a, matrix metallopeptidase 9 (MMP-9), leptin, vascular endothelial growth factor (VEGF), anti-gliadin antibodies (AGA), melanocyte-stimulating hormone (MSH), anti-diuretic hormone (ADH), adrenocorticotropic hormone (ACTH), plasminogen activator inhibitor-1 (PAI-1), anti-cardiolipin antibodies (ACA), Von Willebrand factor, and vasoactive intestinal peptide (VIP). I do not disagree with these biomarkers, but I have found that with about double the amount of biomarker tests, which can usually be obtained at standard commercial labs, and an understanding of the limitations of each test, the accuracy, specificity, and sensitivity of the diagnosis is dramatically increased. More importantly, it will give the treating physician a better understanding and direction of treatment based on the abnormalities instead of following a treatment algorithm. The expanded biomarkers also provide a much better objective measure of treatment success.

TGF beta-1

The biomarker TGF beta-1 plays a vital role in regulating the immune system in chronic infections and illnesses. While potentially beneficial early on in a disease, it becomes a significant player in perpetuating chronic illness. Chronically elevated TGF beta-1 levels occur when there is an overactive Th2/Th17 immune response that is seen in cases of mold illness/CIRS, but also with chronic Lyme disease, parasitic infections, toxin exposure, CFS, fibromyalgia, multiple sclerosis, mast cell activation syndrome (MCAS), IBS, autoimmune disease, immune activation of coagulation, fibrosis; chronic age-related illnesses such as cardiovascular disease, cancer, and infertility; and neurodegenerative diseases, such as Alzheimer's, Parkinson's, ALS, and other inflammatory conditions. Elevated levels are consistent with T cell exhaustion, immunosenescence, a Th1/Treg to Th2/Th17 immune shift, and a highly aged immune system.[224] [225] [226]

New cellular laboratory techniques show that T cell exhaustion (TCE) and immunosenescence are the core underlying pathophysiologic processes causing CIRS. TCE is associated with progressive loss of effector functions of T cells (CD4 and CD8), dysfunctional Th1 immunity, as indicated by a low NK cell function, MCAS, low IL-2, low TNF-alpha in late stages, and an elevated hTGFb, C4a, and IL-10, along with the Th1 to Th2/Th17 immune shift.[227] [228] [229]

Exhausted T cells cannot eradicate intracellular pathogens or mycotoxins or repair toxin-induced damage due to immune-induced mitochondrial dysfunction and other damaging mycotoxin effects while causing excessive inflammation. This sets off a vicious cycle of immune dysfunction, causing mitochondrial damage, which excretes excessive ROS and inflammation and creates more damage and immune suppression, which then causes more mitochondrial damage. The severity of TCE correlates with the level and length of antigen stimulation and the amount of thymic dysfunction. TCE is reversible (distinct subsets of T cells can have different potentials of having the possibility of regaining function) and typically occurs in a few weeks to months, while immunosenescence is not reversible (must eliminate the senescence cells as should naturally happen if the Th1 immunity, such as NK cell function, is robust enough to eliminate them). This generally takes longer to occur (months to years) than TCE. Although most of the data suggest that TCE and senescence are distinct mechanistic processes, there can be a blurring of characteristics. Both processes can coincide and often do.[230]

This immune dysfunction results in numerous additional vicious cycles that include pineal-hypothalamic-pituitary-hormone dysfunction; mitochondrial dysfunction, GI abnormalities, cognitive dysfunction, sleep disorders, increased permeability of the gut ("leaky gut") and the blood-brain-barrier, immune activation of coagulation (hypercoagulability), leptin and insulin resistance, dysfunctional detoxification, and other multisystem abnormalities.[231] [232]

Thus, targeted therapy that addresses this core immune dysfunction, which includes LDN and a variety of immune-modulating peptide therapies, will help normalize the immune system, the resultant multisystem dysfunctions, and subsequently the symptoms of CIRS, allowing the potential for a much more rapid improvement than is seen with current CIRS protocols.

C4a

Biomarker C4a, like TGF-beta, is a marker of a dysfunctional immune system that is shifted from a healthy Th1/Treg dominant immune system, exemplified in young, healthy individuals, to a Th2/Th17 dominant immune system that is exemplified in aged and chronically ill individuals. It helps activate a specific inflammatory process of the innate immune system known as a complement cascade. As a biomarker, C4a correlates with the degree of illness and can help serve as an objective measure of disease and improvement with treatment.[233] An elevated C4a can occur with multiple infections and reactivating infections associated with immune dysfunction, CFS, fibromyalgia, MCAS, autoimmune disease, and many diseases of aging. Again, elevated C4a levels, demonstrating a Th1/Treg to Th2/Th17 shift, can trigger immune activation of coagulation, breathing difficulties, fatigue, impaired detoxification, and cognitive function, all of which are hallmarks of mold illness/CIRS. Still, they are not specific for mold illness or CIRS. Shoemaker reports that mold illness/CIRS patients with high C4a levels suffer from decreased blood flow into the capillaries, which would be expected to be the case with many chronic illnesses and potentially a contributing cause of cognitive dysfunction as is common in CIRS and other chronic immune-related diseases.

A robust Th1 immunity is required to detox from mycotoxins. For instance, Lyme patients with low Th1 immunity function cannot convert weak IgM antibodies to more powerful complement-activating IgG antibodies. On a personal note, I originally only had a single Lyme Western blot and an IgM 41 kd band, which is technically a negative test. After modulating my immunity and improving Th1 activity, I converted to having seven IgG antibodies on the Lyme western blot (a clear positive). With low Th1 immunity, the mycotoxins are not recognized via pattern recognition receptors and are not eliminated, along with the lack of tagging and elimination by IgG antibodies and phagocytic cells. Also, the immune-induced mitochondrial dysfunction results in cells that do not have enough cellular energy to eliminate intracellular and transmembrane heavy metals and mycotoxins.[234]

Matrix Metallopeptidase 9
Biomarker Matrix Metallopeptidase 9 (MMP-9) is a general inflammatory marker that helps break down cell membranes in the walls of blood vessels, enabling inflammatory compounds to travel from the blood vessel walls to various organs and tissues, including in the brain, lungs, joints, and muscles, and peripheral nerves. In mold illness/CIRS-WDB, cytokines cause various white blood cells to dump MMP-9 into the bloodstream, resulting in an increase of inflammatory biochemicals in the tissues, causing inflammation throughout the body. MMP-9 is an enzyme activated by macrophages inducing inflammatory cytokines that destroys the basement membrane of endothelial cells, which serves as a barrier between substances in the blood, allowing inflammatory compounds to penetrate tissue. It is also shown to increase blood-brain barrier permeability, allowing inflammatory substances, cytokines, and

cells to enter the brain.[235] High MMP-9 contributes to the destruction of connective tissues and increases Lp(a), increasing the risk of immune activation of coagulation, cardiovascular disease, and cardiomyopathy.

Cytokine testing can be problematic. A prechilled SST tube is essential to use. Following the lab draw, the specimen should be immediately centrifuged and frozen. This step will prevent the release of MMP9 from the white blood cells into the blood specimen, which can double or triple at room temperature in as little as 30 minutes. Unfortunately, this is often not done in a busy commercial lab, making MMP9 an unreliable marker.

Leptin
Fat cells produce Biomarker Leptin to help regulate hunger and fat stores. With weight gain, increased leptin is secreted, which should feedback on the hypothalamus and tell the body to decrease appetite, increase metabolism, burn fat, and increase thyroid production. In cases of excess inflammation, whether from mold, chronic infection, or diabetes, the inflammatory cytokines block the leptin receptors, so the brain thinks the body is starving and tells the body to store fat, increase hunger, and decrease metabolism and thyroid levels. A number of chronic illnesses and aging can result in leptin resistance.

Much like the elevated levels of insulin seen in patients with insulin resistance, elevated leptin levels indicate leptin resistance. The normal range for leptin in men is listed as 0.5-13.8 ng/ml and 1.1-27.5 ng/ml in women, but these laboratory ranges include obese people and those with chronic illnesses who have significant leptin resistance. A healthy leptin level should be between 1 and 10 ng/ml. Levels above 10 ng/ml are leptin resistance markers and are often seen in people who have difficulty losing weight. Leptin is also needed for the pituitary to produce and secrete TSH. Thus, with leptin resistance, the TSH is not a reliable marker to determine the presence of hypothyroidism. It is also a marker for low thyroid despite having a normal TSH and is often seen in those with insulin resistance. Still, a person can suffer from significant leptin resistance without having any insulin resistance.[236] [237]

Vascular Endothelial Growth Factor

Biomarker Vascular Endothelial Growth Factor (VEGF) is a signaling protein. It plays a vital role in cells responsible for growing new blood vessels needed to supply oxygen to tissues during diminished blood circulation. Under normal conditions, when capillary blood flow decreases, the resulting reduction in oxygen levels triggers the release of hypoxia-inducible factor (HIF). HIF, in turn, aids in the production of VEGF and erythropoietin (EPO). VEGF increases blood flow by creating new blood vessels, while EPO increases the production of red blood cells. Together, they work to improve the oxygen supply to the cells.[238]

In patients with mold illness/CIRS, VEGF is suppressed due to high cytokine levels. The result is diminished oxygen supply to the tissues, leading to muscle cramps, which Shoemaker feels is the cause of extreme exhaustion following exercise or physical activity. While it very well may play a part, post-exertional fatigue has been shown to mainly be a function of mitochondrial dysfunction and immune activation of coagulation, resulting in a premature anaerobic threshold, which is a hallmark of CIRS, chronic Lyme, CFS, FM, neurodegenerative diseases, and most every age-associated illness.[239] The normal range of VEGF is 31-86 pg/ml. Bartonella will stimulate VEGF. As a side note: my VEGF was off the chart when I was diagnosed with Bartonella in addition to Lyme and Babesia. Due to this elevated VEGF, my vessels were grotesquely enlarged all over my body. They were not varicose veins, just huge. I got them sclerosed for cosmetic reasons, but after I could rid my body of Bartonella, I scarcely had a visible vein to draw blood from or start an IV.

Anti-Gliadin Antibodies

Biomarker Anti-Gliadin Antibodies (AGA) are produced in the body as a reaction to gliadin, a compound contained in gluten. AGA is one of the factors that cause celiac disease. Under normal circumstances, gliadin is broken down into various amino acid chains (peptides). To utilize these peptides, specific epithelial and endothelial cells in the intestines known as tight junctions (because they resemble a tightly sealed interlocking gateway) need to open to allow the peptides to pass through. Once the nutrient or signaling peptide has passed, the tight junctions immediately close in healthy people. In some patients with mold illness/CIRS or other chronic illnesses (as well as patients with celiac disease), the gliadin protein trigger inflammatory and immune reactions that keep the tight junctions from completely closing, resulting in "leaky gut." The normal range for AGA is 0-19 units. AGA levels above this range can be another nonspecific indicator of mold illness/CIRS because it occurs in many chronic diseases, and "leaky gut" is a significant problem for so many chronic diseases due to the associated immune dysfunction, as will be discussed later in this chapter.[240] [241] [242]

Rather than just checking for anti-gliadin antibodies, it is straightforward and inexpensive to check for a hundred or more food sensitivities (IgG antibodies, not IgE, which is an allergy). If you test positive for a significant number of foods, it demonstrates that these large food proteins are getting absorbed when they should not be. This shows that the tight junctions in the gut are damaged, which is called leaky gut. If you have a leaky gut, you can be sure that your blood-brain barrier is also leaky. The good news is that there is a combination of peptides that heal inflammatory gut issues, dysbiosis, IBS, GERD, and specifically heal the tight junctions and leaky gut (discussed later in this chapter).[243] [244] [245]

Melanocyte-Stimulating Hormone
Biomarker Melanocyte-Stimulating Hormone (MSH) helps regulate many other hormones and plays an essential role in the body's inflammation responses to foreign pathogens. It is one of the most anti-inflammatory substances produced in the body.[246] Unlike steroids, however, MSH and its analogs, such as the MSH fragment KPV, do not lower the body's ability to fight infections; rather, they significantly enhance the body's immunological defense against invading organisms and also have potent broad-spectrum antimicrobial effects against bacteria, viruses, mold, parasites, and fungi (discussed later in this chapter).[247] [248] Thus, low levels of MSH will result in multisystem inflammation (i.e., CIRS) and an inability to fight many infections, with MARcONS infection of the sinuses being a specific example. MSH acts as a guardian of the

skin and mucous membranes, killing fungi and coagulase-negative staphylococci. With normal MSH, MARCoNS will not survive.[249] [250]

MSH and leptin have reciprocal stimulating effects on each other. Under normal conditions, increased leptin levels result in a corresponding increase in MSH and vice versa. However, inflammatory cytokines interfere with leptin receptors, causing leptin resistance and high leptin levels, which is associated with low MSH because the leptin signal does not reach the receptors in the brain. Low levels of MSH are evident in patients with mold illness/CIRS and can remain low even after treatment. When this happens, leptin production increases without a corresponding rise in MSH levels, resulting in leptin resistance and unhealthy weight gain. A rise in leptin levels in healthy people would trigger the brain to create more MSH, which does not occur in CIRS patients.

MSH is also involved in the opening and closing of tight junctions in the intestinal tract. Diminished MSH levels can prevent tight junctions from closing correctly, leading to a leaky gut.[251] In addition, some research has reported that approximately 80 percent of patients with low MSH levels also have MARCoNS (multiple antibiotic resistant coagulase negative staph, usually concentrated in the sinuses). This creates a vicious cycle because MARCoNS produces toxins that suppress MSH production.[252] Treating MARCoNS can be necessary to restore MSH levels to normal levels. There are, however, much better ways to deal with and treat low MSH and MARCoNs than what is recommended for this in the CCSCP, as we will see.

Anti-Diuretic Hormone
BiomarkerAnti-DiureticHormone(ADH),alsoknownas vasopressin, is produced by specialized nerve cells in the hypothalamus. It helps maintain blood pressure, blood volume, and tissue water content by controlling the amount of water your kidneys reabsorb as they filter out waste from your blood. ADH signals the kidneys to conserve water and produce a more concentrated urine, diluting your blood, lowering the blood's osmolality (particle concentration), increasing blood volume, and increasing blood pressure. Conversely, suppose you produce too little ADH. In that case, your body loses too

much water in the urine, potentially resulting in excessive blood osmolarity, frequent urination, dehydration, low blood pressure, extreme thirst, fatigue, mental confusion, muscle aches and pains, frequent migraines, and postural orthostatic tachycardia syndrome (POTS), whereby your blood pressure drops and heart races when standing, and which is associated with high blood sodium levels. This is called diabetes insipidus.[253] Such patients will often "drink like a fish and pee like a racehorse."

If your body produces too much ADH, water is retained, producing highly concentrated urine, high blood volume and blood pressure, and low serum sodium levels. This is called the syndrome of inappropriate ADH (SIADH). Symptoms can include nausea, headaches, disorientation, and tiredness or lethargy.

CIRS patients will typically have low ADH levels due to inflammation or damage in the hypothalamus, hippocampus, or amygdala.[254] The normal range for ADH is 1.0-13.3 pg/ml, and normal blood osmolality is 275-298 mOsm/kg. You can order the blood osmolarity level via a blood test, or it can be easily calculated by using several websites where you enter your lab values for sodium, BUN, and glucose. In CIRS patients, there will often be a high normal blood osmolarity, with ADH being low normal.

Adrenocorticotropic Hormone
Biomarker Adrenocorticotropic Hormone (ACTH) plays a vital role in how the body responds to stress. ACTH is produced in the pituitary gland, and its production stimulates the production and release of cortisol from the adrenal glands. In healthy people, cortisol levels rise during the early morning, usually peaking by 8 AM, and then decrease during the evening. However, this process is negatively impacted by chronic inflammation and chronic illness, including mold illness/CIRS. Under such circumstances, cortisol production is interfered with, diminishing the body's ability to deal with stress.

In a state of good health, the production of ACTH is adjusted in response to the rising or lowering of cortisol levels. But in patients with mold illness/CIRS and other immune-related illnesses, this process is often disrupted, causing fatigue, interfering with healthy sleep, and triggering a variety of other symptoms, including hypoglycemia (low blood sugar), fatigue, nausea, weakness, dizziness, weight loss, muscle aches, diarrhea, irregular periods, and inability to handle stress. The normal range for ACTH is 8-37 pg/ml, and the normal ranges for cortisol are 4.3-22.4 ncg/dl (morning) and 3.1-16.7 ncg/dl (evening).

Inflammation induces the secretion of corticotropin-releasing factor (CRH) from the hypothalamus, which then stimulates the pituitary to produce ACTH, which stimulates the adrenals to make cortisol. The problem is that the pituitary can become resistant to CRH and cause ACTH resistance in the adrenals with significant inflammation. This results in high levels of CRH, which is a potent stimulator of inflammation and mast cell activation, but it may not stimulate cortisol due to ACTH resistance.[255] This results in low cortisol, further increasing inflammation and mast cell activation and an inability to handle physiological stress. In addition, there can also be suppression of CRH in the hypothalamus, which results in low levels of ACTH and cortisol, resulting in increased inflammation and mast cell activation and an inability to handle stress.

Plasminogen Activator Inhibitor-1, Anti-cardiolipin Antibodies, and Von Willebrand Factor

Biomarkers Plasminogen Activator Inhibitor-1 (PAI-1), Anti-cardiolipin Antibodies (ACA), and Von Willebrand Factor (VWF) comprise the standard coagulation panel recommended in the current CIRS treatment algorithm but are inadequate to consistently identify those who are hypercoagulable and have immune activation of coagulation. Only doing these three tests according to the CSSPC will miss up to 90% of CIRS patients that suffer from immune activation of coagulation, which is shown to occur in up to 90% of CIRS patients, depending on the sensitivity of the testing panel done.[256]

The common understanding of CIRS holds that PAI-1, ACA, and VWF can cause blood clots and are biomarker indicators of abnormal bleeding conditions. Mold illness/CIRS and other inflammatory diseases cause PAI-1 to rise, increasing blood clotting and the risk of fibrosis. ACA antibodies target normal body tissues, negatively impacting phospholipid proteins in cell membranes. Elevated

ACA levels are involved in connective tissue disorders such as scleroderma and lupus and can cause miscarriages. PAI-1 and ACA in combination are a significant risk factors for heart attack and stroke, and deep vein thrombosis (DVT). Mold illness/CIRS patients are also at risk for a type of acquired Von Willebrand Syndrome, a condition that prevents proper blood clotting and which can result in frequent or heavy nosebleeds and, in women, excessive bleeding during menstruation.[257] [258]

The HUPRTOC recommends a much more extensive and comprehensive hypercoagulation panel because the standard hypercoagulation panel recommended in the current CIRS protocol will miss 60-90% of those suffering from immune activation of coagulation. Missing this abnormality will often result in multiple levels of treatment failure and a frustrating protracted illness (see Immune Activation of Coagulation later in this chapter).[259]

Vasoactive Intestinal Peptide
Biomarker Vasoactive Intestinal Peptide (VIP) is a neuropeptide produced in the hypothalamus, pancreas, gastrointestinal tract, and other places in the body. VIP is an interesting substance; it has many beneficial anti-inflammatory effects but can vigorously promote immune dysfunction. VIP plays a vital role in regulating the body's inflammatory responses; however, studies are inconsistent, with some showing a worsening of inflammation and autoimmunity and others showing anti-inflammatory effects.[260] [261]

VIP is also involved in regulating blood flow and the response of the pulmonary artery during exercise. Low VIP levels are thought to cause pressure to build in the pulmonary artery during exercise and strenuous physical activity, resulting in shortness of breath. I have found that immune activation of coagulation is likely a more frequent cause of shortness of breath or air hunger and that symptoms resolve with treatment. Both scenarios can, however, certainly be contributing symptomatically. Shoemaker has reported that nearly all (98 percent) mold illness/CIRS patients have low VIP levels.[262] This may be influenced by the fact that this test requires complicated processing and to immediately be placed in dry ice, which is often not done correctly at standard labs. If not processed correctly, which frequently happens, it becomes undetectable. This is often mistaken for a suppressed VIP level due to mold toxins.[263]

The CSSPC considers normalizing VIP levels essential for helping CIRS patients fully recover. It must be given only after all other parts of the CSSPC are successfully completed in their entirety, which can take years, if ever.[264][265] The normal range for VIP is 23-63 pg/ml. VIP can be very beneficial, but it has a high failure rate and can make someone chronically worse and more difficult to treat. While VIP has many beneficial pleiotropic immune-modulatory effects, if there is any inflammation present, VIP becomes a potent inducer of Th2 and Th17 and a suppressor of Th1, which is the opposite of what you want with CIRS, chronic Lyme, CFS, fibromyalgia, autoimmune disease, and any chronic disease of aging. Th17 is a potent stimulator of autoimmunity, and the low Th1 and elevated Th2 are markers for T cell exhaustion and immunosenescence.[266][267][268] If you don't have any inflammation, VIP typically has anti-inflammatory effects, but if it is given in an inflammatory environment, such as in the presence of C4a and especially hTGFb (major hallmarks of CIRS), it will drive the immune system into more of a T cell exhaustion, immunosenescent, and aged immune system phenotype, further stimulating inflammatory Th2, and Th17 immunity and suppressing Th1.[269][270]

This is why Dr. Shoemaker states (and very astutely, I might add) that VIP should not be given unless you have dramatically cleaned up the immune dysfunction and inflammation.[271] This also explains why some people feel better from it while others worsen and become more difficult to treat. It has also been shown to reduce metabolism and suppress NK cell activity.[272] Thus, you dramatically inhibit your body's ability to destroy pathogens and toxins. This reduction in killing may make you feel better for a short time, as inflammatory cytokine levels may temporarily be reduced, but you will be at risk of worsening symptoms, the inability to fight off pathogens and cancer, and be more prone to toxic exposure, as your ability to eliminate these substances is diminished. There is concern that it stimulates breast and prostate cancer, potentially due to the suppression of NK cell function, and has been associated with an increase in PSA.[273] It has been shown that VIP stimulates substance P, a potent inflammatory marker associated with allergies.[274] As observed in a 2022 study in the *Journal of Immunology*, "Down-regulation of IL-21 by VIP could also diminish differentiation and activation of NK cells whose cytotoxic activity is augmented in the presence of IL-21".[275] Considering the potential stimulation of substance P, the stimulation of Th2/Th17, and the suppression of NK cell function and Th1, it is not surprising that the standard protocol takes a long-time to see beneficial effects and that patients never seem to recover fully, and they seem to always remain hypersensitive to future exposures to mold.[276][277] While VIP has many beneficial anti-inflammatory effects and can result in beneficial effects at a particular time, it must be given at the correct time, not too early, and not too late because its underlying immune-modulatory effect is opposite to that is what is needed for a speedy and complete recovery and may have the opposite effect you want or are expecting.

Problems With the Standard Treatment of Mold Illness/CIRS
The biggest problem with any treatment of mold illness/CIRS is that most physicians never look for this condition, or they use inappropriate treatments intended for other conditions based on symptomatic treatment, such as antidepressants and antianxiety, antiseizure, and pain medications. As a result, unless patients are aware of or suspect their symptoms are due to mold or other biotoxin exposures and seek out knowledgeable physicians in this area, they will typically suffer for months and even years without their symptoms being adequately addressed. At the same time, their overall health continues to worsen. Even if a mold patient finds a doctor knowledgeable about mold-associated illness and CIRS, the current standard of care, the CSSPC, often takes months or years to see improvement, if any. The few physicians in the U.S. who recognize, screen for, and treat mold illness/CIRS, usually do so by following the CSSPC. It consists of twelve steps, which need to be administered in sequential order and do not directly address the core dysfunctions of CIRS, but rather utilize a prolonged, expensive, and inefficient therapy that has a high rate of side effects and failure or often only results in partial improvement. The HUPRTOC

immediately addresses the underlying core dysfunctions seen with CIRS and mold-associated illnesses, as well as directly protecting the body from the toxic effects of the myco- and other enterotoxins.

The CSSPC process often requires multiple years to achieve improvement, if it does at all. Additionally, much like the diagnosis of Lyme disease, the diagnosis of CIRS is not precise. While Shoemaker has done significant work and research regarding the diagnosis, pathophysiology, and treatment of CIRS, he has tried to piece together a diagnosis based on visual contrast and Neuroquant® testing, genetic susceptibility, biomarker analysis, symptom grouping, and most recently, genomic analysis. While a detailed review and critique of each of these modalities are beyond the scope of this chapter, it is clear that many of these modalities are either difficult to get, expensive, complicated, and most importantly, not specific for CIRS. This is not surprising, as the underlying pathophysiology of CIRS is not specific, although most doctors think of mold when they think of CIRS.

This is not an attack on Dr. Shoemaker or the CSSPC because it suffers from the same lack of sensitivity and specificity as the diagnosis of chronic Lyme disease. While I diagnose many patients with chronic Lyme disease, I try to explain to the patients that while Lyme (*Borrelia burgdorferi*) may very likely be present and a significant cause of their symptoms, the actual problem and reason for their symptoms are multifactorial. While Shoemaker clarifies that chronic Lyme disease can cause CIRS, I argue that mold can be a significant contributing cause of the symptoms of Lyme disease, and mold may need to be addressed to be able to treat many patients with chronic Lyme disease successfully. Much like the problem with chronic Lyme disease, it is often a mixture of unknown infections and external and internal etiologies that result in a vicious multi-system dysfunction cycle. The same is true of CIRS, and no wonder the method of diagnosis is imprecise.

The good news is that they all have common pathophysiology, which Shoemaker agrees with, of immune dysfunction that then results in a vicious cycle of multisystem illness, which can be detected with a high degree of certainty. If a patient appears to have both mold and Lyme disease, the peptides can usually treat both simultaneously, so you don't have to decide which to treat first. The even better news is that with a greater understanding of the underlying pathophysiology associated with CIRS, HUPRTOC addresses more of the underlying physiologic abnormalities of both conditions than the old CSSPC, so you often see significant improvement much more quickly than with the current method of treatment, and it is effective when the current protocol is not. HUPRTOC does not, however, throw the baby out with the bathwater. It is an enhanced protocol that builds on the CSSPC, usually leading to a much faster and more effective recovery than with the CSSPC.

Based on the common pathophysiology, so many conditions can be looked at as variations of the same processes that involve chronic, often unknown infections (primary and reactivating), immune dysfunction, including T cell exhaustion, immunosenescence, and Th1 to Th2/Th17 shift, thymic and pineal involution, mitochondrial dysfunction, excessive mast cell activation, pineal-hypothalamic-pituitary-hormone axis abnormalities (including thyroid deficiency not detected by standard blood tests and other hormone deficiencies), immune activation of coagulation, cancer, rapid aging, GI dysfunction, leaky gut and blood-brain barrier, brain inflammation, obesity, cognitive dysfunction, insulin resistance, endothelial dysfunction, inflammation, autoimmune disease, neurodegenerative disease, cardiovascular disease, toxic overload, abnormal temperature and vascular regulation, anxiety or irritability, sensitivities, sleep disturbances, muscle or joint pain, CFS, fibromyalgia, chronic stress, depression, migraines, diabetes, PCOS, PMS, neuropathies, chronic kidney disease, and potentially a number of often unexplained or misdiagnosed symptoms and conditions. The population may be living longer, but it is also sicker. In 2013, just one in twenty people (4.3%) had no health problems, with a third of the population experiencing more than five ailments.[278] People lose more "years of healthy life" to illness now than they did in the 1990s; the Global Burden of Disease Study published in *The Lancet* showed that older Americans are sicker compared to ten other high-income counties despite the universal coverage that

Medicare provides. Older Americans had the highest rate of having three or more chronic conditions and required help with activities of daily living (36% in the U.S to a low of 13% in New Zealand.[279]

On a personal note, during a particularly stressful period of my life, I became progressively sicker to the point of being mostly bedbound for months with severe fatigue, anxiety, panic attacks, a severe sleep disorder, profuse sweating, neuropathy, complete inability to handle stress, allodynia (skin hurts with regular touch), along with many other symptoms. I then went into heart failure and intermittent a-fib. I could not stand upright or walk upstairs, and I developed autoimmune kidney disease and antiphospholipid syndrome. I was diagnosed with Lyme disease, Babesia, Bartonella, and a number of reactivating viruses and mold toxicity. I initially tried massive doses of antibiotics and the CSSPC, doing four to seven intravenous antibiotics simultaneously at many times the maximal doses for close to four years, and yet had no improvement. My immune system was barely functioning (my natural killer cell function ran between 0 and 3 LU (normal is > 30 LU); no wonder the antibiotics didn't work. I remember being in the ICU with sepsis and overheard the nurses talking outside my room, stating, "This is the AIDS patient that keeps coming up negative for HIV." I luckily found the power of immune modulation and directed pathophysiologic treatment with peptides and LDN.

After trying peptides, I felt different within a few days, and by the six-month mark, I was a different person. To the astonishment of my cardiologist, I walked into his office and was shown to have a normal cardiac function test about a year later after he said that I could maybe improve 10% in 10 years if I did intense cardiac rehab. He had never seen such a recovery. I also found a number of therapies that were very synergistic with the peptides, including LDN, T3, ozone, stem cells, plasmapheresis, IVIG, and oligonucleotide therapy.

Diagnosis of CIRS

One can certainly use the CSSPC for the diagnosis of CIRS, but we have found that simple antibody levels to toxic molds, which is a straightforward test to get from standard commercial laboratories and an inexpensive method to determine exposure to toxic molds, is shown to have a high sensitivity and specificity. This can also be done at a number of specialty labs. A significant number of studies show that this simple test is accurate, sensitive, and specific, especially when combined with positive symptoms and biomarkers.[280] [281] [282] These tests can easily be ordered by standard labs and done at a fraction of the cost and time called for by the standard CIRS protocol. It has also been shown that all patients with mold exposure (positive antibodies to toxic molds) also have autoantibodies to neurologic tissues, with over 80% showing abnormal nerve conduction studies.[283] The most specific neural autoantibodies need to be done at specialty labs.

Most CIRS patients, especially those who have Lyme disease, will also have antibodies against brain structures called PANS.[284] This is associated with significant neuro-psychiatric dysfunction that seldom gets correctly diagnosed. The combination of symptoms and toxic mold antibodies and/or a simple, inexpensive home or business mold testing (can do more expensive versions); an expanded group of biomarker testing that includes the Shoemaker biomarkers plus additional easily obtained (but rarely ordered) tests, along with a number of the following symptoms can make the diagnosis much quicker and more accessible and much less expensively than what the current protocol calls for. The symptoms include significant fatigue, sleep disturbance, post-exertional fatigue, memory or cognitive dysfunction, ADD/ADHD, OCD, addictions, GI disturbance, flushing, excessive sweating, light sensitivity, unexplained weight gain or loss, excessive thirst or urination, joint pain, headaches, rashes, muscle pain or weakness, anxiety or depression, neurologic symptoms, including neuropathy, numbness or tingling, shooting pains, sensitivities, shortness of breath or poor endurance, histamine intolerance, static shocks, arrhythmias or palpitations, chronic cough, mast cell activation symptoms, or diagnosis of chronic Lyme disease or associated infection, CFS, fibromyalgia, PTSD, bipolar disorder, infertility, regional pain syndrome, POTS, PANS or PANDAS, Ehlers-Danlos syndrome (EDS), yeast overgrowth, leaky gut, seizers, severe periodontal disease, chronic sinusitis, SIBO,

IBS, IBD, any autoimmune or neurodegenerative disease, and anything not clearly explained by another underlying condition. In a review of 119 patients exposed to mold in water-damaged buildings with positive antibodies to toxic molds and associated symptomatic peripheral neuropathy, 99 out of the 119 mold exposed patients had confirmatory abnormal nerve conduction studies, and, more importantly, all of the patients had highly significant increases in autoantibodies against neural antigens compared to healthy controls. Of the nine antineuronal autoantibodies tested, the most significant were anti-myelin basic protein, myelin-associated glycoprotein, anti-tubulin, and anti-neurofilament antigen.[285]

Immune Dysfunction and CIRS

CIRS, "chronic Lyme disease," CFS, fibromyalgia, autoimmune disease, toxin exposure, aging, neurodegenerative disease, inflammatory illness, and much more are associated with significant immune dysfunction, which includes T cell exhaustion and immunosenescence with resultant Th1 to Th2/Th17 immune shift, and a reduction of natural killer cell (NK cell) activity in the majority of people with chronic mold exposure.[286] [287] [288] In a review article entitled "The Neurological Significance of Abnormal Natural Killer Cell Activity in Chronic Toxigenic Mold Exposures," the authors state:

> In the light of this review, it is concluded that chronic
> exposures to toxigenic mold could lead to abnormal NKC
> activity with a wide range of neurological consequences,
> some of which were headache, general debilitating pains,
> fever, cough, memory loss, depression, mood swings,
> sleep disturbances, anxiety, chronic fatigue, and seizures.
> Depression, psychological stress, tissue injuries, malignancies,
> carcinogenesis, chronic fatigue syndrome, and experimental
> allergic encephalomyelitis could be induced at very low
> physiological concentrations by mycotoxin-induced NKC
> activity...[289]

Low NKC activity is also an objective marker for severe disability in patients with CFS and is associated with worse overall symptoms and increased cancer risk in CIRS patients.[290] [291] [292] Most labs test CD57 NK cells, which are more mature but less active than CD56 NK cells. An elevated CD57 NK cell number may be a marker for immunosenescence. It is always better to check the activity rather than the number, as the cells may be there, but they have poor surveillance and cytotoxic activity.[293] [294] [295] We recommend getting the natural killer cell function through Quest (special send out) and a total CD57 and CD56 as part of an extensive immune panel, or CD56 and CD57 number from LabCorp. Also, Cyrex Laboratories has a test panel called the Lymphocyte MAP that can be very helpful in determining immune dysfunction. CIRS patients have an increased incidence of autoantibodies to neural structures, including but not limited to microtubule-associated protein-2, myelin basic protein, tau, glial fibrillary acidic protein, tubulin, and S-100B. The mycotoxins also directly inhibit thymic, NK cell, and mitochondrial function.[296] [297] [298]

NK cells are thought of as cytotoxic lymphocytes critical to the innate immune system and function as a marker for Th1 immunity, but they serve immunoregulatory functions, with low NK cell activity being associated with significant atopy and IgE levels and clinically worse autoimmunity, inflammation, and the multisystem symptoms of CIRS, chronic Lyme disease, CFS, fibromyalgia, neurodegenerative disease, MCAS, and diseases of aging.[299] It makes sense, as it is shown to be an accurate downstream marker of Th1 immunity, so a low Th1 immunity would be expected to be associated with worse Th2/th17 inflammation and autoimmunity.[300] [301] [302]

There is almost always a combination of a triad of chronic stress, chronic infection, and chronic toxin exposure in those suffering from mold-associated illness/CIRS.[303] [304] We have found that most CIRS patients have a predisposing cause, a chronic infection (such as Lyme disease), physiologic stress, or an environmental factor (or factors) that make them dramatically more sensitive to the toxic effects of mold, mycotoxins, or other enterotoxins. It is rare, except in extreme cases of sizeable toxic exposure, for a previously healthy person with a robust, balanced immune system to suffer from mold sensitivities or CIRS.[305] [306] It appears that the majority of CIRS patients were predisposed to CIRS because of an already compromised immune system, with a low NKC function, mitochondrial dysfunction, T cell exhaustion, immunosenescence, or if they suffer from immune-related conditions, such as autoimmunity, chronic Lyme disease, or other infection, CFS, fibromyalgia, sleep disorder, physiologic stress, autoimmunity, obesity, MCAS, neurodegenerative diseases, atopy, aging, depression, diabetes, and any age-related or inflammatory condition.[307] [308]

In a recent review entitled "Mold, Mycotoxins and a Dysregulated Immune System: A Combination of Concern?" the authors conclude, "There is growing evidence that mycotoxins are of specific concern for individuals with pre-existing immune system impairment."[309] This further exemplifies the core dysfunction in mold-associated illness/CIRS and why LDN, immune-modulatory peptides, and other immune-modulatory therapies are the critical first-line therapy for CIRS, which the current CIRS treatment protocol fails to adequately address and only in a very indirect way.[310] [311] [312]

Mold can exacerbate sensitivities and conditions in at least eight main ways:

One: mold components, including spores, mycelium molecules, B-1,3 glucans, glycoproteins, and hyphal fragments, have been shown to act as allergens, increasing inflammation and sensitivities via the increased production of histamine, mast cells, and IgE.

Two: the immune-modulating effects of mycotoxins previously discussed, including suppression of NK cell function, thymic function, pineal-thymus axis, Th1 immunity, IL-2, IL-12, MSH, and VIP, stimulation of thymic involution, Th2/Th17 immunity, and subsequent inflammatory cytokines TGFb, C4a, C3a, IL-6, MMP-9, and others (see T Cell Exhaustion and Immunosenescence).

Three: the stimulation of autoantibodies, including a wide range of anti-neuronal, antimitochondrial, and many other autoantibodies, triggers PANS and worsening of most autoimmune disorders.

Four: mycotoxins have direct toxic effects on mitochondria.

Five: direct damage to mucosal and other tissue barrier functions, including gastric, pulmonary, and BBB integrity and the function of tight junctions.

Six: mycotoxins alter the gastrointestinal microbiota, causing a dysbiosis via direct antimicrobial effects, mucosal inflammation, and effects on the enteric immune system, altering gastrointestinal function, secretions, and immunity.

Seven: suppression of the pineal-hypothalamic-pituitary-(multi-hormone axis), including adrenal, thyroid, gonadotropins, growth hormone, ADH, estrogen, progesterone, aldosterone, DHEA, melatonin, oxytocin, MSH, etc.

Eight: immune activation of coagulation (more on this to follow).[313] [314] [315]

T Cell Exhaustion and Immunosenescence

When T cells are exposed to persistent antigen and/or inflammatory signals, such as the case with chronic infections, cancer, chronic mycotoxin, or other toxic exposure, you can see a deterioration of T cell function: a state called T cell exhaustion. "Exhausted" T cells (ETC) lose robust effector functions, express multiple inhibitory receptors, and are defined by an altered transcriptional program. TCE is often associated with inefficient control of persisting infections and tumors, but the revitalization of exhausted T cells can reinvigorate immunity.[316] As stated, TCE is associated with progressive loss of effector functions of T cells (CD4 and CD8) and phenotypic and functional defects, thymic dysfunction and involution, dysfunctional Th1 immunity, as indicated by a low NK cell function (activity), low IL-2, and elevated hTGF-b, C4A, IL-10, and IL-6 (high Th2/Th17), and immune activation of coagulation.[317] [318] [319]

Exhausted T cells lose their ability to kill pathogens as well as their proliferative capacity first; then, they lose the ability to secrete a number of cytokines. The severity of TCE correlates with the level and length of antigen stimulation. Again, TCE is reversible (distinct subsets of T cells can have different potentials of having the possibility of regaining function) and typically occurs in a few weeks to months, while immunosenescence is not reversible (must eliminate the senescence cells, which should naturally occur but does not with chronic inflammation and many chronic illnesses) and occurs in months to years. Although most of the data suggest that TCE and senescence are distinct mechanistic processes, there can be a blurring of characteristics. Both processes can occur and often do at the same time.[320] [321] Exhaustion develops more rapidly, and the responding T cells do not recover function if the infectious loads are not contained or the toxic exposure is not eliminated. TCE and its multisystem vicious cycle of repercussions, such as mitochondrial dysfunction, immune activation of coagulation, pineal-hypothalamic-pituitary-hormone axis dysfunction, etc., make the body unable to eliminate the chronic infection or eliminate the toxic burden.[322] [323]

As a sidenote that at the time of writing is currently in the news, T cell exhaustion is shown to occur with COVID, particularly Long COVID.[324] [325] [326] Researchers in the United States and Turkey found that two-thirds of patients with Long-COVID have a reactivated Epstein-Barr infection due to (TCE) compared to only 10% of controls.[327] Similarly, other researchers have shown reactivation of Lyme disease, Bartonella, Mycoplasma, and Toxoplasmosis in Long-COVID patients secondary to TCE.[328] [329]

Cellular senescence is defined as a stable growth arrest that is induced when cells reach the end of their replicative potential or are exposed to significant cellular stress or insult, DNA damage, inflammation, metabolic stress, or tissue damage signals. Cellular senescence, especially immunosenescence (immune aging), is a significant determinant of the degree and level of physiologic aging and disease. Immunosenescence contributes to the progressive inability to defend against infectious diseases, cancer development, autoimmunity, inflammation, and cardiovascular and neurodegenerative diseases. A significant cause of immunosenescence is the progressive involution of the thymus from about age ten until it functions at less than 10% in your 40s.[330] [331] It is not a coincidence that diseases of aging start accelerating after the nadir of thymic function. The immune system is usually balanced between the division that fights intracellular infections, called Th1, which enables self-tolerance, called Treg. The division that fights extracellular infections and induces inflammation is called Th2 and Th17. Excess Th2 and Th17 lead to excess inflammation, autoimmunity, degenerative diseases, diseases of aging, multisystem illness, and rapid aging. As what occurs with T cell exhaustion, immunosenescence is also synonymous with a Th1 to Th2/Th17 shift, which in normal aging is primarily caused by the lack of thymus function and thymic peptides, but any chronic illness exacerbates it, aging, stress, obesity, depression, anxiety, EMFs, chronic infections, and toxins, which, as you would expect, cause rapid aging. As with TCE, immunosenescence is a significant contributor to autoimmune disease, CFS, neurodegenerative diseases, diabetes, obesity, cardiovascular disease, gastrointestinal (GI) dysfunction (due to the gut-brain-immune axis), hypothyroidism, mast cell dysfunction, and neurodegenerative diseases.

Mycotoxins are shown to suppress thymic function directly, cause thymus involution, suppress IL-2 and natural killer cell function, and stimulate inflammation, Th2 and Th17 immunity, IL-6, and TGFbeta.[332] [333] Giving thymic and/or pineal peptides, including thymosin alpha 1, thymogen/vilon (Thymogen alpha 1), thymosin beta-4 (TB4), TB4 active frag, BPC-157, and KPV, as well as DSIP, LDN, mitochondrial peptides, and Cerebrolysin, are shown to reverse and prevent mycotoxin induced thymic involution and loss of thymic effect and subsequent immune dysfunction, inflammation and damage, thus protecting the body from and reversing these damaging effects of mycotoxins.[334] [335] [336]

This establishes a vicious cycle of cause and effect with chronic illness. The abnormal immune balance promotes immuno- and cellular senescence, resulting in poorly functioning cells and senescent cells that secrete significant amounts of reactive oxygen species and inflammatory mediators, which recruit additional senescent cells, causing rapid aging and multisystem illness and diseases. This worsens the immune imbalance, causing progressive illness and deterioration rather than reverting to a repair and rejuvenation mode. It becomes a "chicken or the egg" conundrum: does immunosenescence result in the inability to clear senescent cells, resulting in an accumulation of senescent cells and inflammatory secretions with associated inflammation, or does the excess accumulation of senescent cell production of inflammation suppress the immune system, resulting in immunosenescence, which then results in the inability to clear the senescent cells, resulting in the accumulation of senescent cells, with resulting inflammation?

According to the U.S. Center for Disease Control (CDC), approximately 80% of aged individuals are afflicted with at least one chronic disease due to declining thymic-related immune function.[337][338] Many things negatively affect thymus involution, pineal dysfunction, and subsequent immunity, including age, genetics, inflammation, lifestyle, obesity, EMFs, diet, exercise, stress, pregnancy, toxins, hypothyroidism, low growth hormone, chronic infections, and zinc deficiency.[339][340][341] EMFs are shown to speed up thymic and pineal dysfunction dramatically and involution, resulting in rapid multisystem aging and an increased risk for CIRS, other multisystem diseases, and neurodegeneration previous felt to be diseases of the old.[342]

Knowing this, one would not think it a giant leap to assume, "Why not give back the missing thymic and pineal peptides causing the core dysfunction of CIRS that occur with age and cause or contribute to almost all diseases of aging?" Yet, that is precisely what integrative, functional, and precision medicine doctors are doing. Such supplementation can reverse T cell exhaustion and immunosenescence, proving to be the core abnormality of most chronic inflammatory illnesses.

Thymic and Other Immune Modulatory Peptides for CIRS

Immune modulatory therapies are proving to be ideal therapies for CIRS, which include thymosin alpha 1 (the TA1 replacement is considered by many to be oral vilon/thymogen "Thymogen alpha-1"), thymosin beta 4 (TB4), TB4 frag, thymulin, BPC-157, KPV, mitochondria peptides, Cerebrolysin (oral CerebroPep), epitalon, pinealon, stem cells, exosomes, LDN, glutathione, NAC, zinc, ozone, and vitamin D. All are significant immune-modulators that can reverse the core dysfunction that results in numerous multi-system diseases, including CIRS.[343][344][345]

Additionally, the short peptide bioregulators thymogen/vilon (Thymogen alpha 1), TB4 active frag (Ac-SDKP), and KPV suppress a core issue in the underlying immune dysfunction present in CIRS: an elevated TGFb.[346][347][348] The nice thing is that supplementation with thymic and other peptides have been shown to be extremely safe, with studies unable to find a toxic dose, even at 1000 times the usual therapeutic amount. This is unheard of and in contrast to the small therapeutic window typical of medications.[349] [350]

TCE can be reversed, and immuno- and cellular senescence cells can be eliminated, which naturally occurs with a healthy Th1 immune system. When that is not the case, peptides, LDN, and other T cell stimulators and modulators can achieve the same result by restoring thymic function, blocking upregulated inhibitory receptors, such as PD-1, giving specific senolytic therapies (not addressed due to the limited scope of this chapter), and reducing the Th2 and Th17 associated cytokines, IL-10, IL-6, IL-7, and hTGFb.[351] [352] [353] Immune modulatory peptides and LDN are ideal for this role, resulting in subsequent improvement in most all of the biomarkers and symptoms of CIRS much faster and more efficaciously than utilizing the current CIRS protocol (CSSCP), which only indirectly and minimally affects the impaired functioning. Thus, the standard protocol only slowly normalizes the physiologic abnormalities over an extended period of time.[354] [355] [356] Simply removing antigen does not reverse TCE or restart the memory T cell differentiation process unless it happens early in the process.[357] [358]

Several thymic and pineal peptides modulate immunity to establish a healthy, balanced Th1/Treg-Th2/Th17 immune system, but they have differing effects. Thymosin alpha-1 (TA1) is approved in over 30 countries for various infections and cancer therapy. To achieve a broad overview of thymic peptides, think of TA1, thymogen, and vilon as increasing Th1/Treg, thymosin beta 4 (TB4), thymulin, and TB4 active frag (Ac-SDKP) as increasing Th1 and reducing Th2/Th17 along with providing additional rejuvenating properties. In contrast, BPC-157, KPV, and DSIP (not thymic peptides) reduce Th2/Th17 with additional healing, anti-inflammatory, rejuvenating, and antiaging effects, acting directly on tissues and through the gut-brain-immune axis.[359] [360] [361]

TB4 active fragment (Ac-SDKP) is a small part of the TB4 peptide that provides the majority of healing and immune-modulatory effects and removes a part (domain) of TB4 that can have a negative impact of stimulating mast cells, which cause inflammation.[362] The full-length TB4 is 43 amino acids long, so it cannot be absorbed orally. In comparison, TB4 active fragment (Ac-SKDP) is only four amino acids in length and is orally bioavailable, being orally absorbed intact. It is also approximately ten times as potent per weight as the full-length TB4 and is available as a supplement. It is a potent inhibitor of TGF-beta 1, a central player in CIRS.[363 364 365] The combination of thymogen/vilon (Thymogen Alpha-1) are potent immune-modulators and is considered an oral replacement for TA1 based on their mechanism of action and effects (potent Th1 stimulators) with confirmatory metabolomic testing.[366 367 368]

In one study, seventy-six five-month-old female rats were divided into two groups and were treated with only 5 mcg per rat of thymogen (44 rats) or saline (32 rats) five times per week for 12 months. The animals were monitored up to their natural death, and all the tumors discovered were studied microscopically. The study found that the maximal life span of thymogen treated group was 4.6 months longer than the control group and slowed aging from 0.007082 days^{-1} to 0.004123 days^{-1}. The occurrence of tumors and malignant neoplasia was 1.5 and 1.7 times lower, respectively. The authors concluded, "The ability of thymogen to inhibit spontaneous carcinogenesis and prolong life span has been established."[369] Thymogen has consistently slowed aging, extended lifespan, normalized immune dysfunction, reduced inflammation, and prevented and treated inflammatory diseases, infectious diseases, and carcinogenesis.[370 371 372]

Oral vilon is also a potent Th1 stimulating immune modulator, much like thymosin alpha-1, and is shown to suppress and prevent malignancy, reduce inflammation, and prevent and treat inflammatory conditions, chronic infections, autoimmunity, and atopy.[373] Vilon, as are TB4 active frag and thymogen, is a particularly potent inhibitor of TGF-beta, which is a main biomarker and core issue with CIRS.[374 375 376] Vilon can also normalize multiple hormones and neurotransmitters, leading to improved sexual and thyroid function, fertility, and resistance to emotional stress.[377 378] Vilon can also inhibit hypertrophy of the adrenals, involution of the thymus, and raises plasma albumin levels, which is a biomarker for overall health.[379 380 381]

Both vilon and BPC-157 tend to have a homeostatic effect on the body's systems. They both tend to lower blood pressure if it is high but will raise it if it is low, which works well for POTS and other conditions associated with mast cell activation and autonomic dysfunction. In a study looking at the thymomimetic effects of vilon on the immune status and coagulation hemostasis in elderly patients with type I diabetes, who, almost without exception, suffer from various degrees of immune dysfunction and hypercoagulability, the authors summarized their results: "It was found that the administration of vilon resulted in optimization of coagulation hemostasis, which was manifested in the increased content of natural anticoagulants: antithrombin II, and protein C, as well as the stimulation of fibrinolysis."[382]

They also noted a reduction in the amount of insulin needed and a normalization of T and B lymphocytes and IgA levels, pointing to a stabilizing hemostasis effect.[383] TB4 active frag, thymogen/vilon (Thymogen alpha-1), BPC-157, and KPV are orally bioavailable using unique oral delivery methods and available as supplements with strict manufacturing and regulatory requirements in conjunction with the production of extensive quality and safety data. Oral LDN and injectable peptides are available at specialty compounding pharmacies with a valid prescription.

Peptides and LDN (What is a Peptide?)

If you've investigated ways to improve your health, you've probably come across the term "peptide" and wondered what it is. A peptide is a compound made of two or more amino acids linked in a chain. Essentially, peptides are short chains of amino acids linked together. By definition, if the chain is longer than 40 amino acids (AAs), it is called a protein. If it has fewer than 40 AAs, it is called a peptide. You may also hear the term "oligopeptide," which is a term sometimes used for short peptides with fewer than twenty AAs. The simplest peptides are dipeptides (two AAs), followed by tripeptides (three AAs), tetrapeptides (four AAs), and so on. Meanwhile, a polypeptide is a long, continuous unbranched peptide chain.

Peptides control and modulate most systems in your body in a tissue and cell-specific manner, including hormone production, immune function, the sleep cycle, the production of inflammatory mediators, DNA replication, cell division and renewal, cancer cell destruction and apoptosis, libido, and sexual arousal, weight loss, lean muscle gain, mitochondrial function, cognitive function, mood, energy and other metabolic activities, tissue healing and specific biological functioning of the brain, skin, eyes, urinary and reproductive systems, aging and longevity, and many more.

Compared to medications and hormones, peptides tend to be more selective and less likely to be associated with serious adverse side effects. Peptides are generally cell surface signaling molecules that indirectly affect cellular activity via a cascade of secondary messengers. Hormones work on specific receptors in the nucleus, affecting protein synthesis, generally being slow on and slow off, less selective, and, in general, higher risk. Peptides have pleiotropic effects (no single effect) that are generally like those of supplements but more potent and selective and are quick on and quick off but can have lasting epigenetic changes. Peptides are very synergistic with other peptides, supplements, hormones, antibiotics, and most other therapies.

Small natural peptides have a long history of safety and effectiveness, being used in European countries for over 40 years, having hundreds of thousands of patient-years (hundreds of thousands of patients using for almost half a decade) that demonstrate their excellent safety and effectiveness. However, despite the many obvious clinical advantages, including unprecedented safety and efficacy and decades of commercial successes in Europe, the full potential of peptide therapeutics has yet to be unleashed in the United States. A significant reason is that they have surpassed their patent potential, making them undesirable to the pharmaceutical industry. In addition, the high cost of manufacturing has hindered their widespread use.

Peptides are naturally produced in the body by linking amino acid residues together through peptide bonds in an end-to-end fashion; each amino acid carries a unique functionality that adds a specific property to the peptide. The different amino acid residues target specific physiologic effects. As a result of their being bioidentical to what the body produces, the peptides are used to target and optimize particular physiologic functioning of the body's systems as "optimization and replacement therapies" that add back or supplement peptide levels in cases where endogenous levels are inadequate or absent. This is much like the incredible breakthrough in the 1920s, where the isolation and therapeutic use of the peptide/protein insulin was used in people with diabetes.

Based on peptides' extensive track record of safety and effectiveness over decades, and the fact that it has finally been realized that they have significant advantages over most drugs and protein therapeutics (including their small size, which gives them the ability to penetrate cell membranes, the blood-brain barrier, biofilms, mitochondria, gastrointestinal membranes, avascular tissue, and much more), their therapeutic potential has seen a significant explosion of interest. They also have high potency, specificity, activity, and affinity. In addition, they have a huge therapeutic index (the effective dose divided by the toxic dose), which is many-fold higher than even over-the-counter medications and supplements.

Peptides have an incredibly low likelihood of drug or supplement interactions other than positive synergistic effects. Being small and water-soluble, they are naturally degraded by the body and don't accumulate in specific organs, such as the kidney or liver, further increasing their safety profile. In addition, many popular peptides have no known toxic level, meaning researchers have not been able to elicit any toxicity effects no matter how high the dosage (consult your physician).

General Classes of Peptides

A detailed review of all the different classes of peptides is well beyond the scope of this chapter, but, in general, one way to classify peptides and small molecules is by location of origin and main activity.

Immune Modulating Peptides

Immune modulating peptides are secreted by or affect the pineal-thymic-immune axis and, ultimately, the immune system. These peptides, almost without exception, help normalize a dysfunctional immune system, which is consistently shown to be a shift from a healthy Th1/Treg dominant system to an unhealthy Th2/Th17 dominant system that is dominated by inflammation; autoimmunity; mitochondrial dysfunction; inability to fight intracellular infections and convert IgM antibodies to IgG; thymic dysfunction; T cell exhaustion; cellular and immunosenescence; inability to detoxify; low adrenal, thyroid, and growth hormone levels and effects even though standard lab tests look normal; and low or low-normal levels of the sex hormones, antidiuretic hormone, MSH, and VIP. This multifactorial immune dysfunction usually involves three things: stress, chronic infections, and significant toxic exposure.

This results in a vicious cycle that can involve a multitude of multi-system diseases, including CIRS, CFS, FM, autoimmune disease, allergies and sensitivities, excessive mast cell activation, sleep and mood disorders, fatigue, neurodegenerative diseases, GI disorders, cognitive disorders, rapid aging, and much more. These peptides include thymosin Alpha 1 (TA1), vilon/thymogen (Thymogen alpha-1), thymosin Beta 4 (Tβ4), TB4 active frag (Ac-SDKP), BPC-157, KPV, TB4 active frag (AGES), and Zn-thymulin.

Pineal Peptides
Pineal peptides include epitalon, pinealon, melatonin, and delta sleep-inducing peptide (DSIP). These potent antiaging peptides modulate thymus function, increase telomere length, and modulate immunity, sleep, and the hypothalamic-pituitary-hormone axes. These peptides, especially when combined with the thymic peptides listed earlier, have significant antiaging properties, increasing lifespan and healthspan, preventing malignancy formation and spread, and preventing and treating most of the all-too-common age-related diseases. The synergistic combination of thymic immune-modulators and pineal peptides protect against a wide range of toxic insults, whether from a drug overdose or an environmental toxin, including heavy metals and myco- and other enterotoxins. Pinealon and epitalon and BPC-157, TB4 active frag, KPV, DSIP, and Cerebrolysin protect the brain from the toxic effects of excitotoxins, such as myco- and other endotoxins. Short regulatory peptides were studied under oxidative stress conditions caused in animals by hypobaric hypoxia. The authors concluded, "Our results suggest

that pinealon has a pronounced antihypoxic effect. The pinealon capability of increasing the neuronal resistance to hypoxic stress is complex; it is based not so much on the inhibition of ROS increase in cells in response to stress as on limiting the excitotoxic effect of NMDA. The pinealon effect on brain metabolism in stress-sensitive animals is expected to be the most pronounced."[384]

Removal of the pineal gland results in the destruction of the thymus gland and impairment of the immune system accompanied by wasting diseases.[385] Given that the pineal peptides epitalon and pinealon can reset and reverse the damaged pineal-hypothalamus-pituitary-hormone axis so commonly seen in CIRS, chronic Lyme disease, and many chronic illnesses and diseases of aging, they, incredibly, can normalize thyroid hormone levels in hypophysectomized (lacking a pituitary) animals.[386] Being that the pineal-thymus axis is bidirectional, thymic peptides in turn influence the pineal gland secretions, including melatonin and circadian rhythm.

The pineal peptides epitalon and pinealon and the thymic bioregulator vilon are shown to increase telomere length, melatonin levels, exercise tolerance, and mental working capacity and prolong life span.[387] Vilon and epitalon reduced the HER-2/neu (breast cancer) gene expression by 2.0-3.6-fold in transgenic mice.[388] As stated, the oral use of pinealon increases telomere length, but it also stimulates serotonin production and promotes normalization of the antioxidant system, improves exercise tolerance, promotes and maintains a "trained status," and improves energy metabolism in athletes.

There is some evidence that one mechanism that pinealon and vilon appear to realize their geroprotective and exercise-stimulation effects is by upregulating the irisin gene.[389] The pineal gland is smaller in obese patients, insomniacs, and those with significant environmental toxin exposure. The amount of calcifications in the pineal gland "brain sand" correlates with pineal malfunction and is associated with various neurodegenerative disorders, such as Alzheimer's disease, MS, schizophrenia, and other pathological conditions.[390] The pineal gland can also directly stimulate thyroid secretion. Surprisingly, the highest amounts of melatonin are produced in the GI tract, but the thymus gland and the spleen also secrete it. In turn, melatonin also stimulates thymocyte maturation and thymic peptide release. Melatonin also stimulates SIRT1, leading to further anti-inflammatory and antioxidant effects, as well as mitochondria, and modulates mitophagy via mitochondria melatonin receptors. Based on the current literature and safety profile, the combination of a pineal and a thymic peptide appears to be a potentially potent option to provide an insurance policy against rapid aging, chronic illness, and the disorders that accompany the aging process. Further well-done clinical trials are needed in this exciting area to elucidate such therapies better.

In one study, the geroprotective effects of thymic and pineal peptides were investigated over six to eight years in 266 elderly patients after being treated for two to three years. The authors concluded:

> The obtained results convincingly showed the ability of
> the bioregulators to normalize the functions of the human
> organism, i.e. to improve the indices of cardiovascular,
> endocrine, immune and nervous systems, homeostasis and
> metabolism. Homeostasis restoration was accompanied by a
> 2.0-2.4-fold decrease in acute respiratory disease incidence,
> reduced incidence of the clinical manifestations of ischemic
> heart disease, hypertension disease, deforming osteoarthrosis
> and osteoporosis as compared to the control. Such a significant
> improvement in the health state of the peptide-treated patients
> correlated with decreased mortality rate during observation:
> 2.0-2.1-fold in the Thymalin-treated group; 1.6-1.8-fold in the
> epitalon-treated group and a 2.5-fold in the patients treated
> with thymalin plus epitalon as compared to the control.[391]

A separate group of patients was treated with the peptides annually for six years, and their mortality rate decreased 4.1 times the rate of the controls.[392] Pinealon and epitalon were shown to restore melatonin secretion in aged individuals to that of healthy controls, with multivitamins having no effect.[393]

A major part of the vicious cycle of CIRS is that the immune dysfunction causes mitochondrial dysfunction, which then feeds back, causing more immune dysfunction, pineal-hypothalamic-pituitary-thyroid, and other hormone deficiencies, which further contribute to the downward spiral. The key is to target the underlying abnormalities and stop or rewind the vicious cycles that are causing such difficult-to-treat multi-system illnesses such as CIRS. The combination of vilon and epitalon changed the expression of five of thirteen mitochondrial genes, improving mitochondrial function by increasing the expression two to sixfold in four of the genes and reducing one by 55%. The combination also inhibited pro-oncogenic genes and activated anticarcinogenic genes.[394]

Gastrointestinal/Leaky Gut/Inflammatory Bowel Disease/Gut-Brain Axis Peptides

BPC-157 is a naturally occurring peptide in human gastric fluid. It has enhanced stability compared to other peptides, is resistant to enzymatic hydrolysis and stomach acid breakdown, and is orally bioavailable, which is surprising due to its size (15 amino acids in length). It is the most popular peptide and is undoubtedly considered the "go-to" peptide for treating gut issues.

BPC-157 has a wide range of healing, rejuvenating, and antiaging effects, which include the up-regulation of growth factors and genes involved with proangiogenic effects (stimulates capillary formation to deliver more oxygen and nutrients to tissues), modulation of nitric oxide (NO) synthesis, modulation of the serotonergic and dopaminergic systems, as well as exerting significant beneficial effects on leaky gut, the gut-brain axis, and the microbiome. It has similar effects as TB4, TB4 active fragment, and KPV, but it has a different mechanism. This makes them very synergistic and a powerful rejuvenation combination.[395] [396] [397]

BPC-157 reduces inflammation and promotes healing in most tissues and systems in the body, including the gut (it probably has the best track record for leaky gut, but TB4 active frag and KPV are key combinations with BPC-157), the brain (improves mood, cognitive function, traumatic brain injury), skin, muscle, degenerative joints, the heart (prevents and treats arrhythmia, heart failure, and Lyme myocarditis), peripheral nerves (neuropathic pain), the bladder (incontinence), the immune system (inflammatory conditions, mast cell activation, and autoimmunity) and is protective against neuro-, myco- (mold) and endotoxins, improves insulin resistance and is antimicrobial, outperforming the antiviral acyclovir for the herpes class of viruses at 1/1000th the dose, making it an ideal therapy for CIRS.[398 399 400]

While many physicians consider oral BPC-157 to be a gut-healing peptide, it has been demonstrated to protect and heal a wide range of both gastrointestinal and systemic tissues and organs. It is clearly shown to be equally efficacious and equipotent when injected for systemic conditions as when given orally (i.e., a dose given orally or via injection is equally effective for systemic disorders).[401 402 403]

Every study that has tested the oral form against injectable BPC-157 for systemic conditions, such as MS, muscular-skeletal damage, central and peripheral nervous system damage, metabolic issues, and other body systems, has shown that oral administration works equally well at the same dose. There might be a slightly better result if injecting intraarticular, but other than that, the studies show that oral BPC-157 will have the same efficacy as an injectable for systemic issues. We have found that some people prefer capsules, mouth sprays, or oral strips, while others prefer injectables. We also do it intravenously.

TB4 active frag (Ac-SDKP) is also resistant to enzymatic degradation and absorbs whole, as does the melanocyte-stimulating hormone MSH fragment KPV. They both have a selectivity of the tight junctions in the GI mucosa, the pulmonary mucosa, and the blood-brain barrier, making the BPC-157, TB4 active frag, and KPV trio an effective therapy for GI issues, including leaky gut, dysbiosis, IBS, inflammatory bowel disease, and SIBO (especially when the antimicrobial peptide, LL-37, is added). DSIP is produced in the gut and where its highest levels are found. It is also very anti-inflammatory and appears to absorb sublingually, but we have not directly tested it. In a recent study, oral antimicrobial peptide LL-37 was shown to significantly improve COVID symptoms compared to placebo.[404 405]

One key aspect of treating the gut with the peptides listed above is that they work on the gut-brain axis and the brain-gut axis. It is a bidirectional system. For instance, treating SIBO with antibiotics often results in relapse because the systemic condition causing an unhealthy gut via the brain-gut axis is not addressed. Peptides treat both sides of the loop. I usually add a good spore-based probiotic, oral IgG, and sometimes butyrate or digestive enzymes.

Mycotoxins destroy the gut mucosa and damage the tight junctions throughout the body, causing significant inflammation with the immune dysfunction, as discussed above, directly and indirectly damaging mitochondria, causing pineal-hypothalamic-pituitary-hormone axis dysfunction, immune activation of coagulation, inability to detox, autoimmunity, and a multitude of other dysfunctions. One of the many nice things about peptide therapy for CIRS is that the peptides protect the body from the toxic effects of mold and mycotoxin exposure while they correct the dysfunctions and stimulate healing and rejuvenating. In an extensive review of BPC-157's effects on the gastrointestinal tract, the authors summarized their findings, "Stable gastric pentadecapeptide BPC 157 is an anti-ulcer peptidergic agent, safe in inflammatory bowel disease clinical trials and wound healing, stable in human gastric juice, and has no reported toxicity. Particularly, it has a prominent effect on alcohol-lesions (i.e., acute, chronic) and NSAIDs-lesions (interestingly, BPC 157 both prevents and reverses arthritis)… and acts as a free radical scavenger and exhibits neuroprotective properties."[406]

There are two critical aspects of the GI system that influence health and disease pathogenesis: the microbiome's effects on the neurologic system, inflammation, and health, and the brain's influence on the microbiome and overall GI functioning (intestinal mobility, mucous secretion, secretory functions, blood flow, etc.). Additionally, a "leaky gut" means there is a "leaky brain" (the blood-brain barrier (BBB) is not able to keep out toxins, infectious agents, and inflammatory molecules and cells). There is also brain inflammation due to this gutbrain connection if there is gut inflammation.

Numerous studies show that BPC-157, TB4 active frag, KPV, and DSIP reduce gut inflammation and promote healing of the gut, the brain, BBB, and other tissues in the body. Additionally, TB4 active frag and KPV promote healing of the GI and BBB tight junctions, which are core abnormalities that result in leaky gut and leaky brain, making them a powerful combo for leaky gut and cognitive, mood, and neurodegenerative diseases. The power of the effectiveness of these peptides in the treatment of leaky gut and diseases of the central nervous system is that they have the rare ability to work on both sides of the gut-brain axis, positively affecting the gut's health and its influence on brain health and the brain's health and its influence on gut health, and their influence on the overall body's inflammation and functioning via the gut-brain-immune-inflammatory connection.

Additionally, these peptides will also bind to mycotoxins and protect the body against the effects of numerous toxins, including mycotoxins, making them an ideal therapy for CIRS. Additional immune-modulatory peptides, including vilon/thymogen (Thymgen alpha-1) and thymulin, will further reduce the inflammation caused by a leaky gut, which prevents the system-wide damage caused by leaky gut and will subsequently help heal excessive brain inflammation and leaky brain. This will, in turn, help heal the leaky gut and GI dysfunction via the brain-gut axis and all of the body's inflammation and functioning via the gutbrain-immune-inflammatory connection.

EMFs and CIRS

There has been a massive increase in electromagnetic radiation (EMF) exposure in the last few decades, which continues to increase exponentially. We are exposed to 1018 more EMFs (1,000,000,000,000,000,000) than we experienced as recently as 1917.[407] Over the last twenty years, a robust body of independent science has emerged showing significant negative biological impacts from exposure to EMFs, including evidence of developmental delay, neurological and cognitive dysfunction, neurodegenerative diseases, heart abnormalities, thyroid, and other hormone deficiencies, reproductive effects, accelerated aging, diabetes, autoimmunity, fatigue, cancer, and much more.[408 409 410] EMFs cause increased ROS and inflammation, immune dysfunction, mitochondrial dysfunction, epigenetic disruption, abnormal activation of voltage-gated ion channel, leaky gut, and BBB, among other serious health problems.[411 412 413]

EMFs, in particular, are shown to dramatically speed up thymic and pineal dysfunction and involution, resulting in rapid multi-system aging and increased risk for multisystem diseases and degeneration previously felt to be diseases of the old.[414] This was well recognized very early in the seventies by Dr. Robert O. Becker (twice nominated for Nobel Prize), who said, "I do not doubt in my mind that, at the present time, the greatest polluting element in the earth's environment is the proliferation of electromagnetic fields (EMFs)."[415] EMFs are shown to significantly increase brain inflammation, including the hypothalamus, hippocampus, and amygdala, causing significant neurologic and cognitive defects and neurodegeneration. EMF sensitivity is common in CIRS, chronic Lyme disease, CFS, fibromyalgia, neurodegenerative diseases, autoimmunity, chronic Lyme disease, mast cell activation syndrome (MCAS), and many diseases of aging. They share the same immunological phenotype: Th1/Treg to Th2/Th17 shift with mitochondrial dysfunction, pineal-hypothalamic-pituitary-hormone dysfunction, leaky gut and BBB, immune activation of coagulation, GI dysfunction, brain inflammation, and neurodegenerative diseases, and other diseases of aging, all set off by immune dysfunction.

Calcium-gated channels are located throughout the body, especially in the gut, heart, and brain. They are a core component of the Cell Danger Response (CDR), which causes immune dysfunction, abnormal cell signaling, pathological mitochondrial metabolism, significant inflammation, cell toxicity, and death.[416 417 418] EMF toxicity occurs in everyone to different degrees.[419]

The following are a few studies that demonstrate the potential hazards of the typical levels of EMF exposure experienced by most people in the United States, which is greatly enhanced with CIRS and other chronic illnesses secondary to preexisting abnormalities.

- Prenatal exposure to 900 Mhz EMFs resulted in offspring with a high degree of a dysfunctional thymus and spleen, as well as mitochondrial and immune dysfunction (thymic dysfunction and T cell exhaustion with Th1/Treg-Th2/Th17 shift), decreased glutathione and SOD, reduced NK cell function and number, gut dysbiosis, increased GI and BBB (brain) permeability, pineal-hypothalamic-pituitary-hormone dysfunction (resulting in multiple hormonal deficiencies that are not detected by standard blood tests.[420] [421]

- Aldad et al. exposed pregnant mice in utero to a mobile phone on active call mode throughout gestation. The offspring were shown to have memory impairment and hyperactive behavior compared to unexposed mice.[422]
- Tang et al. chronically exposed rats to 28 days of mobile phone EMFs. They found significantly altered neurobehavioral performances, impaired spatial memory, and damaged BBB permeability by activating the mkp-1/ERK pathways. It was also shown that the rats experienced impaired special learning and reference memory. Morphologic changes were found in the rats' hippocampus.[423]
- Saikhedkar et al. exposed rats to cell phone radiation for 4 hrs/day for 15 days, which induced deficits in learning and memory. They also found hippocampal neuronal degeneration.[424]
- Pregnant rats exposed to cellphone RF-EMF throughout gestation drastically affected learning acquisition and memory retention, EM67, and further study also showed hippocampal morphological changes.[425]
- Numerous studies have shown that rats exposed to cellular phone RF-EMR for various periods result in increased long-standing subsequent anxiety. One study found reduced GABA and aspartic acid in the cortex and hippocampus.[426] [427]

The good news is that peptide combinations, such as LDN, thymogen/vilon (Thymogen alpha 1), BPC-157, TB4 frag, KPV, selank, semax, MOTSc, humanin, SS-31and Cerebrolysin (IV and oral-available as a supplement) can mitigate and prevent a significant amount of EMF toxicity. BPC-157 is shown to block the abnormal activation of voltage-gated ion channels caused by EMFs. BPC18, BPC23, BPC45, BPC61, BPC66, BPC-157, and thymosins modulate the immune system to maintain a healthy a Th1/Treg-Th2/Th17 as opposed to the pathogenic, inflammatory TH2/Th17/Th9 immune system caused by many things, including EMFs.[428] [429] [430]

Thymic peptides, such as TB4 active frag, thymogen/vilon

(Thymogen alpha-1), BPC-157, KPV, and oral Cerebrolysin (CerebroPep) have a wide range of mechanisms that protect the body against the damage of EMFs. This includes a general decrease in EMF-induced inflammatory cytokines.[431][432][433]

Biomarkers

TGF beta-1, C4a, and MMP-9 are markers of a high Th2/Th17. The immune system is like a seesaw in that one side usually dominates; high Th1 immune activity suppresses Th2 and Th17 immunity, while high Th2 and Th17 immunity suppress Th1 immunity-depending on the condition and health of the system. The typical immune abnormalities seen with CIRS are not specific to CIRS but are extremely important. Because immune dysfunction lies at the core of CIRS, additional testing should be done. This should include NK cell function testing as a send out through Quest Diagnostics, though not all draw stations perform the test, and even then, they often only do it at particular times of the day since NK cell number is not as sensitive as activity. For instance, approximately 75% of CFS patients have low NK cell function, and 25% have low NK cell numbers. Other recommended tests that demonstrate immune dysfunction include CD4/CD8 ratio (< 2.5), NK cell function <30 LU, increased hTGFb-1 (TB4 frag, KPV, and vilon are potent suppressors of TGFb-1), increased C4a, tT3/rT3< 12, tT3/T4 ratio < 3, leptin >12, immune activation of coagulation, autoimmunity, toxic mold antibodies, low DHEA, AM cortisol < 12 with an ongoing chronic infection, low vitamin D, low pregnenolone, low testosterone, low GH or estrogen, increased CMV, EBV titers or H-pylori, low IgG subclasses (adequate Th1 immunity is required to convert IgM antibody to IgG), hyperlipidemia, high (high normal) eosinophil cationic protein (ECP), ACE > 30, and a low WBC (this can be useful, and is, of course, very easy to get, but it is not very sensitive).[434][435][436] Conditions associated with immune dysfunction include ongoing chronic infections, SIBO, IBS, PMS, cardiovascular disease, kidney disease, cognitive dysfunction, CFS, fibromyalgia, PTSD, traumatic brain injury, diabetes, obesity, hypothyroidism, chronic dieting, depression, osteoporosis, MCAS, frailty, depression, CIRS, allergic conditions, autoimmunity, aging, stress, anxiety, neurodegenerative diseases, inflammatory diseases, and most chronic illnesses.[437] [438] [439]

You will find that close to all CIRS patients have significant immune dysfunction. Treatment usually entails LDN, TB4 frag, thymogen/vilon (Thymogen alpha-1), BPC-157, and KPV as a starting point, usually pairing LDN with a thymosin peptide or peptide combination along with a modulator and suppressor of Th2/Th17, which would be BPC-157 as a staple and KPV as a great choice, especially if the patient has any mast cell activation issue. I would then add pinealon or epitalon to improve the immune dysfunction and the pineal-hypothalamic-pituitary-hormone axis, which will improve hormone production. Other effective therapies include stem cells, exosomes, glutathione, NAC, zinc, ozone, vitamin D, and others.

While both the standard CSSPC and the HUPRTOC recommend that patients remove themselves from the mold source as a common-sense first step, the peptides BPC-157, TB4 active frag, KPV, epitalon, pinealon, oral Cerebrolysin, MOTSc, and SS-31 are essential at protecting the body against the toxic effects of the myco- and enterotoxins. You can use sequestrants (binders), but a properly functioning cell and the system will be able to eliminate the mycotoxins. However, if there is low cellular energy, another major issue with CIRS, the body cannot eliminate the toxins. The same is true for heavy metals. Due to the damaged pineal-hypothalamic-pituitary-thyroid axis and systemic inflammation, all but a small percent of CIRS patients will have low tissue levels of thyroid even though the standard thyroid function tests, including the TSH, look normal. They will usually have a low normal TSH, a normal free T4, a low normal free T3, and a high normal reverse T3, along with an SHBG level less than 80 in women and 30 in men.[440] [441] [442] Supplementing with T3, in addition to immune modulators and mitochondrial peptides (such as MOTSc and SS-31), is shown to significantly improve mitochondrial function and cellular energy and reverse the dysfunctional mitochondrial cell danger response.[443] [444] The increased cellular energy will facilitate the ability of the cells to detoxify and eliminate mycotoxins and will also enable cellular and tissue resistance to the toxic effects of mycotoxins and heavy metals. I believe oral and intravenous phosphatidylcholine and polyMVA outperform cholestyramine (CSM) for biotoxin removal if combined with the above.

ACTH, Cortisol, and Stress

Stress and CIRS can result in significant mast cell activation (MCAS). As stated above, both conditions stimulate CRH, which is a potent stimulator of mast cells. When this is combined with the stress and CIRS T cell exhaustion and immunosenescence-induced immune dysfunction, MCAS is often a significant problem. While direct mast cell inhibitors, the standard protocol for MCAS, can be helpful, upstream regulation via reversing the out-of-balance immune system, which includes reversing the Th1 to Th2/Th17 shift with LDN, pinealon, epitalon, TB4 frag, thymogen/vilon (Thymogen alpha-1), BPC-157 and KPV, is a much more effective method as a sole therapy or in combination with direct mast cell inhibitors for controlling excess mast cell activation. I would then consider the pineal peptides, pinealon, or epitalon. You will often notice many of the biomarkers improving as the immune dysfunction improves and the pineal gland, the hypothalamus, and pituitary inflammation decrease. Cerebrolysin (IV or oral), selank, semax and humanin reduce activation of microglial (brain mast cells) and brain inflammation.

Using ACTH and centrally acting agents for cortisol stimulation tests, a study published in the *Brazilian Journal of Infectious Diseases* demonstrated that HPA axis dysfunction could be determined accurately using basal cortisol levels in individuals with chronic infections. They found that a basal cortisol below 11.5 ug/dl had a 94% specificity for HPA axis dysfunction. It is not uncommon for such patients to have a high ACTH, which correlates with a high CRH.[445] So, in addition to therapy with LDN and the peptides mentioned above, you want to give a low physiologic dose of cortisol, 5-15 mg per day, to help optimize cortisol levels and improve the body's ability to handle stress and avoid another vicious cycle. This will also bring the ACTH and CRH down, a potent mast cell activator. Also, any condition associated with inflammation or stress, including EMF-induced inflammation, will result in the Th1/

Treg to Th2/Th17 shift, increasing the risk of MCAS, autoimmunity, and most every disease of aging. This HPA axis dysfunction should be treated with physiologic doses of cortisol 5-15 mg/day to optimize the cortisol level in physiologically stressed individuals and bring down CRH, a potent stimulus of mast cells and associated with a significant Th1/Treg to Th2/Th17 shift.

In a review article that I published, "Diagnosis and Treatment of Hypothalamic-Pituitary-Adrenal (HPA) Axis Dysfunction in Patients with Chronic Fatigue Syndrome (CFS) and Fibromyalgia (FM)," it was demonstrated that while both CFS and FM patients are shown to have central HPA dysfunction, the dysfunction in CFS is at the pituitary-hypothalamic level. In contrast, the dysfunction in FM is more related to dysfunction at the hypothalamic and supra-hypothalamic levels.[446] Because treatment with low physiologic doses of cortisol (<15 mg) is safe and effective and routine dynamic ACTH testing does not have adequate diagnostic sensitivity, it is reasonable to give a therapeutic trial of physiologic doses of cortisol to the majority of patients with CFS and FM, especially to those who have symptoms that are consistent with adrenal dysfunction, such as low blood pressure or have baseline cortisol levels in the low or low-normal range.[447]

Peptides were not available when the review article was published, so it describes the appropriate treatment as giving cortisol if a patient's morning cortisol level is below 12. Now, this can be rectified through the use of peptides. Some cortisol may be beneficial for some patients for a time. Most specialists in the treatment of mast cell disorders strictly focus on direct mast cell inhibitors and don't understand how it is a disease of immune dysfunction, not mast cells. The mast cells are not abnormal; they are being inappropriately stimulated. Thus, while direct mast cell inhibitors have benefits, treating the upstream cause of the mast cell activation is more appropriate and effective. While most of the peptides will improve MCAS and associated symptoms, BPC-157 and especially KPV (a fragment of melanocyte-stimulating hormone (MSH) which like MSH) have very potent anti-inflammatory effects, including mast cell inhibition. KPV is, however, about a hundred-fold more potent anti-inflammatory and mast cell inhibitor by weight. Also, KPV does not stimulate melanocytes, so there is no risk of hyperpigmentation. Its small size and stability make it orally bioavailable, whereas the large MSH peptide is not orally absorbable. Additionally, it has significant broad-spectrum antimicrobial activity.

MSH and KPV

MSH and KPV help regulate many other hormones and play an essential role in the body's inflammation responses to foreign pathogens, one of the most anti-inflammatory substances produced in the body. Unlike steroids, however, MSH and its analogs do not lessen the body's ability to fight infection; rather, it enhances its immunological defense against invading organisms and has potent broad-spectrum antimicrobial effects against bacteria and viruses, mold, parasites, and fungi. Thus, low levels of MSH will result in multi-system inflammation (i.e., CIRS) and an inability to fight many infections, with MARcONS infection of the sinuses being a specific example.

MSH and leptin have reciprocal stimulating effects on each other. Under normal conditions, increased leptin levels result in a corresponding increase in MSH and vice versa. However, when leptin receptors are interfered with by inflammatory cytokines, causing leptin resistance, high leptin is associated with low MSH because the leptin signal does not reach the receptors in the brain. Low levels of MSH are evident in patients with mold illness/CIRS and can remain low even after treatment. When this happens, leptin production increases without a corresponding rise in MSH levels, resulting in leptin resistance and unhealthy weight gain. A rise in leptin levels in healthy people would trigger the brain to create more MSH, which does not occur in CIRS patients.

MSH is also involved in the opening and closing of tight junctions in the intestinal tract. Diminished MSH levels can prevent tight junctions from closing properly, leading to a leaky gut. In addition, research has established that approximately 80 percent of patients with low MSH levels also have MARCoNS (multiple antibiotic resistant coagulase negative staph, usually concentrated in the sinuses).[448] [449] This creates a vicious cycle because MARCoNS produces toxins that suppress MSH production. Treating MARCoNS is therefore vitally important to restore MSH levels to normal levels. The normal range for MSH is 35-81 pg/ml.

It is not practical to give MSH due to its poor bioavailability and short half-life. Commercially available MSH analogs have been developed, including Melanotan I & II and PT-141. Melanotan I & II have been known as the "Barbie Doll" peptide because it stimulates weight loss, libido, and activation of skin melanocytes (in other words, it makes you tan). However, tanning is a double-edged sword, as it works well for younger individuals, but older individuals will often develop dark spots as areas of sun damage darken. PT-141 works for erectile dysfunction in men and is FDA approved for sexual dysfunction in women. While effective, it has a significant side effect of nausea and vomiting and can stimulate skin melanocytes, although less than Melanotan I & II.

It has recently been found that the C-terminal tripeptide of MSH, KPV, is much more anti-inflammatory (many times as potent) than its parent compound MSH; it is orally bioavailable, while MSH is not; it promotes healing of the gut and numerous other organ systems; is organoprotective; prevents cellular stress-induced toxicity; is very effective for excess activation of mast cells, as in mast cell activation syndrome (MCAS) and activated microglia in the brain (neuroinflammation); results in no stimulation of skin melanocytes; is very non-toxic; and has a broad spectrum of antimicrobial and antibiofilm properties, having both direct antimicrobial effects against fungi, mold, bacteria, viruses, and parasites, as well as indirect effects mediated through the immune system, even at very low (picomolar), concentrations.[450] [451] [452] MSH is potentially the most potent inhibitor of mast cell activation. The best part is that it does not suppress the ability to fight infections; rather, it improves it.[453] [454] A review article that examined the direct and indirect antimicrobial and immune-modulatory effects of MSH and its fragments found that MSH and its C-terminal fragment demonstrated potent antifungal, antibacterial and immune-modulatory activity, stating, "The C-terminal region (KPV) of α-MSH demands special attention for several reasons. It exhibits in vitro and in vivo anti-inflammatory activity similar to that of the parent peptide without the metabotropic effect. Moreover, this essential anti-inflammatory sequence, C-terminal tripeptide (KPV) of α-MSH, is also essential for its direct antimicrobial efficacy. Therefore, this short molecule KPV appears to have tremendous potential to be developed as a therapeutic agent as it is more suitable for clinical use…"[455]

PAI-1, ACA, and VWF

Plasminogen Activator Inhibitor-1 (PAI-1), Anti-cardiolipin Antibodies (ACA), and Von Willebrand Factor (VWF) comprise the standard coagulation panel recommended in the current CIRS treatment algorithm. The HUPRTOC recommends a much more extensive and comprehensive hypercoagulation panel because the standard panel will miss 60-90% of those suffering from immune activation of coagulation. Missing this abnormality will often result in multiple levels of treatment failure and protracted illness.

There are over 60,000 miles of blood vessels in the body, of which 80% are capillaries. Inflammation from mold, bacteria, parasites, viruses, mycotoxins and other toxins, mast cells, and immune and mitochondrial dysfunction can trigger the clotting cascade, causing fibrin to be laid down on the capillary walls and thick, sluggish blood. This combination causes the body to suffer from diminished ability to deliver nutrients, medications, and oxygen to the cells and remove waste products from the cells.

The internal width of a capillary is 8-10 microns (a human hair is 50-100 microns in diameter), and a red blood cell is about 7 microns wide. The sludge-like fibrin layer formed during a hypercoagulable state is about 1 micron thick. The red blood cells are also less flexible, making it difficult to flow through the narrowed capillaries. The fibrin-coated capillary walls also impair the ability of nutrients, supplements, and medications to penetrate the cells and the capability of waste products to exit the cells. This often leads to treatment-resistance in patients and is one cause of thyroid resistance.

The oxygen that usually takes approximately two seconds to diffuse into the cells can take up to 5 minutes to penetrate the thickened capillary walls, potentially causing cellular hypoxia, mitochondrial dysfunction, and extensive need to utilize anaerobic metabolism with even minimal physical or mental stress or stimulation. In addition, with fibrin coating the vessel walls, the endothelial cells can no longer release heparans, the body's natural blood thinner, perpetuating the cycle. Typical symptoms include air hunger, shortness of breath, poor endurance, fatigue, muscle pain, and POTS, where the fibrin-coated vessels become stiff and unable to compensate with positional changes quickly. Patients may sometimes notice mottled (blotchy), lace-like purple discoloration under the skin (often on thighs and lower legs), called livedo reticularis. This is most commonly seen with Bartonella infections but can occur with other causes of immune activation of coagulation.

The coagulation system can also contribute to the innate immune system by trapping invading organisms and secreting antimicrobial peptides into the space between and below the platelet aggregates-fibrin fibers-red blood cell complex.[456]

However, certain molds and bacteria have developed ways to use this stimulation of coagulation to increase virulence. The invading organism can either secrete substances that can activate clotting or hinder the coagulation pathway at the fibrin monomer formation state to hide under and amongst the fibrin monomers or by encasing themselves in a shield of fibrin that effectively blocks phagocytosis.[457] A study investigated the interplay of the complement and coagulation systems in host defenses. The authors found that complement activation and coagulation support cellular immune responses lead to the direct killing of bacteria via assembly of the Membrane Attack Complex (MAC). The coagulation system can entrap bacteria inside clots and generate small antibacterial peptides, but pathogenic bacteria have developed numerous strategies to modulate and evade these defensive mechanisms. They write, "Borrelia burgdorferi expresses a variety of plasminogen receptors on their surface, including the outer surface proteins (OspA and OspC) and Erp proteins (ErpA, ErpC, ErpP), to establish plasmin formation during all stages of infection," This allows Bb to break down and be free of any potentially entrapping fibrin monomers.[458]

Like many processes in the body, immune activation of coagulation is initially beneficial, but as it continues, it becomes detrimental, which is often the case with unresolved chronic infections, including Lyme disease and other bacteria, viruses, parasites, and mold. Toxins can also induce coagulopathy, including mycotoxins and heavy metals. This is often seen in cases of CIRS, CFS, fibromyalgia, chronic inflammation, autoimmunity, GI dysfunction, and many chronic illnesses. You can see herxheimer reactions when starting vascular enzymes or heparin, as the toxins and infections are released.[459] A number of studies have found that 60-90% of CIRS, CFS, fibromyalgia, Gulf War syndrome, and Lyme disease patients have abnormal immune activation of the clotting system. In comparison, 75% have a genetic predisposition for thrombophilia, which is a fourfold increase over the general population.[460]

The HUPRTOC Immune Activation of Coagulation Panel is much more extensive than the one used in the CSSPC. The HUPRTOC panel includes D-dimer, soluble fibrin monomer (SFM), fibrinogen, prothrombin fragment 1+2, thrombin antithrombin (TAT) complex, factor II activity, PAI-1, anti-Xa, anti-phospholipid antibodies, lupus anticoagulant, anti-B2GPI antibodies, Sed rate <5, low normal PTT, elevated fibrinogen, increased LP(a), PAI-1 4G/5G genetic polymorphism, an elevated or high-normal eosinophil cationic protein (especially when provocated with an antiparasitic, this has a high sensitivity for the detection of Babesia and associated hypercoagulability), factor V Leiden deficiency, and elevated homocysteine. This panel is exponentially more sensitive at detecting abnormal coagulation. If you miss immune activation of coagulation, which is so common with CIRS, and fail to treat the hypercoagulation, the patient is less likely to respond to therapy. A study examined the relationship between the level of activated partial thromboplastin time (PPT) within the normal range and the risk of venous thromboembolism in 13 880 individuals over 13 years. The study found a 5.5-fold increased risk of idiopathic venous thromboembolism for those with a PTT level below the mean. The authors concluded, "A single determination of the activated partial thromboplastin time below the median increased the risk of future venous thromboembolism. Findings were independent of coagulation factor levels, and a low activated partial thromboplastin time added to the risk associated with other risk factors."[461]

Immune Activation of Coagulation (Hypercoagulation) treatment includes:

- Low dose heparin is typically started and titrated up to 5000 iu SQ bid (safer than aspirin). Heparin also binds inflammatory cytokines and is an immune modulator. Low dose heparin binds extracellular histones produced in sepsis and CIRS, blocking their cytotoxic effects, it blocks Babesia's entry into the red blood cell, and its immune-modulatory effect lowers inflammation and helps with herxheimer reactions, which are all separate benefits apart from heparin's anticoagulatory effects. In addition, it can artificially raise the level of free T3 and free T4.[462 463 464]
- Lumbrokinase 400,000 LU twice daily on an empty stomach. This directly activates TPA, degrades fibrin and works intravascular and in intracellular space, and reduces Lp(a)).
- Nattokinase 1000 FU twice daily on an empty stomach. This indirectly acts on TPA and degrades fibrin only in the intravascular space. You can get both in Fibrinix.
- Melatonin 20 mg per night is a much higher dose than usually given. It is shown to improve hypercoagulability in a dose-dependent manner.[465]
- BPC-157 500-1000 mcg orally twice daily. It breaks down fibrin and clots, treats hypercoagulation, reduces bleeding time in hypocoagulation and in heparin overdose (without affecting heparin effects), reduces mortality in heparin, warfarin, and aspirin overdose, and prevents heparin-induced thrombocytopenia.[466]
- The immune modulators LDN, TB4/TB4 frag, thymosin, thymogen/vilon (Thymogen Alpha-1), KPV, DSIP, Thymosin alpha 1, epitalon, and pinealon improve hypercoagulability through their immune-modulatory effects and their ability to stimulate melatonin levels.

The response to treatment can be dramatic; treatments that previously had no effect become effective, as the therapeutics, oxygen, and nutrients can now enter the cells much easier, and waste products can more readily be removed. Heparin, BPC-157, TB4 frag, KPV, and vascular enzymes are biofilm busters, and immune modulators. Heparin, BPC-157, TB4 frag, and KPV are significantly antimicrobial (heparin inhibits Babesia invasion of erythrocytes).[467] The newer anticoagulants and warfarin don't work very well for this type of hypercoagulation), though low molecular heparin is okay.

VIP

As discussed earlier, the CSSPC emphasizes that normalizing VIP levels is essential for helping patients fully recover. It must be given only after all the other parts of the CSSPC are successfully completed. The normal range for VIP is 23-63 pg/ml. VIP can be very beneficial in the short run, but it has a high rate of failure and can make someone chronically and physiologically worse and more difficult to treat in the long run. VIP will usually normalize with immune-modulatory treatment and lowering hypothalamic inflammation; effective therapies include LDN, TB4/TB4 frag, thymogen/vilon (Thymogen alpha-1), BPC-157, KPV, epitalon, pinealon, DSIP, AOD, growth hormone, and growth hormone secretagogues. Additionally, you don't have to wait until the other aspects of CIRS are successfully treated with the peptide therapy above, as is required with the current CIRS treatment algorithm; it can be done as initial therapy. As briefly discussed above, VIP has a dark side if given with TGF-beta or inflammation.

VIP stimulates Th17 and down-regulates NK cells in the presence of TGFb-1. One study found that the combination of VIP and TGFb-1 resulted in a thirtyfold increase in the T cell production of IL-17, resulting in a vicious cycle of autoimmunity and T cell exhaustion, which is precisely what you don't want for long-term resolution.[468] Pointing out this fact, the authors of one study state, "These results indicate that VIP plays an unanticipated permissive and/or proinflammatory role in propagating the inflammatory response in the CNS, a finding with potential therapeutic relevance in autoimmune neuroinflammatory diseases such as multiple sclerosis." Thus, enhancement of the relative contribution of VIP-VPAC1 axis signaling can skew the CD4 T cell response toward a Th17-rich proinflammatory type." [469]

VIP treatment substantially reduces the number of CD4 cells producing IL-2 and TNF-alpha and increases IL-10 and TGFb-1, all of which are a major driver of TCE.[470 471 472] An additional concern is that while the half-life of VIP is only two minutes, but the physiologic results, such as TCE are long-lived.[473] The problem is VIP is essentially transforming T cells into the dysfunctional immobilized state of TCE.[474 475] This short-term gain of reduced inflammation and symptom relief is associated with a longer-term worsening of the condition.

New cellular laboratory techniques show that T cell exhaustion (TCE) is a significant issue with many chronic illnesses, infections, and cancer. You typically see TCE with continued antigen exposure and/or inflammation, especially chronic infections and cancer. TCE is associated with progressive loss of effector functions of T cells (CD4 and CD8) and phenotypic and functional defects, sustained upregulation and co-expression of multiple inhibitory receptors, lack of availability of CD4 T cell help, increased levels of CD43, altered expression of key transcription factors, metabolic derangements, and failure to acquire antigen-independent memory and responsiveness, dysfunctional Th1 as indicated by low NK cell function, low IL-2 and low TNF-alpha in late stages, and elevated hTGFb and IL-10, with a high Th2/Th17.[476 477 478]

Earlier, we discussed the core dysfunction of CIRS being an elevated hTGFb, a Th1/Treg to Th2/Th17 shift, and a low NK cell function. It is no surprise that giving VIP in the presence of hTGFb is a bad idea. It will dramatically increase the potent proinflammatory cytokine responsible for most autoimmune diseases. In addition, if given with an elevated TGFbeta-1, VIP appears to induce a particular T cell phenotype of long-term immunosuppression called T cell exhaustion, which is associated with the inability to clear chronic infections and cancer with an increased risk of autoimmunity. The immune-modulatory peptides listed above will lower inflammation, normalize the abnormalTh1 to Th2/Th17 immune shift.TB4 active frag, KPV, and vilon are, in particular, ideal therapeutics for CIRS, as they directly address the core components of CIRS immune dysfunction and inflammation. They are potent inhibitors of TGFb and stimulate NK cell function, Th1 immunity, IL-2, and TNF-alpha, reversing T cell exhaustion. They can also be used to reverse those who have suffered from negative immunologic aspects of VIP.[479] [480] [481] With TCE being perhaps the core pathophysiology of CIRS, which leads to a vicious cycle of multi-system dysfunction, these peptides should be an initial first-line therapy for CIRS. Treatment can potentially prevent or reverse the subsequent abnormalities slowly treated over time with the CSSPC. Additional peptides are shown to protect the body from the damage caused by myco- and other enterotoxins, which can be given along with the immune-modulatory peptides discussed above, being a much better strategy than the CSSPC. Patients will not likely need VIP, but if there appears to be a need to use VIP, patients should be treated with these peptides before starting VIP. They can also be given concomitantly with VIP to help prevent VIP therapy's potential long-term adverse effects.

There are numerous clinical trials underway investigating ways to reverse TCE because it is a significant reason individuals cannot clear chronic infections and cancer and suffer from autoimmune disease and most of the inflammatory diseases of aging. The good news is that some of the new therapies introduced in this chapter are shown to be able to reverse TCE. While VIP can improve CIRS patients' symptoms for some time under the right conditions (i.e., low TGFb) by causing paralysis to parts of the immune system, I would be cautious in using VIP at any time for extended periods or in anyone with a chronic infection.[482] [483] [484]

Anti-Diuretic Hormone (ADH)

The old CIRS protocol recommends using DDAVP, an analog of ADH, which can be used. With immune-modulatory and directed therapy to reduce inflammation of the hypothalamus, hippocampus, and amygdala, ADH abnormalities will often significantly improve or resolve. Those who suffer from POTs usually respond well to such therapy This includes the use of oral, sublingual, or nasal

BPC-157, TB4 frag, thymogen/vilon (Thymogen alpha-1), LDN, oral Cerebrolysin (CerebroPep), delta sleep-inducing peptide (DSIP), epitalon or pinealon, or even better, a combination of the above from a doctor knowledgeable in the use of peptide and LDN therapy.

Testosterone and Other Hormones

For CIRS and many chronic illnesses and inflammatory conditions, including aging, all the hormones need to be evaluated with the understanding that, as discussed, the pineal-hypothalamic-pituitary-hormone axis is dysfunctional secondary to the immune and mitochondrial dysfunction seen in many chronic illnesses, which results in multiple hormonal deficiencies that are not detected by standard blood tests because 95% of endocrinologists and other doctors do not take into account the suppressed hormonal axis and just assume that it is healthy despite hundreds of studies to the contrary. For instance, such patients can have deficient tissue levels of thyroid throughout the body, but the standard measure of hypothyroidism, an elevated level of thyroid-stimulating hormone (TSH), doesn't happen because TSH secretion is suppressed, this results in a misdiagnosis of normal thyroid activity greater than 95% of the time.

Adhering to this oversimplistic view of thyroid function because it is simple is intellectually wrong and immoral, as it leaves so many patients misdiagnosed as euthyroid (normal thyroid) when their lives can be profoundly changed for pennies a day. In CIRS and with many chronic illnesses, doctors rely on a diagnosis based on TSH secretion from a suppressed and physiologically dysfunctional pineal-hypothalamus-pituitary axis to appropriately sense low tissue thyroid levels and then properly respond with the secretion of increased levels of TSH from the pituitary. Therefore, it is low, not high, which is the standard simplistic definition used by most endocrinologists and other doctors as the gold standard for diagnosis despite its glaring well-documented shortcomings and the hundreds or thousands of published peer-reviewed journal articles demonstrating such.[485] [486]

CSSPC/Shoemaker Protocol

This section will summarize the Shoemaker protocol and compare and contrast it with the HUPRTOC.

Step 1. Remove the Patient from the Exposure Source. This is a vital step in both protocols. If the patient is not removed from the source of mold (most often water-damaged buildings), the other steps will, at best, only provide limited symptom relief and, at worst, fail altogether. In some cases, mold exposure occurs in both the patient's home and place of work. In cases where water damage is not apparent in the home or workplace, testing by an accredited lab may be necessary. You can pay for expensive testing, but I have found that inexpensive plates can be purchased online, which after being placed around the house for an hour, then closed and left to sit for a few days per directions, can be sent in for identification. More sophisticated tests can be used, or a mold specialist could be enlisted. One that is worth considering is the Environmental Relative Mold Index (ERMI) test kit, which scientists at the Environmental Protection Agency originally developed. Current versions of the ERMI test use DNA testing to detect over 36 mold and other fungal species and provide rapid and accurate results. These tests are available from EMSL Analytics, Inc. (see their website for more information, including how to order). If mold is present, a mold remediation specialist should be utilized to repair the problem and assess the indoor air quality.

The adage "better safe than sorry" certainly applies to mold in your home. Therefore, it is highly advisable to regularly inspect indoor environments for mold, especially in homes and other buildings that have been subject to water leaks or further water damage. Examine basement walls and areas around sinks, bathtub and shower, washing machine, and dishwasher for visible mold. Touch these areas with your hands, feeling for moisture or cold spots, indicating hidden moisture.

Step 2. Use Binders to Lower the Circulating Toxic Burden. This is the primary, most vital, lengthy, and cumbersome step in the Shoemaker protocol. However, with the HUPRTOC, this step usually becomes unnecessary and is replaced with the LDN and peptide immune-modulatory and mycotoxin protection therapies discussed earlier. With such treatment, the body is protected from the toxic effects. It can naturally remove the toxins with improved immune function, reduced inflammation and cellular stress, suppressed Cell Danger Response, increased cellular energy and mitochondrial function, improved hormone levels and gastrointestinal function, rescued T cell exhaustion and elimination of immunosenescence, inhibited immune activation of coagulation with a renewed ability to suppress chronic infections, improved brain, and cognitive function, and a return to homeostasis. Also, it should be noted that like mycotoxins, thyroid hormones undergo enterohepatic circulation, so giving binders will also bind up and eliminate thyroid hormone, whether or not you are on supplemental thyroid replacement. Thus, thyroid levels should be overseen if on binders, and a knowledgeable doctor should consider judicious use of T3 replacement. Binders are so efficient at lowering thyroid levels we use them as first-line therapy to stabilize patients with hyperthyroidism, such as Grave's disease until we can treat the underlying cause.

Step 3. Eradicate MARCoNs: The replacement of low MSH with KPV and improvement in immune function from LDN and peptide therapy will almost always eradicate the MARCoNs. If not, a combination of nasal KPV, BPC-157, TB4 frag, and the antimicrobial peptide LL-37 will usually finish off any residual cases. Nasal ozone can also be effective.

Step 4. Correct Anti-Gliadin (AGA) Antibodies: It is easy and inexpensive to check for a hundred or more food sensitivities (IgG antibodies, not IgE, which is an allergy). If you test positive for a significant number of foods, that demonstrates that these large food proteins are getting absorbed and should not be. The combination of LDN, BPC-157, TB4 active frag, and KPV is the most effective therapy for gut inflammation and leaky gut, with TB4 active frag and KPV specifically targeting dysfunctional tight junctions. This will also help heal a leaky blood-brain barrier. The addition of oral IgG and a potent spore-based probiotic can also benefit, as can avoiding gluten and taking high dose digestive enzymes with betaine to improve stomach acid. It is a good idea to check for H-pylori and intestinal parasites.

Step 5. Correct Abnormal Androgens: This step should be called Correcting All the Hormones, which generally are low secondarily to the pineal-hypothalamic-pituitary-hormone axis, as discussed in this chapter. The thyroid is probably the most important and can reap the most significant benefit with proper treatment even if the TSH is normal. T3 is the treatment of choice (see review articles listed in this chapter). Also, consider growth hormone or growth hormone secretagogues, low dose cortisol, injectable testosterone, and the nonaromatizable androgen, nandrolone, which does not convert to estrogen or DHT is less androgenic, so it has fewer side effects than testosterone. You can adjust the ratio to keep the estrogen level optimal. Giving the pineal peptides pinealon and/ or epitalon will often repair this dysfunctional axis and bring the hormone levels back to normal levels except for the thyroid. It will improve thyroid levels, but there are additional thyroid transport problems into the cells in the periphery, so T3 should also be given. Fixing the immune system and the inflammation will usually fix the issue of excessive aromatase activity. Shoemaker recommends DHEA and HCG, which I do not because it will likely dramatically increase estrogen levels.

Step 6. Correct Antidiuretic Hormone (ADH) and Osmolality Problems: Shoemaker recommends that treatment with desmopressin (DDAVP) be a synthetic form of ADH. However, this is seldom needed, as this is corrected (along with POTS if present) with the therapy discussed in this section.

Step 7. Correct Matrix Metallopeptidase 9 (MMP-9). are an indication of chronic inflammation. To reduce MMP-9, Shoemaker recommends the omega-3 essential fatty acids and a no amylose diet. This is very difficult to maintain and usually doesn't have a significant effect. MMP-9 will come down with the therapies discussed in this section.

Step 8. Correct Low Vascular Endothelial Growth Factor (VEGF). The standard protocol was once erythropoietin (EPO) to increase VEGF, but that is no longer recommended due to the risk of side effects. Shoemaker recommends using omega-3 fatty acids and following a no amylose diet, as mentioned in the previous step. Again, this is unlikely to improve VEGF levels. However, several peptides are shown to be potent stimulants of VEGF, and activation and upregulation of VEGF receptors without the side effects of VIP, including TB4, TB4 active fragment (Ac-SDKP), and BPC-157 (modulates). TICD92.[487] [488] These peptides modulate the immunity beneficially, as opposed to VIP, and are shown to be extremely safe even at doses 1000 times the typical therapeutic doses. Vitamin D, melatonin, baicalin, and exercise also stimulate VEGF.

Step 9. Correct Elevated Levels of C3a: This is a marker of immune dysfunction. Shoemaker recommends using statin drugs in conjunction with Co-Enzyme Q-10 (Co-Q10). Statin drugs are toxic to the mitochondria, and the fact that mitochondrial dysfunction is a core abnormality in the overwhelming majority of CIRS patients, taking a statin doesn't make sense. This can result in muscle pain and weakness, fatigue, memory loss, diabetes, leptin resistance, neuropathy, neurologic issues, heart failure, rhabdomyolysis (muscle breakdown), and hormone abnormalities. All of which is not good for anyone, let alone a CIRS patient. The immune-modulatory therapy discussed earlier will lower the C3 and C4 levels.

Step 10. Correct Elevated Levels of C4a: This is a marker of immune dysfunction. In the past, Shoemaker recommended using the drug Procrit (erythropoietin) to correct C4 levels. However, since the FDA gave the drug a black box warning, he now recommends that patients and their physicians follow the rest of his protocol, including vasoactive intestinal peptide (VIP), having to wait until step 12 of the protocol. As discussed, immune dysfunction is the core abnormality in CIRS and is addressed very quickly with HUPRTOC, which will lower both C4a and C3a.

Step 11. Lowering Transforming Growth Factor Beta-1 (TGF-beta-1): TGF-beta-1 is a vital issue, if not the most critical issue, with CIRS, as discussed. This is addressed early in HUPRTOC. Shoemaker recommends using losartan, an angiotensin II receptor antagonist drug (brand name Cozaar), for 30 days. Since losartan's primary use is for treating hypertension, patients must be monitored to ensure their blood pressure levels do not fall too low. Early treatment that utilizes the peptides that lower TGFb, TB4 active frag, thymogen/vilon (thymogen Alpha 1), and KPV will usually significantly lower hTGFb in days or weeks instead of months or years, as is the case when utilizing the CSSPC.

Step 12. Use Vasoactive Intestinal Peptide (VIP) to Restore Immune Balance and Regulation. As stated previously, addressing immune dysfunction is the cornerstone of successful treatment of CIRS and is handled very early with the HUPRTOC instead of waiting until the last step, which is the CSSPC. Unfortunately, many people never make it to this step because they continue to suffer from significant inflammation even though this step is considered to be "the pinnacle of the pyramid." The CSSCP makes VIP seem like the nirvana that you have to reach, but the truth is that some people find symptomatic relief with it as long as there is no inflammation. However, especially if there is a significant amount of hTGFb, it also makes things worse. It is undoubtedly a mixed bag that provides some beneficial effects, but at the same time, potentially makes a full recovery much less likely. The problems associated with using VIP become abundantly clear with a careful examination of its physiologic effects. While it can improve the situation for some time, just looking at its not-so-positive effects, one should be concerned about its routine or long-term use in these multi-system patients. I have found that many patients who are doing reasonably well and attribute their success to VIP are usually very likely to relapse, sometimes worse than before, remain sensitive to mold, or don't feel quite as good as they convince themselves they do.

New Therapy for Mold Illness/CIRS-WPD

The latest research demonstrates that chronic exposure to a toxic mold infection or mycotoxins causes TCE and immunosenescence with a Th1/Treg to Th2/Th17 immune shift with additional direct suppression of NK cell, thymic and mitochondrial function, setting off a deep vicious cycle of multi-system illness. Many CIRS patients have preexisting T cell exhaustion due to stress, chronic Lyme or other infection, autoimmune disease or other chronic illness, other toxic exposures, etc. This makes such patients much more prone to established mold, fungus, viral, bacterial, and parasitic infections because their immune system is too weak to fight the infection and unable to detoxify the mycotoxins. This makes them much more likely to develop severe sensitivities and excessive mast cell activation with excessive production of reactive oxygen species (ROS) and inflammation with a mold exposure that wouldn't bother a healthy person. This further contributes to a vicious cycle of progressive illness and deterioration rather than reverting to a repair and rejuvenation mode.

The current standard of care protocol for CIRS hopes to ultimately fix the immune system via a lengthy 3 phase (12 steps) process that tries to treat the various associated biomarkers that all have their origin in mycotoxin-induced T cell exhaustion rather than directly treating the immune dysfunction, which then corrects the resultant abnormalities. Patients can get better much faster by addressing the core abnormality early in the treatment protocol. With the current CIRS protocol, doctors are taught to address each dysfunction caused by T cell exhaustion. Only then should they use a weak immune-modulating peptide, VIP, to try and finally normalize the immune system and hopefully see significant symptomatic improvement. Doctors with substantial knowledge of specific immune-modulating peptides and other immune-modulating therapies, such as LDN, peptides (including immune-modulating, anti-inflammatory, pineal-pituitary-hypothalamic-hormone axis normalizing (including thyroid, adrenal, estrogen, progesterone, testosterone, MSH, melatonin, ADH, growth hormone, oxytocin, neurotransmitters, secondary messengers, and gastrointestinal), mitochondria, endorphin, brain nootropics, sleep inducers, mood and pain center modulators, antimicrobial, and much more), ozone and other IV therapies, ozone plasmapheresis, stem cells, and exosomes, will usually understand how targeting the core abnormality, T cell exhaustion, will be much more likely for CIRS patients to see improvement with therapy. They will often see CIRS patients get better in weeks or months, not months to years, as with the current CIRS protocol.

Knowing this, you might ask, "Why not give back the suboptimal thymic and other peptides that occur with age and cause or contribute to almost all of the diseases of aging?" Thankfully, the concept of peptide and small molecule supplementation and optimization to reverse this immunosenescence is catching on. It had always been assumed to be an inevitable part of aging with resultant disease and degeneration. The nice thing is that supplementation with thymic peptides is extremely safe, with studies unable to find a toxic dose, even when 1000 times the average therapeutic amount. This is unheard of and in contrast to the small therapeutic window typical of medications. Water would be lethal at such dosing extremes.

As with other poorly understood conditions, such as chronic fatigue syndrome (CFS) and fibromyalgia (FM), mold illness/CIRS-WDB is frequently ignored or misdiagnosed, leaving the vast majority of patients who suffer from this condition helpless to find effective resolutions for their problems.

It is well established that molds and mycotoxins negatively impact the immune system because of their immunotoxic and cytotoxic effects. Dr. Shoemaker has provided excellent service for the many patients suffering from CIRS and mold-related illnesses. He has done a tremendous amount of research to prove (to those who will listen) that this is a significant problem. CIRS and mold-related illnesses will, in my opinion, likely skyrocket due to the increasing exposure to immunosuppressing environmental substances combined with the expansion of 5G, which will significantly stimulate the growth and toxicity of the majority of toxic molds.

I hope you found this chapter helpful on your road to recovery from CIRS, or if you are a healthcare practitioner, I hope it helps you understand the pathophysiology of CIRS better and that it gives you additional practical tools to combat this multi-system illness and other illnesses. Linda Elsegood and all the volunteers and doctors with the LDN Research Society have a passion for learning, teaching, and helping those with complex, poorly treated illnesses. They are here for you. I hope you found this chapter interesting or at least helpful, that it changed the way you look at CIRS and other inflammatory illnesses, and that you derived some benefit from your time spent reading this book.

SEVEN

Ophthalmic Conditions

SEBASTIAN DENISON, BSc. (PHARM), RPh

Every few weeks it seems another paper or case study is published regarding the success of low dose naltrexone. This chapter focuses on its ophthalmologic uses, based upon the amazing research and clinical work undertaken by many others. As a compounding clinical pharmacist who has worked with naltrexone and seen its use and the science surrounding it grow for more than twenty years, I have been asked to compile this information and will do my best to make it applicable for both scientists and patients.

As a 2019 world report on vision from the World Health Organization attests:

> Globally, at least 2.2 billion people have a vision impairment or blindness, of whom at least 1 billion have a vision impairment that could have been prevented or has yet to be addressed. Tens of millions have a severe vision impairment and could benefit from rehabilitation which they are not currently receiving. The burden of eye conditions and vision impairment is not borne equally: it is often far greater in low- and middle-income countries, among older people and in women, and in rural and disadvantaged communities.[489]

Although sight is one of the most depended upon senses in the animal kingdom, preserving sight is not such an easy task. This chapter will explore the anatomy and immunology of the eye, a selection of ophthalmologic disease states, and some of the common underlying mechanisms that cause these diseases. Finally, we will explore how naltrexone may be of benefit for patients.

Anatomy of the Eye

The eye is arguably the second most complex structure in the body, second only to the brain. Understanding its structure and function is necessary to also understanding the difficulties in treatment. This overview is discussed with a patient in mind.

There are seven main components that serve to create vision in the human eye: the cornea, iris, pupil, aqueous humor, lens, vitreous humor, retina, and optic nerve. For a visual representation I would suggest searching for an image from a reputable source online with the search parameters "HUMAN EYE STRUCTURE" and select image. There is much more detail to the structure, but for the purposes of this chapter we may not go into as much detail.

When light reflects off an object it enters the eye through the cornea. The cornea's main functions are primarily to focus that light into the pupil through to the lens, and to protect the eye. The cornea is not vascularized, meaning it does not contain the same blood vessels as other tissues in the body, as the blood and the network of blood vessels would interrupt the passage of light through it. This is an important detail that carries through much of the structure of the eye, as lack of vascularization also limits normal immune function.

The area between the cornea and the pupil is filled with the aqueous humor. The aqueous humor is produced and replenished by the ciliary bodies and provides support and nutrients behind the cornea. The aqueous humor prevents drying of the cornea, provides oxygen and nutrients to the cornea, and washes away both debris and invading pathogens.

The light then passes through the pupil (aka the dark middle spot), which focuses the light toward the lens. The pupil is controlled by the iris and ciliary body, which serve to limit the amount of light coming into the eye. The light then passes through the lens, which focuses the light onto the retina, a thin film of tissue on the back of the eye. The retina is made up of thousands of photoreceptors called rods and cones. Rods and cones receive light in different ways. Rods tend to need much less light; they help you see at night and are also responsible for detecting movement. Cones are much more concentrated at the back of the eye (called the macula, which contains the fovea), and use much more light than rods, and are responsible for seeing both color and detail. Different animal species have differing amounts of rods and cones, though mammals and many other animal species share the overall structure of the eye and macula with only minor differences. These rods and cones then convert light into electrical impulses that travel along the optic nerve to the brain.

The interior of the eye is filled with vitreous humor, which although it is more gel-like than aqueous humor and not continuously replenished, serves a similar function to the interior of the eye, for both nutrient and oxygen delivery. Its other main purpose is to allow the light to pass from the lens to the retina as clearly as possible and maintain proper eye volume and shape.[490] Other parts of the anatomy of the eye not directly related to sight but to the function of the eye are the conjunctiva, sclera, and choroid. The conjunctiva covers the sclera (i.e., the white of the eye) and surrounds the eye except for the cornea, and is responsible for the immune barrier for eye, producing mucous and secreting tears.[491] The choroid is another layer of tissue between the retina and the sclera. This layer is very highly vascularized and brings blood and nutrients to the sclera and retina. The combination of these three tissues is called the uvea and is the main barrier, known as the blood-ocular barrier, between the rest of the body and the interior of the eye.

All parts of the eye are both highly specialized and unique in structure and must be maintained in perfect balance. When they are not, we notice loss of function in our vision.

Immune System in the Eye

Understanding the immune system specific to the eye not only aids understanding of disease and treatment but also the difficulty in delivery of medications. The immune system in the eye is equally complex but also has its own discrete intricacies and revolves around the structures described in the previous section. It overlaps with the immune system in the body but also has discrete properties that make it highly specialized and protective of the eye and is also known as ocular immune privilege.[492] Our ocular immune privilege relies on the surrounding tissue and the ability of immune cells to pass into specific areas of the eye. The passage of anything found in the blood to the eye is tightly regulated by the blood-ocular barrier and prevents a majority of cellular components from entering into the actual eye. This divides the eye immune function into two specific areas we can focus on: both the ocular surface (the exterior and surrounding tissue of the eye) and the ocular tissue and structure of the interior of the eye.

This section is meant to provide an overview, discussing specific details that pertain to the use of naltrexone. There are of course physical barriers to the eye that prevent injury, such as the eyelids and surrounding bone, but the main barriers are the external facing tissues, the conjunctiva, sclera, and cornea. Highly vascularized (containing lots of blood vessels) tissue surrounding the eye serves to provide not only nutrients but the full activity of the immune system to these tissues. The conjunctiva is a mucous-like membrane that surrounds the eye, along with the sclera, the retina and the optic nerve, which have all of the same immune cell function seen throughout the rest of the human body.

Normal immune function activity involves the body's response to microbes (living organisms) that may or may not be foreign, turning pathogenic (causing disease) due to entry into areas not normally occupied by microbes. There is an innate system (non-specific) and an adaptive system (specific). An innate response is responsible for the initiation of an inflammatory response, as well as the recruitment of other immune cells for both the initial attack on the invading pathogens, as well as the appropriate signaling for a pathogen-specific response. These pathogen-associated molecules (called pathogen-associated immunostimulants) stimulate two types of innate immune responses—inflammatory responses and phagocytosis (engulfing and digesting) by cells such as neutrophils and macrophages. These responses can occur quickly, even if the host has never been previously exposed to a particular pathogen. This can include histamine release, cytokine release, and the attachment of antibodies to the foreign microbes.

Macrophages reside in tissues throughout the body and are especially abundant in areas where infections are likely to arise, including the lungs, eyes, and gut. They are also present in large numbers in connective tissues, as well as the liver and spleen. Leukocytes such as neutrophils, eosinophils, and basophils are rapidly recruited to sites of infection both by activated macrophages and, in some cases, by pathogens. Natural killer cells (NK cells) are present throughout the body and have both cytotoxicity (killing) and cytokine-producing (signaling) functions.[493]

All these different immune cells and other cellular surface tissues have a specific receptor family that recognizes the pathogenic nature of the invading microbe, known as toll-like receptors (TLRs). TLR activation on any of the innate immune cells stimulates the expression of molecules that both initiate an inflammatory response and help induce adaptive immune responses. TLRs are abundant on the surface of macrophages and neutrophils, as well as on the epithelial cells throughout the different tissues in the body.[494]

Unlike innate immune responses, adaptive responses are pathogen-specific. Pathogenic material or antigens, such as the broken-down bacterial cell wall components, allow for recruitment and activation of a different arm of the immune system responsible for previous encounters with the invading microbe. The function of adaptive immune responses is to destroy specific invading pathogens. Since these responses are very destructive, it is crucial that they be made only in response to molecules that are foreign to the host and not to the molecules of the host itself. The ability to distinguish foreign pathogens from the self is a fundamental feature of the adaptive immune system; failure of this feature is what is considered an autoimmune disorder.

Adaptive immune responses are carried out by white blood cells called lymphocytes. There are two broad classes of such responses: antibody responses and cell-mediated immune responses. There are also two different classes of lymphocytes, called B cells and T cells. B cells are activated to secrete antibodies, which are proteins called immunoglobulins. B cells make antibodies to specific pathogenic material such as bacterial or viral structures, and unfortunately can also make antibodies to the body's own normal tissue. T-cells, such as CD 4+ helper T-cells and CD 8+ cytotoxic T-cells, react directly against a foreign antigen that is presented to them on the surface of a host cell. The same type of signaling molecules, cytokines, are produced with different versions creating a symphony of cellular function. Through a tightly controlled, cytokine-signaling cascade, this can either lead to a greater recruitment and amplification signal, or can direct a continued pathogenic destructive action.[495]

These immune responses are what protects the tissue surrounding the eye itself, with that barrier between the eye highly protected by the uvea interface. The same interface we see between the exterior of the eye and the interior of the eye allows for the transfer of nutrients and immune components and white blood cells, predominantly neutrophils. The immune privilege of the eye is also the main reason that use of oral and topical medications for eye disorders is extremely complex, why the eye is so dependent on the innate system for protection, and why recognizing inflammation early is important to eye health.[496]

As described earlier, the cornea's main function in addition to focusing incoming light is to protect the eye from direct contact with harmful debris and microbes. The cornea covers the pupil and iris directly, and is made up of a thin, flexible, strong collagen matrix that provides the light-focusing structure; it also has distinct cellular components that protect the rest of the eye.[497] The structure of the cornea is so precise that any dysfunction—including inflammation, damage, or excessive growth—leads to a negative impact on vision. Since the cornea is not vascularized, it has its own immune components in the form of tears, the corneal epithelium, keratocytes, and polymorphonuclear cells. All of these have specialized immune functions and contain specialized signaling products, such as immunoglobulins and cytokines.[498] Tears prevent drying of the exterior of the cornea and also support the nourishment of the eye. In addition, tears flush away foreign particles from the surface. Tears are supplied by the lacrimal glands and have discrete immunological components that may also be a factor in the activation of the innate system—proteins that attach to pathogens such as immunoglobulin-A (IgA) or immunoglobulin-G (IgG), which attach to invading microbes, and proteins that degrade bacterial cell walls, such as beta-lysin.[499] [500] Corneal epithelial cells also participate in protecting the ocular surface by secreting cytokines to activate immune defenses to protect against microbial invasion. Most commonly, cytokine interleukin (IL)-1 is released when the cell membrane is ruptured by infectious agents or trauma. IL-1 and the associated IL-receptor are primarily responsible for the initiation of the innate inflammation response to signal that there is a problem in the tissue.[501] IL-1 production must be tightly controlled during both injury and infection as it is a key initiator and mediator of inflammation; with chronic production and release of IL-1 the inflammatory cascade is continued and can lead to dysfunctional immune response, usually caused by natural killer cells, and both CD+4 and CD8+ cellular-mediated tissue destruction. This then leads to microbial invasion, neovascularization, and the subsequent destruction of cornea structure.[502] [503] [504] [505] [506]

The ability to secrete the cytokine IL-1 is also shared by keratocytes, another corneal derived immune cell. This cell type remains quiet or inactive until damage such as a scratch or injury, then springs into action. Keratocytes also have a defensive capacity during microbial invasion. Under the influence of IL-1 and tumor necrosis factor (TNF)-α, keratocytes synthesize both IL-1 and cytokine interleukin 6 (Il-6). IL-6 interacts synergistically with IL-1 and TNF-α to amplify and specify immune responses, but when uncontrolled can also be a factor in uncontrolled inflammation, tissue destruction, and pain.[507] [508] The polymorphonuclear leukocytes (neutrophils, eosinophils, and basophils) are a type of white blood cell and the main effectors of the innate immune system, initiating inflammation in response to foreign microbe invasion, but again, overactivation may lead to tissue destruction and structure changes that lead to vision degradation or loss. There is also a subset of specialized immune cells, called Langerhans cells. These come in contact with invading pathogens, engulf them, migrate out of the eye and through the lymphatic system to your lymph nodes, and present the pathogenic-antigen material for further adaptive immune activation and specific response. Langerhans cell migration to the lymph nodes results in the adaptive antibody-mediated response that changes the immune cell access. This cascade then allows change in the blood-ocular barrier and the infiltration of macrophages and leukocytes into the interior of the eye. This can lead to significant changes as well as tissue destruction if improperly controlled.[509]

The rest of the interior of the eye relies primarily on the same inflammatory cascades with similar cells found throughout the eye. The same TLRs are present on the cellular surface of the in the ciliary body, iris, and retina.[510] [511] To summarize, both in the body and directly in the eye, the inflammatory response is a coordinated, directed response to pathogens and follows the same series of steps, starting with cell surface pattern receptors (for example the TLR or IL receptor recognizing pathogenic material), followed by the activation of inflammatory pathways such as the production of IL-1, IL-6, IL-17 and TNF- α, which are then released to both recruit and amplify the signal that a greater immune response is needed. This normal innate and adaptive function of the immune system due to pathogens or microbes, when controlled, not only prevents and fights infection, but also clears cells that are not healthy, via initiating cellular apoptosis (cell death) and direct cytotoxic effects on cells that are becoming cancerous. When the immune system becomes dysfunctional, in either direction (either too little or too great a response), people become sick. The inability to fight infections or clear cancers are instances of low function, but too much inflammation or cellular destruction result in chronic diseases or autoimmune disorders.

Infections, Injury, Insult, and Inflammation

The average person touches their eyes upwards of fifty times a day. Everything we touch, we then transfer to what we touch next. This is known as Locard's exchange principle, the basis for forensic sciences and also the reason we introduce so many irritants and pathogens into our own eyes.[512] Ambient air circulation and wind, liquid splashes, solid material, and accidental introduction of irritants into our eyes is common and normal, yet these can all become a threat if not for our immune system and its ability to resolve problems quickly.

It is easy to tell when you have an irritant or microbial contaminant in your eye as you may experience blurry vision, lots of discharge in the corners of the eye, red discoloration in the eye. Tear production can be excessive or decreased, and irritation for many people includes the sensation of grit or sand in the eye. There is usually swelling and in some cases pain. Very common mild or superficial causes like an allergic reaction or minor infection (conjunctivitis, or pink eye) are something many people are familiar with. More serious issues involve the need for specialists.

The underlying mechanism behind these symptoms is the immune system's innate response as described in the previous section. In response to something as simple as allergens or dust, excess tears and redness are considered normal, as cytokines are produced to be on guard for invading microbes. Without this primary response, you would not see a protective response, allowing microbes to create a toehold infection. Once established, a minor infection could quickly turn into a vision-altering event, and even threaten vision loss. The same inflammatory reaction takes place when injury or insult occurs. A scratch of the cornea or an abrasion of the sclera have a similar inflammatory cascade that helps prevent an infection and also sets in motion a healing cascade that ensures repair of the damaged tissue.[513] [514] This same inflammatory response can also occur due to any type of surgery to repair damaged ocular tissue, such as cataract surgery, retinal damage, or laser eye surgery. The same inflammatory mechanisms that we see in the response to allergens and microbes are also initiated by tissue damage, but again mediated by cells in the eye.[515] [516]

Normally, allergies, superficial injury, and infections can be treated with anti-inflammatories, antihistamines, and antibiotics that control the inflammation, but after injury or surgery, extreme care must be taken to prevent infection as well as to prevent further damage due to an uncontrolled inflammatory process. Usually after surgery there are distinct combination antimicrobial/anti-inflammatory medications with consistent monitoring to catch when problems occur.

In many cases, eye inflammation can occur with a direct irritant or microbial infection, which if left undiagnosed or untreated leads to damage. One of the most common forms of inflammation in the eye is uveitis, a group of disorders of the uvea. The clinical presentation is noted as inflammation in the middle layer of the eye, very red and potentially painful, with the usual cause being infection, injury, inflammatory disease, or a distinct non-ocular autoimmune disorder. In all of these cases controlling inflammation to prevent further damage is the primary effort of treatment, along with appropriate identification of cause.[517] There are multiple other diseases of the eye that relate to uncontrolled inflammatory damage. Depending on the level of inflammation and duration, diseases like keratitis and age-related macular degeneration can be linked to dysfunctional chronic inflammatory signaling.[518] [519] Keratitis, if left untreated, can become a vision-threatening disease, with causes from bacterial, viral or fungal infection, or injury. When the corneal epithelium tissue becomes damaged from an infection this can lead to inflammation of the layers of the cornea, or keratitis. If the infection is in the back or posterior of the eye, complications from that infection cause inflammation and swelling in the retinal area, again threatening vision; this is known as endophthalmitis. Macular degeneration is when the retina is damaged and starts to thin, which leads to blurry vision and eventually full loss of vision. There are two types, dry and wet, with dry being most common and slowly progressive, while wet is rapid and usually accompanied by new blood vessels growing on the retina.[520]

These amongst other eye disorders are all considered inflammatory mediated, which means preventing chronic inflammation will prevent or slow the progress of these vision- threatening conditions. To prevent progression from acute inflammation to persistent, chronic inflammation, the inflammatory response needs to be altered to prevent tissue damage and to change the immune system recruitment of immune cells to the area. What many have found, however, is that the same cascade repeats itself. We start to notice the same pattern emerging. IL-1 both types, IL-2, IL-4, IL-6, IL-8 IL-12, IL-17, TNF-α, IFN-γ, TGF-β1, and TGF-β2 are all examples of the primary cytokines of inflammation and tissue damage in other chronic disease progression.[521] Inflammation is also a primary cause of autoimmune diseases. In practice we see many of the same inflammatory cytokines present in most patients with autoimmune disorders for whom, when overlapping the disease underpinnings, we can start looking at similar treatments and options.[522] [523]

We have known for a while that the major autoimmune diseases, including rheumatoid arthritis, psoriasis, lupus, multiple sclerosis, and irritable bowel syndrome, all share the same underlying immune dysfunction, similar clinical presentation, and the same response to therapeutic interventions: "In each of these diseases, chronic and often intermittent inflammation contributes over time to the destruction of target organs that house inciting antigens or are the sites of immune-complex deposition."[524]

What we are also noticing is that the same signaling pathway that is responsible for activation is also responsible for the chronic over-activation signaling. The same TLR family that is the critical link between the innate and the adaptive immune responses is now considered the linchpin in developing these chronic inflammatory pathways, with continuous activation or dysregulation of TLR signaling.[525] With the recent understanding of the link between these receptors and disease, more research has been conducted and found the same receptors are uniquely present and responsible for the same chronic inflammation in the eye. For example, the TLRs are present in uveitis, age-related macular degeneration (both dry and wet types), keratitis, and dry eye.[526] [527] [528] [529] [530] [531] [532] The same TLR family also mediates the overlapping chronic inflammation and destruction of the lacrimal glands (tear production) either as a secondary effect of autoimmune disorders or as a distinct Sjogren's syndrome.[533] Chronic dry eye and Sjogren's syndrome result in reduced tear production; since tears are required to wash away debris or microbes, their reduction can be a direct cause of increased infection of the eye. This infection once established, then causes an adaptive response that has its own complications.[534] [535] But also, and very importantly, these same receptors (TLR) that cause so many problems may be a target of therapeutic intervention.[536]

What we do now

The standard of care developed for the treatment of inflammation in the eye is similar to almost every other inflammatory or autoimmune condition: corticosteroid eye drops (such as prednisolone) for rapid decrease in inflammation, and non-steroidal anti-inflammatory eye drops (such as diclofenac). But if these do not control inflammation we may step to a different option.[537] [538] Clinically, we are now seeing the move to include a new class of medications called "biologics" for the treatment of uveitis, neurotrophic keratopathy, Graves' disease, and age-related macular degeneration.[539] [540] But this is where it gets interesting— where we observe overlap in both disease progression from immune system dysfunction and the treatment standard of care, we can use the same overlap for new options for additional care. The same cytokines and TLR dysfunction are present in not only autoimmune disorders but also in many chronic disease states, such as cardiovascular disease, osteoarthritis, and Alzheimer's, and are also being researched for their role in cancer initiation and progression. We can use the same research and apply to the ocular disease states in the same way.[541]

In this way the eyes become a part of diagnosis in patients and may be an early warning system for patients not yet diagnosed with an autoimmune disorder. Uvetis and dry eye are actually considered a comorbidity with multiple rheumatoid diseases and are usually treated by an ophthalmologist and a rheumatologist.[542] [543] [544] As we are now seeing cardiovascular consults and dermatology, if we examine the eyes, in many cases they open a window into the underlying immune system. In fact, new standards of practice indicate that common eye exams can indicate or uncover potentially life-threatening illnesses. The same underlying pathophysiological changes we discover in the eye will be present in the rest of the patient.[545]

The Role of Low Dose Naltrexone

Everything I have discussed so far in this chapter is related to humans, but much what concerns us—such as the structure and function of our eyes, as well as our immune systems—applies to all mammals.[546] Our immune system is so highly conserved amongst vertebrates that we can use animal models very effectively to predict how human immune responses will occur. With respect to the TLR family, only the mouse has any appreciable differences (mainly due to their rapid regeneration, they have two extra TLRs not found in humans).[547] Some of the studies that are discussed in this chapter are done in animal models, but it is imperative that this information not be dismissed as inapplicable, as this is the normal progression of understanding, with potential practical application to human health and disease.

Naltrexone is an amazing drug molecule with a lot of potential with regard to underlying mechanisms that we have discussed thus far in this chapter. Naltrexone was originally considered an opioid receptor antagonist drug that directly blocked opioids from interacting with the opioid receptor. This was used to treat people with accidental opioid overdose, but it was discovered later that it also interacted with another family of receptors.[548] It was found that the molecule interacted in the TLR 4 receptor, the TLR 9 receptor, *and* in the opioid growth factor receptor axis (OGFr axis).[549 550 551 552]

Tissue growth (proliferation) can be both positive and negative, but again given the functionality of the eye, must be tightly controlled and discrete; we do not want excessive structural blood vessel growth due to the negative impact on vision or the inability of the eye to regenerate healthy structure. Any time we observe that abnormal growth of tissue is occurring in the eye, it is accompanied by vision changes. When chronically and excessively activated, the same immune system receptors (TLRs) that are responsible for that initiation cascade of inflammation and thus the healing lead to excessive growth, or abnormal tissue growth.[553] As mentioned earlier, excessive chronic inflammation can cause direct damage to tissue beds (for example, retinal damage (macular degeneration)) but when it crosses a threshold of damage, we then notice a change in blood vessels in the retina. This chronic inflammation and ongoing damage induces an excessive growth of new, abnormal blood vessel on the retina. These blood vessels unfortunately alter the ocular barrier and end up "leaking" excess fluid into the eye.

This is where things get interesting: it's not only the immune system inflammatory response that affects tissue growth. This normal healing cascade works in conjunction with another receptor and signaling system to control cell growth, called the opioid growth factor axis, made up of the receptor and the opioid growth factor signal molecule. The opioid growth factor (also known as (Met-5)-enkephalin) has many functions, including pain response, GI function, and regulation of tissue growth, and is one of the originally discovered opioid peptides.[554] In this specific discussion we want to focus on its "negative" or inhibitory effect on tissue growth, meaning it prevents an overgrowth or hypertrophy of tissue when it is normally produced. When it becomes unbalanced (too much or too little of the OGF is produced), it causes either too much growth, or disorganized growth, or it inhibits normal regrowth or repair. It has to maintain this delicate balance of enough activity to prevent uncontrolled disorganized growth, but still allow healing. When a patient has other complications such diabetes or immune system dysfunction, this system becomes very unbalanced. In the case of diabetes, poor wound healing, disorganized healing, and tissue degradation occur.[555] In the case of immune dysfunction or constant inflammation, hyperproliferative growth can occur, such as hypertrophic scars, contracture scars, and finally cancer and metastasis.[556] This system, first discovered and originally discussed in 1975, is slowly becoming better understood and appreciated. Dr. Zagon and his team should be lauded for their continued discovery and understanding of the OGF-OGFr system and its substantial effects on tissue growth and regulation, but also, some of the more interesting and related information pertaining to the role of naltrexone in this same system. In the team's earlier papers, they found that the OGF-OGFr axis "plays a role in cell proliferation and tissue organization during development, cancer, cellular renewal, wound healing, and angiogenesis."[557] Not long after, the team realized an amazing discovery: naltrexone blocked the same OGFr. This was a stunning development with respect to the potential of naltrexone for everything from wound healing to anti-proliferative effect for cancer treatments.[558] [559] [560] As they unlocked the many applications, Dr. Zagon and his team stumbled upon a twofold effect with respect to the OGFr axis in the eye. It could alter the healing response in the cornea, making it faster, but also improve the structure of the repair.[561] The ability to alter healing and to optimize its effect, in such delicate and functionally important tissue, is an incredibly important and profound therapeutic intervention.[562]

But LDN's true value in the majority of the patients is in its duality of mechanism and function in both of these systems when used for optimization: the direct action on the TLR function induction of inflammation, and its ability to modulate organized growth of healthy tissue. If we can control or modulate both inflammation and growth, we prevent direct damage to tissue, and we retain best possible function of the tissue. In this regard we can potentially offset much of the progression of the most common diseases of the eye, while maintaining vision.

I understand this is a very bold claim, but this is borne out by experiments in many different studies. For example, one paper showed a reduction of inflammatory cytokines with the use of oral low dose naltrexone in ten weeks, "We found that LDN was associated with reduced plasma concentrations of interleukin (IL)-1, IL-1Ra, IL-2, IL-4, IL-5, IL-6, IL-10, IL-12p40, IL-12p70, IL-15, IL-17A, IL-27, interferon (IFN), transforming growth factor. TGF-β, tumour-necrosis factor TNFα , and granulocyte-colony stimulating factor (G-CSF)."[563] These same cytokines are associated not only with autoimmune disorders, but in each of the most common diseases in the eye.[564] This has been widely recognized and pursued by researchers for over a decade now with the understanding that the initial contact through TLR will mitigate much of the damage in ocular diseases due to inflammation, with the overall decrease in the same inflammatory cytokines.[565] It could have a positive impact on everything from allergic conjunctivitis all the way through to dry eye and prevent inflammatory-mediated tissue damage and tissue growth abnormalities.[566] We start to see the OGFr axis effect not only through the TLR mechanism but also in the structural repair and controlled growth of the tissue from all of Dr. Zagon and his team's research.[567]

Of note as a compounding pharmacist, naltrexone is well-absorbed and water soluble, therefore easily passable through the blood-ocular barrier in the same fashion we see it pass the blood-brain barrier. All of the preceding papers are looking for molecules to affect these systems independently and we already have that molecule. We can control inflammation through the TLR system and modulate inflammation and control an immune response to an optimum level. By controlling this process, we may prevent further tissue damage, therefore preventing loss of function. In this process we also prevent any healing cascade dysfunction, whether an inability to heal or a hyper-proliferative tissue response. In all of these negative scenarios, vision is threatened, but with the addition of naltrexone we can restore and optimized immune and repair system. So, the big questions are is it safe and does it work?

Multiple papers have been generated with respect to safety and tolerability of naltrexone, mainly with respect to oral dosing in both adult and pediatric patients. In one large retrospective meta-analysis, oral LDN was shown to be safe with minimal side effects, most commonly, sleep disturbances and vivid dreams, which were the exact same noted side effects from the previous paper.[568] For direct topical application in the eye, another paper explored these same parameters and found it resulted in minimal side effects.[569]

This safety research has opened the door to so many treatments for a number of reasons; what are the diseases of the eye that are immune mediated with structural changes that negatively affect vision? The number of these diseases seems to be endless, likewise the possibilities for safe intervention. And in many patients with other systemic diseases that have the same mechanisms, we are seeing case studies being published showing promise, so what is happening for this area? Dr. Zagon, Dr. McLaughlin, and Dr. Sassani have found recently that both dry eye and corneal sensitivity were resolved with naltrexone eye drops.[570] What we have since seen clinically is an expansion of topical use. We are seeing more use and therefore more case studies undertaken with investigations of macular degeneration (chronic inflammation-mediated) to uveitis, dry eye, to corneal repair and post-surgical repair.[571] [572]

Oral dosing for eye disorders is still an option for a number of reasons. If we return to the previous discussion that many systemic issues present in the eye in the form of uveitis, it lends itself to the resolution of systemic issues that would then resolve the clinical manifestation of inflammation in the eye. In many cases of autoimmune disorders that directly respond to oral LDN, but in this paper, it demonstrates that oral LDN may have benefit in patients that have Sjogren's syndrome.[573] In one case study, multiple patients with a rare neuropathic pain in the cornea had their pain resolved with oral LDN, which was also found to be safe and well-tolerated.[574] The more we discover about LDN, the more applications we find. If we look at one recent paper discussing the extremely complex and difficult ocular fibrosis-type diseases, they all have a similar theme of underlying cause and progression, hyper-inflammatory response mediated by a dysfunctional innate immune system, with the following tissue destruction and complications threatening sight.[575] If we apply what we know with how naltrexone works, combined with an appropriately compounded, well-tolerated dosage form, how much can we achieve?

As pharmacists, we understand not only the drugs, but the delivery of those drugs to patients. I have previously mentioned many of the difficulties in administering medications and the blood-ocular barrier, but we also have to understand the patient preference. The most common and preferred route of administration of eye care is a topical drop or ointment; with improved patient compliance and ease of administration a topical formulation would be the choice for most of this patient group.[576] Unfortunately, there are many factors that need to be considered with making any eye preparation, including drug solubility, preservative compatibility, concentration, etc. There is no commercial preparation of naltrexone for eye administration, and probably not one on the horizon, as patent protection would be limited for commercial purposes, therefore a large-scale commercial manufacturing process may not be financially viable. This means it can only be obtained from a specialized compounding pharmacy that is familiar with not only the appropriate clinical intention of therapy but also the ability to compound the medication according to the correct regulatory standards of that specific site. The second big hurdle is that eye drops must be made in a sterile facility. In most countries, any compounded product designed for administration to the eye must be sterile due to the potential for harm to sight if the eye is infected. In the United States, compounding of eye drops falls under USP <797>, in Canada the NAPRA Model Standards for the compounding of Sterile Preparations, in the UK the equivalent MHRA standards, and in Australia the equivalent Pharmacy Board-compounding medicines guidelines.[577] [578] [579] [580] These requirements are much more stringent than the compounding of non-sterile compounds, therefore there are fewer pharmacies capable of compounding a sterile eye drop or ointment. Ophthalmic ointments can also be prepared with naltrexone at these concentrations to achieve a longer residency in the eye and have discrete lubricant effect, but also must be sterile. Lastly, the dosage for topical administration is significantly lower than what we would typically see orally. Typical average oral doses for LDN range from 0.5 mg all the way up to 6 mg, whereas the current topical dose for the eye is 0.002% or 20 ug/ml up to 0.005% or 50 ug/ml, and this requires specialized training to achieve accuracy. Find an excellent compounding pharmacy that specializes in sterile compounding with which you can establish a relationship, whose team is knowledgeable and will work with you individually to ensure the best possible outcome for you.

It seems like every day we discover new uses for naltrexone, in unique doses and delivery systems, but also through our better understanding of the drivers of disease and the new mechanisms to which we can alter those drivers. This chapter has represented what we know currently, and it's a great place to be. I look forward to future discoveries and how they will positively impact our health.

- Eight -

Long COVID

Angus G. Dalgleish, FRCP FRCPath FMedSci
with Wai M. Liu, PhD

The coronavirus disease that appeared at the tail end of 2019, known best by its acronym COVID-19 (COVID), has caused unprecedented disruption to the lives of people in countries throughout the world. For the past two years, at the time of this writing, more than 290 million cases of COVID (in accordance with the applied case definitions and testing strategies in the affected countries) have been reported, including nearly 5.5 million deaths.[581] The virus that causes the disease gains entry into host cells via the angiotensin converting enzyme 2 (ACE2) receptor, and sets off a chain of events that results in the pathology that has been widely reported and recognized.[582] The ACE2 receptor is found on a variety of different cell types and thus the virus is capable of affecting multiple organ systems at once.[583] This can mean the disease presents in seemingly different ways, with symptoms ranging from mild to severe.[584] For the majority of people, the disease resolves itself in about 7-10 days and active therapeutic intervention is not required.

An area of concern regarding the management of patients with COVID infection has been the persistence of a range of symptoms long after the acute phase of the disease has been controlled. The National Institute for Health and Care Excellence (NICE) has noted the presence of "...signs and symptoms that develop during or after an infection consistent with COVID-19, [which] continue for more than 12 weeks and are not explained by an alternative diagnosis," and defines these long-term sequelae of COVID infection as such. They say "...it usually presents with clusters of symptoms, often overlapping, which can fluctuate and change over time and can affect any system in the body."[585]

This condition is more commonly referred to as "Long COVID" and can be more distressing than the initial infection as the treatment strategy is unclear. Reports have highlighted that the number of symptoms and effects that linger following COVID infection is high and can involve as much as 200 disparate effects.[586] Common ones, as detailed by the Office of National Statistics, that are often mentioned include chronic fatigue, disruptions to cognitive functioning, muscle weakness, shortness of breath, chest pain, myocardial disturbances, and sleep disturbances, which together drastically and profoundly impacts quality of life.[587]

It is already known that various organs are known to be involved in this condition; the common link in these systems is the ACE2 receptor. The symptoms that manifest are in some ways connected to the disturbance in ACE2 receptor functioning in these organ systems, and it has been hypothesized that autoantibodies against the ACE2 receptor may develop the initial COVID infection, which continues to disrupt ACE2 receptor function.[588] Nevertheless, the mechanism(s) contributing to the pathophysiology of Long COVID is unknown. They can be loosely separated into two categories; viz. where COVID has a direct effect on tissue and/or homeostasis; or where it stimulates an inappropriate and/or tissue-damaging effect by the immune system.

Lung Damage/Dyspnea

Shortness of breath is listed as the ninth most prevalent symptom, and is experienced by 4.6% of patients five weeks post-infection with COVID.[589] A series of brief communications in 2021 highlighted this, and one report of note detailed the clinical assessment and tracking of 384 available patients treated for COVID in NHS-Trust hospitals in London found that 53% patients that had been successfully treated for COVID that only required oxygen alone, still reported persistent breathlessness 4-6 weeks after discharge from hospital.[590] [591] A number of other studies have indicated that breathlessness can still be present 8-12 weeks later, which significantly reduced health-related quality of life; indeed, the disease post-acute infection can affect people to the extent that breathing support is required while sleeping.[592] [593]

The pathophysiology of the disease and how it specifically affects the lungs have been widely described, and the signs and symptoms together are clinically identical to acute respiratory distress syndrome (ARDS).[594] Through viral infection of epithelial cells of the airways and lungs, these tissues become damaged as the virus replicates and causes cytolysis of host cells.[595] This in turn often initiates an early immune response that together with the early virus-mediated cellular damaging events causes further destruction to the integrity of airway epithelial and endothelial barrier-interface, which ultimately leads to an immunological response.[596] Interleukin 6 (IL-6) is an early-response immunological driver that is rapidly synthesized at local sites of damage.[597] It can orchestrate the proteins produced at this initial stage of inflammation that include C-reactive protein and serum amyloid A. If these acute-phase proteins persist, it can lead to a chronic inflammatory state and disease through amyloidosis.[598] These fibrotic deposits can subsequently increase the likelihood of developing secondary infections that contribute to the pathology of COVID infection within the lungs. Furthermore, their presence has been found in post-mortem examinations of COVID patients.[599]

Persistent Fatigue

Persistent fatigue is, according to ONS data, the most prevalent symptom experienced by patients post-acute-COVID infection. About 11.5% patients experience it at least five weeks after recovery; but this may be an underestimation, as there have been many reports that about a half of long COVID patients experience some form of fatigue.[600] The term can have a range of meanings; it can in some people represent a generic feeling of malaise and low mood that are difficult to measure objectively, whilst in others be assessed by tests and connected with weakness, exhaustion, and reduced energy levels that can be crippling.[601] This latter type of fatigue is of particular concern, and management of it has been surprisingly controversial.[602] The fundamental issue may be the lack of clarity regarding the pathophysiology of the complex condition.

This type of fatigue has been described by many to mimic myalgic encephalomyelitis/chronic fatigue syndrome (ME/CFS), a disabling and complex illness.[603] Again, although the underlying cause of long COVID has yet to be fully elucidated, there is evidence to suggest that the rebounding of the immune system following an acute challenge to the virus contributes to the pathology. Specifically, in a similar way that viral illnesses can lead to ME and or CFS, the inappropriate stimulation/correction of the immune system and subsequent attempts to rebalance immunity can exhaust the function of the immune cells.[604] However, a direct relationship between ME/CFS and the persistent fatigue experienced in some patients post-COVID infection is complex and remains unclear. A review of patients experiencing fatigue that was managed at a post-COVID outpatient clinic showed there was no association between the fatigue and standard markers of inflammation, including IL-6.[605] This suggests the etiology of the fatigue is multifactorial and can include in some cases physical events such as microvascular thrombosis, or perturbations to energy processing at the mitochondrial level.[606 607]

ME and CFS have been associated with changes in the levels of key cytokines such as tissue necrosis factor alpha (TNF-α), interferon gamma (IFN-γ), IL-6 and IL-1β that are released by CD3+ T-cells.[608] In fact, the levels can serve as a readout of the status of these conditions. Not only are the levels of these cytokines important in signifying disease state, but the balance of specific effector T-cells is also important.[609] Additionally, there are studies to show disruption to mitochondria function, as highlighted by changes to mitochondrial membrane potential.[610]

LDN and Long COVID: The Rationale

Low dose naltrexone (LDN) has been used for years in the treatment of many conditions. It has a range of effects that can simply be attributed to a direct effect on the pathology treated, or through modulation of the host immune system. As a number of diseases are intimately linked and attributed to immune dysfunction, the use of LDN to treat them has increased. Using LDN to counteract the effects of long COVID has also been included. This is not without some scientific merit. As we have discussed, ONS data has identified fatigue as the most prevalent symptom of long COVID.

Therapeutic approaches that correct these systems as well as dampening down this ill-placed natural response to a viral infection, may serve to improve the symptoms of long COVID. LDN has potent anti-inflammatory qualities; it appears to modulate and modify different elements of the immune system. In vitro investigations using models of individual components of immunity have described naltrexone altering the intracellular signaling in and subsequent cytokine output of certain immune cells. Although immunity as a whole is more complex, and cannot be simply considered a collection of individual cells working in isolation, it is interesting to note that in patients administered LDN, the systemic levels of cytokines that drive both humoral and cell mediated inflammation, such as G-CSF, IL-4, IL-6, IL-10, IFN-alpha and TNF-beta, were significantly reduced after eight weeks.[611] It is this ability to dampen down cytokines driving key elements of immunity that lends support to the growing view that LDN is immunomodulatory.

Although it is unclear how naltrexone, which is fundamentally an opioid antagonist, can modify the levels of cytokines that influence immune function, what is clear is that opioids such as morphine have been known for some time to be immunosuppressive.[612] Opioid receptors have been found on immune cells, and the role of these receptors in regulating immunity has been described.[613] [614] Crucially, LDN has been successfully used to treat ME/CFS.[615]

More recent work on the mechanisms of action have surprisingly shown LDN impacts the TLR-9 pathway, which can in turn inhibit IL-6 in particular, which is the main cytokine driving inflammation responses associated with COVID.[616] From available data, there is importantly a need to trial LDN in medium- and long-term COVID as there is no other suitable agent. LDN is already accepted as an effective agent to treat ME/CFS as well as fibromyalgia, which has many similarities to the muscular symptoms associated with long COVID.

LDN and Long COVID: The Clinical Perspective

The COVID pandemic officially invaded Britain in late January 2020 but on reflection it was clearly here in the UK as early as November and December 2019. I myself was aware of two clusters of classic COVID symptoms and spread, one of which occurred mid-November and the other in mid-December. In the first one, symptoms gave rise to hospitalization, and doctors confessed they had not seen anything quite like it before as the disease was neither a classic viral infection, nor pneumonia. Fortunately, this patient recovered, but they had contact with a person with severe Parkinson's disease, who eventually succumbed. Overall, there were possibly six cases who had COVID presenting with classic symptoms, although no testing was available at this time. In the second cluster, a couple had both suffered severe respiratory symptoms and shortness of breath, with sweating and, again, the symptoms were different from the usual expected seasonal influenza. On this occasion, COVID was only confirmed retrospectively by an antibody test several months later.

Establishing the origin of the virus is extremely important as it helps to understand the pathogenesis of the disease. This is something in which my colleague Birger Sorensen and I have been active. His team were very quick to note that the charge around receptors binding sites were such that allowed the virus to be more likely to attach to human membranes without necessarily having to engage with the primary receptor that was widely acknowledged as the ACE2 receptor.[617] As described earlier, this is crucially important to the ability of the virus to affect a wide variety of cell types, which reflects in the clinical sequelae. The ability of the virus to interact with olfactory epithelial sustentacular cells that supported olfactory sensory neurons involved in taste and smell gave it the fairly unusual ability to temporarily disconnect these senses; although not in all cases was this to be temporary.[618]

The virus was able to adhere to endothelial and myocardial cells, which gave rise to the myocarditis and cardiac symptoms. Its ability to invade and kill T-cells led to an immune deficiency, making the whole clinical scenario worse. In addition to causing severe respiratory symptoms, the virus also disrupts the clotting pathway, and much of the pathology is caused by micro-clots, which lead to inflammation.[619] This in turn can lead to the shortage of oxygen distribution, which was the forerunner of death in the majority of patients who died from COVID. It is also able to infect muscle cells that would explain the severe muscle pain, as well as the intestinal tract that would manifest as gastrointestinal symptoms and diarrhea.[620] Apart from the loss of taste and smell, COVID patients can often become very confused and complain of great problems concentrating and thinking, with reduced cognitive abilities.

Patients who are very ill, in intensive care, who eventually recovered and were discharged were noted to continue to be seriously unwell, with many of these patients complaining of continued shortness of breath, fevers and fatigue, in addition to cognitive dysfunction. This condition became known as long COVID. However, there were many more patients who got infected with COVID and were ill, but never made it to hospital and were never put in intensive care. Clinically, these patients would complain that many of the symptoms, although they initially improved, would last for 2-3 months, and these symptoms could not be explained by an alternative diagnosis. Sometimes, the symptoms might be considered as a new onset, following the initial recovery from an acute episode, or simply the initial one persisting in a mild form, with symptoms fluctuating and relapsing over time.

It is worth recounting here, a couple of cases of mine (AGD) that highlight the breadth of these symptoms and the way they impact day-to-day living. The first is a patient who had acute COVID but clearly never recovered, having significant shortness of breath, fevers and cough every night for well over a year before successful treatment. His respiratory impairment was such that he had to attend a respiratory clinic, where his poor function was documented and his oxygen-saturations measured on a regular basis. He also had severe myalgia, being in pain on standing up, as well as severe fatigue, whereby he could never really be out of bed for more than one or two hours a day and even then, he had great difficulty in climbing the stairs to go back to bed. He also complained that if these were not enough, but the inability to think clearly, to absorb and recall information and to act on it, was the most debilitating. Such symptoms have been noted by and referred to by many patients themselves as brain fog, had the most dramatic effect on his life as it prevented him running his business effectively. Even now, months after the acute COVID infection, he is still having episodes of being woken at night with shortness of breath and fever, which is very suggestive of an ongoing viral infection that has never been proven by antigen testing.

The second case report is of a young woman who developed symptoms of COVID, most likely from her children, who suffered the common symptoms of a very sore throat, cough, headaches, extreme tiredness, brain fog, but with the addition of severe gastric intestinal symptoms. Although these improved dramatically after a week or so, she was left with severe fatigue, muscle ache, and stomach pains for several weeks afterwards. She was still symptomatic more than two months later, and like the first patient, had tried many self-help treatments that were meant to improve these symptoms but only offered minor transient improvement.

We have already mentioned that these two cases, like all the other descriptions of long COVID, have very many features similar to other post-viral illnesses that have been referred to as ME and CFS. These conditions are often associated with Epstein Barr virus (EBV) infection, which is chronic and is not cleared by the body, as well as having been noted with classical influenza infection in the past. It is worth noting that many patients suffering from long COVID symptoms as described earlier have tried many of the treatments proposed by those suffering and treating CFS. The lack of efficacy of any of these treatments in patients with either CFS or long COVID is very similar. LDN has been used in a number of autoimmune conditions that are associated with some of the features of CFS and has established itself as a routine off-license treatment for the chronic pain and inflammation in multiple sclerosis and fibromyalgia, which indeed, has several shared features of CFS.[621]

I first learnt about the potential of low dose naltrexone in patients with ME/CFS when an immunologist colleague confided to me that his CFS practice had been revolutionized by a new drug that worked in over 50% of the cases, without any relapse. I was surprised that he would not tell me what this was until I suggested that one of his associates, who did not have CFS, should try LDN. He was astonished and told me that it was actually the drug he was using for

CFS. It is a pity that these data were never written up as I know that he treated possibly hundreds of patients with this syndrome, which at the time became known colloquially as "Yuppie Flu," which was a condition on which private clinics tended to focus.

I was therefore delighted to see in *BMJ Case Reports* a case series of three patients with long term ill health due to chronic fatigue syndrome, which all improved upon taking low dose naltrexone.[622] The benefit ranged from "life-changing" to a reduction in some symptoms only, and the paper suggested this warranted further clinical trials, with which I would totally agree. Since then, there has been a paper reporting the potential benefit of LDN in CFS, where the researchers measured and investigated the effect of LDN on the activity on the transient receptor potential channel TRPM3 in patients by using a whole cell patch clamp technique and compared them with age and sex-matched healthy volunteers. They reported that all the patients taking LDN had restored TRPM3-like ionic currents in natural killer (NK) cells. TRPM3 is a nociceptor channel that is substantially targeted by certain opiate receptors, and its implication in calcium dependent NK cell immune function has raised the possibility that it could be a target for the treatment of ME/CFS.[623]

What has been impressive is that the patients who have requested to try LDN have had, with only one exception, significant clinical responses, and in most cases maintained an improvement using it. Of particular interest to note is that none of the patients appear to benefit in the first two to three weeks of treatment. Therapeutically, the benefit is associated initially with a clearing of the brain fog, which is a tremendous relief as patients are able to much more quickly return to normal life. One young patient had been so afflicted by brain fog that he was no longer able to continue with his A-level studies as he could not concentrate or remember anything he had read. It was most remarkable that in his case, this returned within two or three weeks of him taking LDN, and with no residual deficit. Others have reported to me that the chronic fatigue improves but at a much lower rate, but they gradually get more and more energy, and that muscle pain disappears.

The second message I have received from treating these patients is that those who have had symptoms for many months, and subsequently respond to and improve on 3-4 weeks of LDN will not maintain the improvement if they prematurely stop treatment. They require continued administration. Indeed, the fact that several patients have reported that their symptoms relapse when they stop LDN but immediately improve on recommencing, strongly supports that this is cause and effect and not random coincidence, as many are keen to suggest. Those patients who have had long COVID for over a year are not going to maintain improvement unless they are taking LDN for several months afterwards; however, patients who have had symptoms persisting for just 2-3 months have been able to stop LDN after taking it for two months or so.

As we have alluded to earlier, the mechanism of action of LDN in these patients is far from clear. However, there are clues. The suggestion that it involves opiate-receptor metabolism and has an effect on the NK cell function is intriguing and may well have a role.[624] However, we know from complex medical conditions and from the drugs that elicit remarkable effects on them, that the mechanisms are usually not singular but involve many different pathways. A good example of this is thalidomide, which was initially developed for sleeping problems and morning sickness associated with pregnancy. It has turned out to be an effective drug in a number of autoimmune conditions, and the drug-derivatives inspired by it, such as lenalidomide, have been revolutionary in the treatment of certain cancers, such as multiple myeloma and lymphoma. Initially, it was accepted that the mechanism of action was inhibiting the TNF-α pathway. However, publication after publication has clearly demonstrated the ability of these drugs to interfere with many different pathways, including inflammation, immune function, and angiogenesis, to name a few underpins its mechanistic diversity.

Whatever LDN does, it clearly has anti-inflammatory activity, which I believe goes beyond its potential modulatory effects on the opiate receptor. This had led my group to look for alternative receptors, and we were able to identify that it also inhibited toll-like receptors (TLR) 7, 8 and 9, as well and to curtail the IL-6 production that occurs when TLRs are stimulated. Inflammation driven by IL-6 is very common in cancer, and as we mentioned earlier in the chapter, IL-6 is a major cytokine involved in both acute and long COVID. Indeed, antibodies to IL-6 have been recommended by WHO for acute symptoms of COVID.[625] It therefore seems natural to me to be a very possible explanation that LDN is able to slowly dampen down the chronic inflammatory drive induced initially by the virus.

Conclusions

It has now become evident that long COVID is a major issue for the general population, with over a million sufferers reported in the UK alone. There is a general consensus that no specific treatments work. Evidence from colleagues and recent publications have confirmed that many patients with ME/CFS have long term benefits after starting LDN. There is no doubt that many of the symptoms of long COVID overlap with ME/CFS. We have reported clinical evidence of cases who have benefited from LDN, some who have suffered symptoms for over a year prior to commencing treatment, and a number have made a full recovery. Given the absence of standard treatments, we feel it is beholden on clinicians to initiate studies that investigate more fully the potential of drugs such as LDN in patients with long COVID.

NINE

Cancer Case Studies

Angus Dalgleish MD, FMedSci; Dr. Wai M. Liu, PhD,
and Dr. Nasha Winters, ND, FABNO

A s I wrote in my chapter on cancer for *The LDN Book: Volume One,* there have been few controlled clinical trials on low dose naltrexone and the treatment of cancer, therefore most of the clinical data with regard to cancer is anecdotal. This chapter begins with my experience of LDN treatment with patients with multiple liver metastases who have failed standard chemotherapy and is followed by case studies presented by Dr. Nasha Winters.

In the cases of patients with multiple liver metastases, LDN treatment has led to both long-term disease-free status and stability of the disease. Early observations of liver metastases that seem to become stable with the addition of LDN suggest a causal link. Scientifically, this makes sense when one considers that naltrexone concentrates in the liver, and probably produces this effect through inflammatory pathways such as the inhibition of key immune-related receptors such as toll-like receptor 9, which results in the production of interleukin 6 (IL-6), a cytokine strongly associated with cancer progression of all tumor types. Indeed, the one property shared by nearly all cancers is that they thrive on chronic inflammation, with many evolving against a background of chronic inflammation over many decades.[626] For example, liver cancers evolve against a background of hepatitis induced by hepatitis B and C viruses[627], colorectal cancers are more likely to occur in inflammatory conditions of the bowel such as colitis and adenoma[628], and aerodigestive cancers evolve in an inflammatory background caused by decades of smoke irritation.[629] Strong indirect evidence of the practical aspects of this come from long term studies of people taking daily aspirin, where the incidence of several common tumor types may be reduced by 20-50% over many years.[630] Aspirin is a major inhibitor of COX-2 inflammatory pathways. LDN clearly works on a different inflammatory pathway (including TLR-9) and may thus play a major role in cancers known to have an active inflammatory component.[631]

One major cancer that does not respond to standard cancer treatments is mesothelioma. Mesothelioma evolves from asbestosis, a chronic fibrotic lung condition caused by exposure to asbestos, whose fibers are too large to be dissolved by macrophages and which cause very low-grade chronic inflammation. Like many other chronic irritative conditions, this is present for decades before the cancer arises. As an oncologist I have been impressed with how poorly this condition responds to standard treatments including surgery, radiotherapy, and chemotherapy. Indeed, I have remarked on several cases where the tumor seemed to take off after being exposed to chemotherapy. I am aware of a case where a gentleman developed bilateral mesothelioma who decided against debulking surgery and chemotherapy, and instead enquired after alternative treatments. I suggested he maximize his anti-inflammatory treatments including vitamin D3 supplementation and LDN, which I prescribed.[632] As an aside, prescribing LDN along with vitamin D3 has been shown to be effective in inducing long-term remission in a patient with adenoid cystic tongue carcinoma.[633] I also added IMM-101, which is a heat-killed mycobacterium that has shown good responses in melanoma and pancreatic cancer patients.[634] IMM-101 has also been shown to greatly enhance innate immune activity such as NK and gamma delta T cell activity as well as enhancing antigen presentation. It therefore made sense to me to combine such an immune stimulant with an anti-inflammatory agent. This patient exceeded all our expectations and went on to live for another six years with a superb quality of life using this non-toxic combination, before developing peritoneal metastases. To recapitulate, he had been told he would survive about nine months with surgery and chemotherapy.

Chronic inflammation also plays a major role in prostate cancer, and indeed chronic prostatitis caused by a number of infections has been proposed as a major etiological factor.[635] The main systemic treatments for prostate cancer are docetaxel chemotherapy or anti-hormonal. To prolong patient responses to these therapies I started to add in LDN, and in some cases also add in IMM-101 whose precursor, *M. vaccae*, had been reported as inducing PSA responses in prostatic cancers many years before and the observations not taken further. I have now seen a number of prostatic patients who have been stabilized by the addition of LDN with or without IMM-101, both at early hormonal escape and at malignant disease requiring chemotherapy. Clinical responses have been measured in years both for delaying the start of standard hormone treatment and stabilizing lymph node and bone metastases following chemotherapy.

Other cancers that have been reported to respond to LDN include a case of a tongue cancer which responded to LDN and alpha lipoic acid (ALA) alone (ALA is another agent which is often given with LDN in Israel and the United States). I am very impressed by reports of chronic lymphomas/leukemia that respond to LDN when the only alternatives are to watch and wait, or continuous chemotherapy. Confronted with a patient with widespread lymph nodes and blood changes who did not want to undergo chemotherapy without a high chance of cure, I have been able to confirm that LDN has had marked improvement in his measurable disease and blood counts over four years.

These are personal experiences where LDN alone or more usually in combination with another immune-modulating agent has been effective in patients with cancer. There are to date few cases detailed in the literature; however, key ones include:

- Non-small cell lung cancer (past medical history of prostate and lung cancer → prolonged survival and negative for any recurrence after four years).[636]
- Renal cell carcinoma (metastatic disease, unresponsive to conventional treatments → stable disease with disappearance of the signs and symptoms of stage IV RCC, a full nine years following diagnosis).[637]

- Pediatric hepatoblastoma (patients with co-morbidities and complications with conventional chemotherapy → five and ten years disease-free, respectively).[638]
- Pancreatic cancer (metastatic disease, one with a history of prostate cancer → no signs of cancer on PET scanning).[639]

Anti-cancer Properties of Naltrexone

The scientific rationale for LDN as a therapeutic agent in cancer patients is convincing. A definitive mechanism of action (MOA) has yet to be established but is often thought to involve those causing a direct antagonism of tumor growth or modifications to the host immune system.[640] The most commonly discussed MOAs include:

- Inhibition of proliferation

  - Suppression of the PI3-K pathway[641]
  - Increased expression of the cell cycle inhibitor p21[642 643]

- Rebalancing BAX:BCL2 to promote apoptosis

  - Increased expression of the pro-apoptotic BAD and BAX[644 645]
  - Decreased expression of the anti-apoptotic BCL2[646 647]

- Modulating the functions of immune cells

  - Inhibits TLRs and dampens IL6 production, which promotes as anticancer environment.[648]
  - Enhances the maturation of dendritic cells required to mount immune-driven anticancer effects.[649]
  - Anti-inflammatory actions.[650]

Tumor development is a balance of growth and death, and naltrexone—like other opiates and opiate antagonists—is capable of altering this balance. In addition to their universally accepted analgesic qualities, opioids have also been reported to elicit a number of other cellular responses that lead to tumor death. The diversity of these effects also has made it difficult to establish a major cause and serves only to confound the identification of the principal MOA. Indeed, they include those that are pro-survival in nature such as the induction of proliferation and protection against cell death, as well as opposite effects, including growth inhibition and the induction of apoptosis. The ultimate consequences of treatment with naltrexone are determined by dose and schedule. Nevertheless, studies exist to try to best delineate the action of the opioids and their cognate receptors, and in doing so design new therapeutic strategies to best utilize this fascinating class of compound.

To understand the importance and impact of dose, we compared the effect on the gene expression profile of cancer cells of low and high doses of naltrexone, and showed the profiles are completely different depending on the dose used. Specifically, gene ontology analysis showed low doses of naltrexone had a greater impact on genes associated with cell cycle control and the immune responses, and that these effects were unique to this lower dose.[651]. Furthermore, these studies have also highlighted the anticancer action of LDN is associated in part with changes to pERK and PI3-K signalling. These cascades are tightly associated with apoptosis and the mechanisms that regulate it, and so any interference in these would impact the ability of a cell to undergo cell death. We and others have shown that LDN is capable of altering the balance of pro and anti-apoptotic proteins that regulate cell killing. Specifically, our in vitro and in vivo models show how the pro-apoptotic proteins BAX and BAD can be enhanced by a short-term exposure to LDN, which in turn can sensitise cancer cells to the cytotoxic effects of common chemotherapy agents.[652]

There are many reasons for developing LDN as an anti-cancer agent either as an adjuvant or in combination with other agents. Unfortunately, the numerous anecdotes currently reported still require confirmation with properly conducted clinical trials, which are expensive. The cost of clinical trials is the major reason why they have not been conducted to date. But it is hoped that this can be addressed in the near future and that LDN can achieve a licence for adjuvant use in cancer management.

Three Case Studies by Dr. Nasha Winters

Before I met him in person, my colleague Professor Angus G. Dalgleish caught my attention for his chapter on cancer and low dose naltrexone in Linda Elsegood's first volume of *The LDN Book*. I had first used LDN while in medical school under the advice of Dr. Bihari back in the mid-1990s when I worked in an AIDS/HIV center. Later my application of LDN evolved to treating autoimmune disorders, and about a decade ago carried into the cancer world. I didn't understand its mechanism of action at the time, but the patient feedback, lab values, and imaging were compelling enough for me to start using this in nearly every single patient with a diagnosis of cancer.

When I read Professor Dalgleish's chapter in 2016, my wheels really started turning, which led me to have a deeper understanding of the other therapies I seemed to see impressive results from, such as vitamin D3, cannabis, mistletoe, and hyperthermia. His chapter helped answer many of my own questions and validated my choosing to employ LDN in patients with cancer. It has since served to articulate to my colleagues and patients my rationale for such a powerful addition to their treatment plan.

Beyond opiate modulation, Professor Dalgleish highlighted how LDN activates cytotoxic T cells, immune modulates, increases natural killer cells, impacts signaling pathways, antagonizes toll-like receptor-9, combats TNF alpha activity, and is strongly anti-inflammatory. It has also been shown to modulate P13-kinase cascade, which is a highly studied pathway in standard of care oncology research. This pathway plays a role in cancer progression in relationship to metabolism, growth, survival, and motility. Though standard of care treatment is now available to target this pathway, it is often accompanied by terrible side effects and leads to little improvement.

Professor Dalgleish goes on to further elucidate the impact of LDN on the calcium and potassium channel function with the overall effect of disrupting the calcium movement and signaling of cyclic AMP, which also continues to be a focus in much research today. He, like so many others, expresses gratitude to the work of

Dr. Zagon, who has paved the way for this therapy to be utilized in most integrative oncology practices today.

I must say that above and beyond targeting the various hallmarks of cancer, my favorite part of the impact of this medication is on the psychology of the patient and their overall quality of life. The cases I am presenting are perfect examples of how LDN goes beyond addressing tumor burden and progression. You will also note that many of the mechanisms targeted by LDN for cancer spill into other co-morbidities, namely autoimmune disease and chronic viral pathology, taking me full circle back to how I first began using this valuable intervention.

One of the things that struck me most about Professor Dalgleish's chapter was something I noted on many occasions and is particularly relevant today. Optimal levels of vitamin D3 (a hormonal-like nutrient) is necessary for this therapy, and really any immune therapy, to work properly. In a time when we are discussing ways to combat a global pandemic with mass vaccination and masks, little to no regard has been given to what might be the very driver of the vulnerability to the virus and its mutations and the treatment for the virus. Perhaps more attention needs to be placed on this multifaceted, fat-soluble vitamin that impacts hundreds of epigenetic switches and enriches the immune milieu so that many interventions can take root.

The following three cases are examples of immune systems gone rogue and how the well-suited application of LDN brought about better outcomes to mind, body, and soul.

Case #1: EE, 39-year-old Female with Stage IV Breast Cancer
EE was diagnosed at the age of 30 with right sided stage IIB triple-positive breast cancer. Her diagnosis arrived shortly after the birth of her second child and after being misdiagnosed for several months as mastitis.

EE was treated with standard of care including Adriamycin and cyclophosphamide followed by Taxol (all forms of chemotherapy) and was recommended Herceptin (a targeted therapy for HER2Neu positive cancers) for a year along with five years of tamoxifen (a selective estrogen receptor modifier). Between undergoing chemotherapy and radiation, she had a double mastectomy with implants and reconstruction followed by whole chest radiation, given some suspicious lymphovascular invasion.

Basically, she threw everything but the kitchen sink at her cancer from standard of care. She was riddled with debilitating side effects and medical mishaps including surgical complications, radiation burns, dipping blood counts that impacted the timing of her chemotherapy, and loss of range of motion in her right arm. She had to discontinue the Herceptin after four months because of cardiovascular symptoms and cut her tamoxifen dose in half to tolerate the side effects. She was plagued with deep bone pain, hot flashes, insomnia, and weight gain from the treatment, and her anxiety flared.

Prior to her breast cancer diagnosis came a collection of other diagnoses, including rheumatoid arthritis (RA) when she was 22 years old, though she'd been symptomatic since she was 17 following a year of infections—mostly upper respiratory—that resulted in multiple rounds of antibiotics and chest x-rays. She was treated with steroids and methotrexate, and later Plaquenil.

She had been diagnosed with anxiety disorder and used benzodiazepine medications regularly, nearly daily for over twenty years.

She had also been diagnosed with irritable bowel syndrome (IBS) at 16 and had a high ACE (Adverse Childhood Events) score of 8/10, so trauma from her youth played a big role in how she perceived, responded to, and reacted in the world. A study published in 2019 explains further how early childhood trauma could play a role in chronic illness patterns, including cancer, which may be applicable to her case.[653]

Despite her significant medical history, she gave little attention to her health until her cancer recurrence, six years after her initial diagnosis. Her symptom of right hip pain led to imaging, biopsy, and diagnosis of stage IV metastatic breast cancer that went from a triple positive cancer to a triple negative cancer type. She had thought, erroneously, that it was her RA flaring, which had been in remission following her chemotherapy. Her imaging showed extensive metastasis in her right femur, pelvis, lower vertebrae, and right rib cage. She was also severely osteoporotic and her D3 levels were 7 ng/mL! There were also questionable findings on her mastectomy scar line and lymph nodes in her left axilla. Also, the imaging noted that her left breast implant had ruptured.

The stage IV diagnosis was her wake up call to take a different approach. She sought my care for consulting, and I connected her with local resources that could employ the proper testing and treatment. After a deep dive into her blood labs, including autoimmune markers, D3 levels, markers of inflammation, bone marrow, immune function, and metabolic health, we found she was flaring with her rheumatoid arthritis pattern simultaneously with her oncology pattern and that differentiating between the two would be difficult. The most obvious place to start for her was implementing LDN in the standard dosing model of 1.5mg nightly for two to four weeks (she tolerated well, so we were able to move up quicker every two weeks), then 3mg for two weeks, then the top dose of 4.5mg.

We maintained that dose nightly for three months to stabilize her autoimmune flare, paired with high dose D3 to enhance response (50,000iu/d along with K2), with close monitoring of her serum calcium levels for two weeks, then 20,000iu/d for a month, then 10,000iu maintenance. Her levels after eight weeks on this dose went from 7 to 37 ng/mL so we resumed 20,000 units/d. She noted clear improvement in her overall quality of life, pain, and sleep patterns, resolved nearly all her anxiety, and no longer needed to lean on her benzodiazepine medications.

Since her recurrence, she had not resumed her previous RA treatment and despite the urgings of her rheumatologist, refused to go back on steroids, methotrexate or Plaquenil, in favor of spending three months trying LDN and D3 along with significant dietary changes that included carbohydrate restriction and a low-allergen/ low-inflammatory-based diet.

Despite her breast cancer markers remaining very high along with her CRP, her overall symptoms and quality of life improved dramatically, and her imaging showed complete stabilization of her disease process. After her experience with doing "everything" per standard of care her first time around, she was very resistant to employing any with her new diagnosis. Even LDN was a challenge for her as she perceived it as a pharmaceutical, which she strongly wanted to avoid. Within three months of implementing these basic changes, along with some low dose Celebrex (a Cox-2 inhibitor), we were able to get her CRP down from 67 to 6 and her RA Factor back to normal limits. Her IL6 normalized as well.

At that time, we also ran labs on her TNF alpha, which was sky-high. Initially, we assumed this was her RA pattern, yet the improvement of her symptoms and other labs sent us digging more and we uncovered a mold problem in her home as well as got her prepared for and through explant surgery which also harbored mold. Her labs normalized even further, including her breast cancer markers, within four months of her explant surgery.

Following her explant surgery, she was feeling so good that she pulled back on her doctor consults, lab testing, and imaging, and I lost track of her for many months. She also stopped taking her LDN. About six months after that, she reached out in a panic as her symptoms were kicking back in and her labs were on the wrong trajectory again. After resuming her dose at 4.5mg nightly for a month, then four nights on and three nights off thereafter, this patient has since opted to keep this on for the long haul given that her symptoms resolved almost immediately as did her labs.

At the time of publication, she just turned 39 years old, two years out from her recurrent stage IV triple negative breast cancer, with minimal disease burden that doesn't appear to be active in her left axilla and resolved activity in her bone metastasis with no sign of new metastasis anywhere. She is enjoying a life of health and vitality, in her own words "better than I have ever experienced," all the while watching her now 12- and 9-year-olds growing up with a mother, something she and her doctors didn't think possible just a few years before.

The combination of cancer and autoimmunity occurring simultaneously can be tricky to navigate as the therapies for each, can often trigger off the other. The immune modulating impact of LDN is a must in a situation such as this.

Case #2: VR, 66-year-old Male with Renal Cell Carcinoma (RCC)
At age 59, VR, a computer programmer and IT technician, was diagnosed with left sided renal cell carcinoma. Surgery was the only treatment offered and he was considered cured after removal of his left kidney.

I didn't meet him until three years later, when he came to me with end-stage RCC metastasized to his lungs and to the residual left adrenal gland. He was not keen on working with an integrative oncologist, but at the urging of his very persuasive and insistent wife, he agreed. He was not receptive to employing anything that would go against the decision of his standard of care oncology team so I was a bit limited in what we could do but given that his medical team offered him little hope, he was willing to hear me out.

In doing more exploration, toxicity, metabolic imbalance, and chronic stress led to this diagnosis. He was loaded with cadmium (likely from years of working with electronics), as well as mercury, lead, and arsenic. These are all known carcinogens and drivers of RCC. He was also full-bore diabetic, with a HbA1C of 7.4 and insulin of 35, but his wife oversaw all the cooking and took it upon herself to employ a therapeutic ketogenic diet that was high in quality fats, low in protein, and very low in carbohydrate. He was also suffering with hypertension which was causing stress on his remaining right kidney and his creatinine levels were 1.7, which is stage II kidney disease, so imaging and systemic treatments were challenging to employ so as not to destroy his remaining kidney. He also had Hashimoto's autoimmune thyroiditis and his TSH at the time of our evaluation was over 20 and his thyroid antibodies in the thousands, which made him vulnerable to side effects from immune therapies.

His oncology team decided to start with IL2 therapy. I tried to get him to start LDN prior to initiating that in-hospital treatment, but he was resistant. I was able to get him on high dose melatonin, which we knew would enhance and buffer the impact of the IL2 therapy, and the studies I supplied for him and his team were enough for them to give their blessing and for him to acquiesce. It was a bumpy ride through the intensive IL2 treatment, but he made it. Now, the real work began.

They wanted him to wait three months, image, then consider starting one of the checkpoint inhibitor drugs, but his autoimmune thyroiditis was flaring even more, his hypertension was out of control, and his kidney function was still a problem, though slightly improved to 1.4 creatinine levels. That is when I was able to start him on LDN 1.5mg nightly for a week, 3mg for a week, and 4.5mg for a week. He was quite robust and tolerated well enough to titrate up quickly.

My next visit with him, a month into his LDN treatment, shocked me; I couldn't believe it was the same person. His demeanor changed entirely. Before, he sat quietly, arms crossed over his chest, grunting any responses when I pushed him, and relying on his wife to do all the communicating. This time, he was smiling, arms uncrossed, teasing his wife in a sweet way, and answering his own questions. When he stepped out to use the restroom I inquired about this change and his wife, too, stated, she hadn't seen this side of him in years. She was almost in tears noting the transformation that even she had not realized needed to happen. Could it possibly be the LDN?

On his three-month scan to follow up on his IL2 treatment, along with the LDN, D3, mistletoe and dietary changes, the doctors couldn't believe their eyes. They thought they were just going to buy him a bit more time and perhaps slow the progression. What they found surprised us all: no evidence of disease (NED). His kidney function had improved to a 1.2 creatinine, and his thyroid function was now normalized to 3.5 TSH and his antibodies down by 50%. His A1C had gone from 7.4 to 6.1 during that time as well but his blood ketones were running around 2.5-3.0 and his glucose now consistently under 85 whereas before it was well above 100!

We decided to keep on the same plan, and I recommended to maintain it for at least two years and to check in periodically as needed. I didn't hear from him for three years. At that time, his wife reached out again that his scan revealed new growth in his right adrenal gland and suspicious lung lesions. It was revealed that he had "fallen off the wagon" 18 months earlier, returning to some of his old eating habits and discontinuing his supplements and medications. His creatinine level had creeped back up to 1.5 and he admitted to rarely drinking water as well as being highly stressed back in his work environment, something he had greatly reined in when we were last in touch.

Luckily, he knew what he needed to do from an integrative perspective but also felt compelled to do more. He paired an ablative therapy along with a low dose of immune- checkpoint-inhibiting drug after further tumor biopsy revealed his cancer type had a particular target known as CTLA4. We all braced ourselves for the possible side effects that often accompany this approach given his autoimmune history. I feel confident that his response was positive *because* we got him back on LDN, 4.5mg dose, for a full month prior to the ablation and initiation of the CTLA-4 inhibiting drug.[654]

Though he has not been under my care for many years, last I heard, he is six years out from his last recurrence and though not showing NED, he has also not progressed, which is unheard of with this cancer type. He continues to stay committed to his LDN, diet, and mistletoe, and checks in periodically with his labs and metabolic health.

Though billions of dollars are being funneled into modern immune therapies today (known as immune checkpoint inhibitors, or ICPI), they have less than a 20% response rate.[655] And that does *not* mean cure rate. Sadly, the other 80 percent are either non-responders, have terrible side effects, or worse, result in death. The "overshooting" of the stimulation of the immune system on these medications makes this a Wild West process and leaves our patients quite vulnerable. I believe LDN enhances our ability to modulate their response and harness their power to improve clinical outcomes and patient quality of life.

Case #3: 50-year-old woman, 30 years out from Terminal OVCA with a Long Pre- and Post- History of Significant Autoimmune Disease

My own story is another example of autoimmune patterns that comingle with a cancering process. However, I was well in control of my cancering process before employing LDN for my autoimmune issues.

After guiding hundreds of patients on how to bring LDN on

board to help with their autoimmune issues and learning more and more about its impact on cancer treatment and prevention, I finally decided to take my own advice and apply this medication to my own biology.

I was diagnosed with endometriosis at 11 years old, polycystic ovarian syndrome (PCOS) at 14, and irritable bowel syndrome (IBS) at 16. I had cervical cancer twice by the time I was 17 and at 19 was diagnosed with Stage IV OVCA metastasized to my liver and riddled with carcinomatosis and peritoneal implants throughout my entire abdomen. At the time of diagnosis, I suffered from massive fluid accumulation in my abdomen known as malignant ascites and in my lungs known as pleural effusions and even some fluid around the lining of my heart. My kidneys and liver were in complete failure, and I was too ill to tolerate a single dose of chemotherapy and was released to end-of-life care. The rest of that story can be found elsewhere, but for the purpose of this chapter, I want to focus on what has plagued me since.

About a decade after managing to outlive the "un-survivable" cancer diagnosis, I learned I had ongoing wildfires still raging. I was still contending with endometriosis and PCOS but then learned I had also collected into my autoimmune basket Hashimoto's autoimmune thyroiditis, celiac disease (genetic) as well as rheumatoid arthritis (also genetic), all things I had incorrectly attributed to my IBS and injuries from my competitive volleyball days. It would take me another decade of prescribing LDN for my patients before I finally applied it to myself. And it was astonishing to see how much it impacted my autoimmune patterns and seemed to keep my roller coaster ride of rising and falling CA 125 ovarian cancer tumor markers far more stable.

My biggest lesson for this is realizing how much my body relies on it. I have gone weeks on end between doses and found that I can get good management of my RA symptoms (which shows up most in my ankles) as well as my lower limb lymphedema secondary to now calcified lymph nodes throughout my pelvis since my cancer diagnosis. Recently, I did a walking spiritual pilgrimage on the Ruta del Norte of the Camino de Santiago, walking from Irun, France, through five northern Spanish regions, over rugged, mountainous terrain, to Santiago de Compostela, Spain.

This was nearly a thousand-kilometer journey carrying a twenty-pound backpack, walking an average of 8-12 hours every day for five weeks. This was something I dreamed of doing for over a decade to celebrate my fiftieth birthday and my thirtieth year out from a terminal diagnosis. Despite all the thought I put into preparing for this trip, what I didn't do was remember to pack my LDN.

I wasn't that worried given I had taken breaks before over the previous decade, but I didn't account for the accidental exposure to gluten in my first week on the Camino along with an injury to my right ankle and a big flare of my IBS that put me into full-blown autoimmune reaction. What transpired was a frightening and physically challenging five weeks, that made an already difficult physical journey psychologically difficult as well. If you want to read more about my journey as folks are seemingly quite curious, see the entries on my blog (www.drnasha.com/blog/) dated between August and September 2021.

You can't begin to imagine the excitement I felt in resuming my first LDN pill after nearly six weeks! It took about a month to calm my symptoms down, which made me realize that this medication still offers a much-needed insurance policy for my sensitive system. As a health care provider and educator, it still humbles and amazes me that something so simple could be so powerful. I am grateful for the paths laid out before me and the mentors that have guided me to use this medicine for thousands of patients and even for my own wellbeing for over 25 years.

EPILOGUE

YOON HANG "JOHN" KIM MD MPH

Low dose naltrexone has come a long way from its pioneering clinical use by Dr. Bernard Bihari, who initially used LDN for treatment of HIV and later in his career for treatment of late-stage cancer.[656] My first encounter with LDN occurred almost twenty years ago when a patient asked me to research LDN for treating autoimmune thyroiditis. After reviewing the literature on this topic, I determined that the risks of using LDN appeared very low while there may be substantial potential benefit. LDN ended up reversing this patient's autoimmune thyroiditis. Since then, LDN has been the most useful and most prescribed medication in my integrative medicine tool kit for treatment of pain, cancer, and autoimmune disorders.

During my continued research into how LDN works, I came across an article that stated that acupuncture and LDN shared endorphin pathway. The article suggested that acupuncture and LDN could work synergistically.[657] Since I was performing acupuncture as a part of my integrative medicine practice, I began adding LDN to acupuncture treatments for some of my patients with very difficult pain conditions such as trigeminal neuralgia and post-herpetic neuralgia. To my surprise, patients who received LDN no longer needed acupuncture. At this point, it seemed like LDN displayed anti-inflammatory property for the nerves. Later, I would discover Dr Younger's article describing the anti-inflammatory properties of LDN.[658]

Later in my career, while working for an integrative cancer program, I read a case report by Dr. Berkson that described a patient with advanced pancreatic cancer who was treated with a combination of low dose naltrexone and alpha lipoic acid, which showed survival benefits.[659] Later, he published a case series article demonstrating survival benefits for a number of people with advanced cancer who were treated with his protocol.[660] Subsequently, I explored the potential use of LDN within the integrative oncology program, but discovered that the level of existing evidence did not satisfy the institution's requirement for evidenced-based medicine.

The two core concepts for accepting new observations as truth in medicine are reliability and validity. Reliability means repeatability. For example, low dose naltrexone is considered reliable in my integrative pain clinic for treating post-herpetic neuralgia and trigeminal neuralgia when patient after patient shows marked improvement. Without reliability, one cannot claim validity in medicine, though validity is a bit more complex as there are many forms, including predictive validity, internal validity, construct validity, and social validity.

New medical discoveries often involve an initial observation. When a single case is reported in the literature, it is considered a case report. A case series means publishing repeatable observations with different patients. A randomized controlled trial (RCT) is the next step in establishing validity. An RCT design's main advantage is being able to control for known and unknown variables that can result in a wrong conclusion. We are fortunate that the number of RCTs involving LDN is increasing. After a successful RCT, a follow-up RCT with much larger number of participants in multiple geographical locations is conducted to confirm previous observation and strength validity. To date, I am not aware of LDN research in this scale. Thus, in the eyes of conventional medicine, the use of LDN is often viewed with skepticism.

However, today we have many resources in the form of books and review articles which summarize available clinical research findings. An example of an excellent review article on LDN was written by Drs Tojan and Vrooman, titled "Low-Dose Naltrexone (LDN)-Review of Therapeutic Utilization."[661] The article reviews evidence for LDN to treat the following conditions:

- Multiple Sclerosis
- Complex Regional Pain Syndrome
- Fibromyalgia
- GI Tract Diseases
- Cancer
- Skin Conditions

The use of, and interest in, LDN continues to grow.[662] At some level, the popularity and prevalence of use of LDN will begin to achieve social validity arising from society's acceptance of its use. Works such as this publication will help inspire further exploration of new frontiers in LDN and continued interest in the drug, especially in future researchers who will one day help us reach the level of evidence needed to make LDN a standard of care.

Dosing Protocols

SARAH J. ZIELSDORF, MD, MS

Disclaimer: The information in this appendix is intended as a guide only; each patient is unique as is their treatment plan.

Between 2019 and 2021 the LDN Research Trust witnessed an explosion of new research accompanied by the sharing of more knowledge and treatment protocols, and contended with a giant pandemic. When we convened together virtually at the 2021 LDN Conference, our medical advisors yielded a consensus that there are no contraindications to taking LDN during any vaccinations, including DNA vaccines for cancer, and that LDN is especially helpful for both acute viral infections and chronic/reactivated ones. Not only is there not a contraindication between LDN and vaccinations, but the use of LDN may also improve the immune modulatory response toward the vaccine. This may yield a better protective response. And, at the end of 2021, multiple medical advisors (including myself) taught other clinicians our own niche topics and new LDN insights, with still more updates to add, and always more to learn. The bottom line is that the science is ever-evolving. Naltrexone and its myriad effects, uses, and dosing strategies continue both to surprise and challenge my current beliefs and expand my knowledge base.

One of the newest insights I have gleaned comes from integrative naturopathic oncologist Dr. Paul Anderson, who has contributed to our better understanding of dosing strategies for LDN to have the desired effect to help support our patients. We can now say that we are either modulating the immune system, stimulating or stabilizing the immune response, or suppressing dysregulated immune responses. In general, low doses at 1.5mg will provide both stimulation/stabilization, and maximum immune modulation. At high doses of 6mg, the suppression action is strong. Therefore, the 1.5-4.5mg general recommendation is a reasonable approach for most patients desiring immune modulation for chronic autoimmune conditions, for example. But for highly reactive conditions such as mast cell activation syndrome (MCAS), one may need a higher dose that gives a suppressive effect. The LDN Research Trust medical advisors also agree that unless specifically stated, once-daily dosing of LDN yields excellent results, ensures better patient compliance, and reduces expense.

LDN Forms

LDN can be prepared and administered in a variety of forms depending on the needs of the particular patient; all need to be immediate release:

Oral-Liquid LDN allows for titration of dosing from 0.1mg to 16mg.

LDN sublingual drops are best for patients with swallowing difficulties. Sublingual drops are absorbed directly through the oral mucosa for faster absorption and reduce GI issues.

LDN capsules can be made with dosages as low as 0.1mg; fillers vary from pharmacy to pharmacy.

LDN tablets can be scored for easy titration.

LDN topical lotions and creams are normally used for patients with skin conditions, and for children and skin conditions.

LDN troches can be made into any dosage and can be split into four. They dissolve under the tongue in one to two minutes. The benefits are comparable to those of sublingual drops.

LDN eye drops can be compounded as needed for dry eye, autoimmune, and/or inflammatory conditions.

LDN nasal sprays can be compounded for acute immune support or as preferred delivery system for regular use.

Dosing Definitions and Protocols

For reference, naltrexone dosages are described as ultra low dose (1-2 micrograms); very low dose (20-500 micrograms); low dose (0.5-10 milligrams); moderate dose (10-25 milligrams); and high dose (50 milligrams or more). Dosing protocols vary depending on the patient's illness.

Chronic Viral Infections or Long-COVID: Administering 1mg nightly is a reasonable strategy. Some patients may need a higher dose to gain symptom relief and others can only tolerate a lower dose.

Autoimmune Diseases: Start low and increase slowly: 1mg daily for the first 14 days, then increasing by 0.5/1mg every two weeks until maintenance dose is achieved (usually between 3 and 4.5mg).

Cancer: Administer 1.5mg daily for a week, then increase by 1.5mg weekly until at 4.5mg. As per the guidance of your clinician, dose four days on and three days off on a weekly cycle. Take break over the chemotherapy time as directed.

Chronic Pain: Start low and increase slowly: Administer 1mg daily for 14 days, then increase by 0.5/1mg every two weeks until the highest tolerated dose is reached. May need to split dose to twice daily dosing, at maximum 9-10mg daily for best response, especially if there is difficulty absorbing nutrients/medications or for those with a larger body weight.

Fertility/Pregnancy: Start low and increase slowly. Administer 1mg daily for 14 days, increasing by 0.5/1mg every two weeks until the highest tolerated dose is tolerated. Consult with an LDN clinician before taking LDN when pregnant.

Post-Traumatic Stress Disorder (PTSD)/Anxiety/Depression: Most mental health patients respond well to multiple doses of 0.06 mg/kg/bw, about 3 to 6 mg each dose, and many notice no benefit until they reach the 0.06 mg dose level. LDN must be used strategically in a manner that disrupts and suppresses the opioid system-based dissociation underlying these disorders. This disruption/suppression depends on maintaining a relatively constant serum blood level of LDN, which may require up to two or three doses taken during waking hours. The majority of mental health patients can tolerate starting at the full 0.06 mg dose ratio, but it is better to start at half that dose to minimize the possibility of negative side effects. Once a lower dose is well tolerated, the dose can usually be increased rapidly to the 0.06 mg dose range, taking a few days to a couple weeks. If there is a diagnosis of Dissociative Identity Disorder (DID – see pages 159-160 in *The LDN Book: Volume Two*), recent opiate addiction, or a known history of severe early neglect and abuse, one should provide psycho-education and proceed with more caution.

Traumatic Brain Injury (TBI): Recent acute TBI injuries will likely require aggressive treatment with higher doses of naltrexone (>50 mg) for several months or until symptoms improve, followed by a low dose regimen. In some cases, a transdermal application of LDN applied to the carotid artery with the patient lying down to increase the concentration of naltrexone delivered to the brain will be adequate. TBI in an advanced stage of recovery or mid concussions may be treated with the standard MH protocol.

Chronic Fatigue Syndrome/Myalgic Encephalomyelitis (CFS/ME)/Mast Cell Activation Syndrome (MCAS): Once or twice daily dosing could be prescribed, usually standard 1.5-4.5mg.

Allergies: Doses of 8 mg for up to three doses a day have been used by clinicians.

Children: Dosing is calculated by weight. Under 40kg: 0.1mg/kg: 0.1mg initially, increasing over a period of four weeks to optimum dose. Over 40kg: dose as adult.

Note: before prescribing for children, make sure parents/guardians are aware that LDN is an unlicensed medicine.

Opioid Weaning: The recommended dose of ultra-low dose naltrexone (ULDN) is 1 µg given twice daily. The general recommendation for opiate weaning is to taper by 10% monthly if a patient has been taking opiate medications longer than a year. A more aggressive weaning may be considered for a relatively opiate naïve patient (use not longer than weeks to months), such as decreasing by 10% weekly or more— as quickly as five weeks overall. This is a general approach and must be individualized to each patient. This must be done with a multidisciplinary approach utilizing primary care, pain management and other specialists to determine the appropriate treatment plan and closely monitor for adverse effects and need for greater support.

Dosing Time
LDN is generally taken in the evening, although morning dosing works well for those who experience sleep disturbance.

Drug Compatibility
LDN may be compatible with other mediations with the following precautions and caveats:

Biologics: As long as the patient is being monitored and stable before initiation, LDN is compatible with Daclizumab (Zinbryta), Dimethyl fumarate (Tecfidera) Fingolimod (Gilenya), Interferon beta-1a (Avonex, Rebif) Mitoxantrone (Novantrone), Natalizumab (Tysabri) Ocrelizumab (Ocrevus), Peginterferon beta-1a (Plegridy) Teriflunomide (Aubagio), Glatiramer acetate (Copaxone, Glatopa) Interferon beta-1b (Betaseron, Extavia), Tetracyclines, Aminoglycosides, compatible with caveats.

Steroids: Prednisone/Methylprednisolone is compatible as long as the daily dose is <20mg equivalent prednisolone and not being used for organ replacement anti-rejection therapy. Dexamethasone at any dose is compatible as long as it is being monitored by oncology.
LDN may be used with all other prescription only medications and over-the-counter medicines depending on patient disease

state and general clinical patient stability.
If taking short-acting painkillers like co-codamol (acetaminophen or paracetamol with codeine)/tramadol leave four- to six-hour gap before administering LDN. Use with caution with Ketamine.

LDN is **not compatible** with SR Morphines or analogs: MST, oxycontin, dipipanone, and fentanyl. It should also not be taken by patients on active clinical trials. Other incompatible drugs include: anti-rejection drugs, anti-tumor necrosis factor , PD1 inhibitors (Opdivo and Keytruda and all in class), and anti-cancer vaccines— CAR-T and equivalent plus all in class.

Patient Inclusion Criteria
Does the patient have a disease listed on the LDN Research Trust website as currently being treated, or is their disease autoimmune in nature? Blood tests are not required, including liver or renal function, due to the low dose prescribed.

Patient Exclusion Criteria
Concomitant opiate administration increases risk of induced withdrawal. Contraindicated in sustained release opiates or high doses. Switch to alternative pain control and/or leave four- to six-hour gap between opiate and LDN. Cautionary use with short acting opiates. Caution with alcohol and tramadol (Ultram).

Patient Special Considerations
Hashimoto's thyroiditis patients may require closer titration and testing of T3/T4 levels every four to eight weeks during initiation phase.

CFS/ME patients often experience flu-like symptoms and may need slower titration. If exacerbation of symptoms, decrease dose until able to tolerate titrate accordingly. MS patients often experience worsening of MS symptoms in the first eight weeks. This is normal and is often a sign of good long-term response.

Lyme disease patients on multiple antibiotics and DMARD agents should seek careful advice from and work with experienced providers and pharmacists before initiating LDN.

The LDN Research Trust has a list of pharmacies (https://www.ldnresearchtrust.org/ldn-pharmacists) and updated LDN Guides are added annually.

ACKNOWLEDGMENTS

I want to thank all the authors for writing their chapters and sharing their experiences and Michael Metivier and Paula Johnson for their excellent editing. Lastly and not least, thank you for reading it.

CONTRIBUTORS

Angus Dalgleish, FRCP FRCPath FMedSci

Professor Dalgleish is currently the Professor of Oncology at St. Georges, University of London, and Principal of the Institute for Cancer Vaccines and Immunotherapy (ICVI). He qualified in medicine from University College and Hospital with an intercalated Hons BSc in Anatomy with Professor JZ Young, FRS. He spent a year as a flying doctor in Mt. Isa, Australia, before joining the physician training program in Brisbane and then moving to Sydney to specialize in oncology. He returned to the UK to study viruses and cancer with Professor Robin Weiss FRS at the ICR. His research focused on the HIV receptor, pathogenesis, and an effective vaccine candidate in collaboration with Bionor (Norway). Whilst working as an MRC senior clinical research fellow he discovered that Thalidomide had major effects on the immune response which may be useful in HIV and cancer. This led to a long-term collaboration with Celgene, resulting in the discovery of Lenalidomide and Pomalidomide, now licensed for myeloma and lymphoma worldwide. For over twenty years he has researched cancer vaccines and immunotherapy for cancer and noted that *Mycobacterium vaccae* developed for TB corrected the immune deficiency seen in cancer patients. A subsequent development, now known as IMM-101, has shown activity in melanoma and pancreatic cancer and is in trials for these conditions as well as COVID. As a result of these studies, it became clear that good vitamin D3 levels were vital for a clinical response and that several other agents have significant benefit in cancer patients, including LDN.

Deanna Windham, DO

Dr. Windham is a proponent of the innate healing capacity of the human body. We don't heal with traditional approaches, she believes, because they focus solely on disease treatment and symptoms, while ignoring underlying factors that cause disease states to begin with. Another limiting factor to healing is breaking the body apart into isolated systems that ignore how the body works together for health or illness and must be treated as a whole. When all such factors are discovered and treated, healing is a natural state of human being.

Dr. Windham specializes in immune and autoimmune disorders, but treats all concerns with a holistic, integrative approach. She has utilized and is familiar with dozens of treatment modalities that she uses to treat each person individually. Throughout twenty years of practicing medicine, she has earned a reputation among patients and practitioners alike as being compassionate and caring and is sometimes called the Sherlock Holmes of medicine for her thoroughness and ability to investigate and find treatment options for even the most difficult cases.

Elizabeth Livengood, NMD

Dr. Livengood received her Doctorate of Naturopathic Medicine from Southwest College of Naturopathic Medicine and a master's in education from the University of Phoenix. She completed an integrative adult medicine residency where she learned about Low Dose Naltrexone and began teaching at the medical college. Dr. Livengood has also taught science, health, and yoga since 2002.

As a doctor, she has enjoyed work in community clinics, in private practice, and in various teaching capacities. She enjoys educating her patients, lecturing at conferences, and leading yoga classes, workshops, and teacher trainings. Her area of expertise is treating autoimmunity by integrating conventional and natural therapies, which range from cutting edge hair and collagen restoration to foundational nutrition and lifestyle therapies.

Dr. Livengood is a medical advisor for the LDN Research Trust, and an active member in her state association (AzNMA). She contributes regularly to professional publications and has two major writing projects in the works. Recently, she joined two podcasts focusing on a holistic approach to health from a mind/body/spirit perspective.

Yoon Hang "John" Kim, MD

Dr. Kim has been practicing integrative medicine and acupuncture since 1999. As a residential fellow at the University of Arizona, he trained with Dr. Andrew Weil, a world-renowned leader in the field of integrative medicine. His wrote about his decade of work as the director of an integrative medicine practice in the book *Tao of Healing: A Story of Georgia Integrative Medicine*. As an integrative health consultant to hospitals, academic institutions, and clinicians, Dr. Kim has helped to establish integrative medicine practices in many settings.

He is the founder of the Integrative Health Studies Certificate Program at the University of West Georgia, where he has also served as a member of the faculty. He is the author of two books and more than twenty articles on integrative medicine.

During his studies at the Medical College of Wisconsin, Dr. Kim was named a Howard Hughes Medical Research Fellow. After graduating, he undertook a residency in the Preventive Medicine Residency Program at the University of California, San Diego. Dr. Kim completed the UCLA Medical Acupuncture Training Program for Physicians, and holds a master's degree in Public Health (MPH) from San Diego State University.

Kent Holtorf, MD

Dr. Holtorf is the medical director of the Holtorf Medical Group, founder and medical director of the non-profit National Academy of Hypothyroidism, and founder of Integrative Peptides, which is dedicated to training physicians about groundbreaking peptide therapies and bringing doctors and patients the highest quality natural bioidentical peptides as supplements with unique delivery systems.

Dr. Holtorf is an internationally known lecturer, author, and innovator in cutting-edge research and treatments. He has personally trained numerous physicians across the country in the use of bioidentical hormones, thyroid replacement for complex hypothyroidism syndromes, peptide therapies, immune-modulatory strategies, stem cell, exosome and growth factor treatment, hormone replacement for complex endocrine dysfunction, and innovative treatments of chronic fatigue syndrome, fibromyalgia, Lyme disease, and other chronic infectious diseases, CIRS, neurodegenerative diseases, and many others.

He is a fellowship lecturer for A4M. He was the Endocrinology Expert for AOL Health and is a guest editor and peer-reviewer for the medical journals *Endocrine, Postgraduate Medicine*, and *Pharmacy Practice*. Dr. Holtorf has published many peer-reviewed endocrine reviews on complex, multisystem, poorly understood conditions. He has demonstrated that much of the long-held dogma in endocrinology and infectious disease is inaccurate.

He has been a featured guest on CNBC, ABC News, CNN, Fox News (debating the Fox news medical A-team), Good Morning America, The Today Show, EXTRA TV, Discovery Health, The Learning Channel, Glenn Beck, Nancy Grace, Sean Hannity, and more and quoted in numerous print media including the *Wall Street Journal, Los Angeles Times, US News and World Report, San Francisco Chronicle*, WebMD, *Forbes*, among many others.

Nasha Winters, ND, FABNO

Dr. Winters is a global healthcare authority and best-selling author in integrative cancer care and research consulting with physicians around the world. She has educated hundreds of professionals in the clinical use of mistletoe and has created robust educational programs for both healthcare institutions and the public on incorporating vetted integrative therapies in cancer care to enhance outcomes. Dr. Winters is currently focused on opening The Metabolic Terrain Institute of Health, a comprehensive metabolic oncology hospital and research institute in the United States where the best that standard of care has to offer and the most advanced integrative therapies will be offered. This facility will be in a residential setting on a gorgeous campus against a backdrop of regenerative farming, EMF mitigation and retreat, as well as state-of-the-art medical technology and data collection and evaluation to improve patient outcomes.

Pamela Wartian Smith, M.D., MPH, MS

Dr. Smith spent her first twenty years of practice as an emergency room physician with the Detroit Medical Center and then 28 years as an Anti-Aging/Functional Medicine specialist. She is a diplomat of the Board of the American Academy of Anti-Aging Physicians and is an internationally known speaker and author on the subject of Precision Medicine.

She also holds a master's in public health Degree along with a master's degree in metabolic and nutritional medicine. Dr. Smith is in private practice and is the senior partner for the Center for Precision Medicine with offices in Michigan and Florida. She has been featured on CNN, PBS, and many other television networks, has been interviewed in numerous consumer magazines, and has hosted two of her own radio shows.

Dr. Smith was one of the featured physicians on the PBS series "The Embrace of Aging" as well as the on-line medical series "Awakening from Alzheimer's" and "Regain Your Brain." Dr. Pamela Smith is the founder of the Fellowship in Anti-Aging, Regenerative, and Functional Medicine and is the past co-director of the master's program in metabolic and nutritional medicine at the Morsani College of Medicine, University of South Florida. She is the author of eleven best-selling books. Her book *What You Must Know About Vitamins, Minerals, Herbs, and So Much More* was published in 2019. Her newest book, *Max Your Immunity*, was published in 2021. Her new PBS/CNN special will air in fall 2022.

Sarah J. Zielsdorf MD, MS

Dr. Zielsdorf is the owner and medical director of Motivated Medicine, an innovative consultative medical practice in West Chicago, Illinois. She received a BA in microbiology from Miami University, an MS in public health, microbiology, and emerging infectious diseases from the George Washington University, and earned her MD at Loyola University Chicago Stritch School of Medicine. She completed her residency at Loyola University

Medical Center and the Edward Hines Jr. VA Hospital, is an Institute for Functional Medicine Certified Practitioner and board-certified in Internal Medicine.

The Motivated Medicine approach Dr. Z developed is rooted in Translational Medicine, which bridges the gap between current worldwide research and direct clinician care. Dr. Zielsdorf's open-minded approach to treatment is informed by data, advanced diagnostic testing, whole-body wellness, tried-and-true "conventional" medicine, and so much more. As an autoimmune thyroid patient herself, she understands that every individual is biochemically and genetically unique.

Dr. Zielsdorf is an author featured in *The LDN Book, Volume 2* and appeared in Dr. Izabella Wentz's documentary, *The Thyroid Secret*. She lectures nationally at universities and conferences on the subjects of the thyroid, microbiome, autoimmunity, and LDN. Dr. Zielsdorf serves as the education director and a medical and research advisor to the LDN Research Trust and has been a speaker at the International Low Dose Naltrexone Conferences since 2017.

Sebastian Denison, RPh, FAAR

Sebastian Denison received his BS in pharmacy at the University of British Columbia. He worked at Northmount Pharmacy in North Vancouver for eleven years, specializing in HRT, veterinary, pain, and sports compounding. He also was the manager of Pharmacy Operations with the 2010 Vancouver Winter Olympic/Paralympic Games, and then the manager of the Whistler Olympic Village Polyclinic Pharmacy. In addition to his role as a PCCA clinical compounding pharmacist, Sebastian works with both the U.S. and Canadian CORE compounding training education teams and the pharmacy student education team. Sebastian also speaks at physician, pharmacist, and other health care professional education symposiums and events. He has recently lectured for the American Academy of Anti-Aging Medicine on nutrition and pain, pharmacy compounding and collaborative practice, and alternative uses for Naltrexone. Sebastian is currently completing the Metabolic Medical Institute's Fellowship in metabolic and nutritional medicine.

J. Stephen Dickson BSC (hons) MRPharmS

Stephen Dickson has been working with LDN for over a decade in the United Kingdom. Working together with pharma partners in the industry to stabilize the supply chain and standardize methods of obtaining prescriptions in a safe and compliant manner. As well as running the well-established private medical department of Dickson Chemist, he also runs seven NHS pharmacies in Glasgow.

Stephen also works in several other businesses, owning a technology company responsible for dispensing the majority of the methadone in the UK in community pharmacy (MethaMeasure), and one of the largest online controlled drugs systems in the UK (CDRx). Stephen also is an advisor to Canidol pharmaceutics, a company dedicated to furthering the cause for medical cannabis in the UK and helped design the UK Cannabis Clinic Model for use in community pharmacy and primary care.

In his spare time, Stephen plays guitar in several bands (including a Ceilidh band), is on the board of directors of a semi-professional theatre group (where he generally functions as the costume guru), oversees their MethaMeasure North American operation and is a frequent speaker at the LDN conferences internationally.

Wai Liu, PhD

Dr. Wai Liu received his PhD in medical oncology from St. Bartholomew's Hospital, University of London in 2001. During this time, he developed models to assess the effect of combining chemotherapies with other treatment modalities as a way to enhance activity. Dr. Liu has worked in a cancer research environment for over twenty years. He is a prominent scientist in the field of cannabinoid research, an area he has actively engaged for over fifteen years. His team was the first to demonstrate a benefit in combining cannabinoids and irradiation in models of brain cancer. Other interests of Dr. Liu have been to develop new combination strategies that utilize repurposed agents. These have included naltrexone, artemisinins, and the IMiDs. He has also investigated ways of enhancing anticancer activity by modifying the pathological associations between immune and tumor cells by using immune-targeting drugs. He has over 60 publications in the field on cancer research, and worked in collaborations with pharma including GW Pharma, Celgene, AstraZeneca, and Novartis to develop new agents and to perform pre-clinical work. A number of these have continued successfully into Phase I and II trials. He is a Key Opinion leader on the use of cannabinoids as a cancer treatment, and he is regularly contacted by the media for his opinions on this fast-moving area.

Yusuf M. (JP) Saleeby, MD

Dr. Saleeby is a functional & integrative physician with offices in South Carolina. He is a graduate of the Medical College of Georgia and finished post-graduate training at East Carolina University School of Medicine. His first career was in emergency medicine and for his journey into integrative, holistic and functional medicine he embarked on a self-designed curriculum including memberships in A4M, ACAM, and AAMG.

He has been published in medical and fitness trade journals and has contributed chapters in a couple of books on preventive medicine and thyroid disorders. He also published a book on adaptogen herbs in 2006. Dr. Saleeby is a noted regional speaker on topics of functional medicine, autoimmune diseases and tick-borne illness. He is a medical advisor board member to the LDN Research Trust. Dr. Saleeby is a member of ILADS, AARM and IFM to name a few.

In 2018 Dr. Saleeby founded and is current director for the non-profit Priority Health Academy. The Academy's main goal is to educate advanced providers in functional medicine as well as host an annual symposium (in its fourth year as of July 2021). The academy also offers sub-internships to PAs and NPs. Dr. Saleeby has been at the forefront of telemedicine offering this type of virtual service since 2013. Dr. Saleeby and his team of highly trained advanced practitioners are available at the Carolina Holistic Medicine centers in Murrells Inlet, SC and Charleston, SC.

NOTES

Chapter One

1   H. Mørch and B. K. Pedersen, "Beta-Endorphin and the Immune System--Possible Role in Autoimmune Diseases," *Autoimmunity* 21, no. 3 (1995):161-71, https://doi.org/10.3109/08916939509008013

2   Ian Zagon and Patricia J. McLaughlin, "Endogenous Opioids in the Etiology and Treatment of Multiple Sclerosis," In: *Multiple Sclerosis: Perspectives in Treatment and Pathogenesis*, ed. Ian S. Zagon and Patricia J. McLaughlin (Brisbane (AU): Codon Publications; November 27, 2017), Chapter 8, https://doi.org/10.15586/codon.multiplesclerosis.2017.ch8

3   Salwa Refat El-Zayat, Hiba Sibaii and Fathia A. Mannaa, "Toll-Like Receptors Activation, Signaling and Targeting: An Overview," *Bulletin of National Research Centre* 43, no.187 (December 2019): https://doi.org/10.1186/s42269-019-0227-2

4   Editor - Linda Elsegood, "The LDN Book: How a Little-Known Generic Drug, Low Dose Naltrexone, Could Revolutionize Treatment for Autoimmune Diseases, Cancer, Autism, Depression, and More," (2016): White River Junction, Vermont: Chelsea Green Publishing.

5   A Benjamin Srivastava and Mark S Gold, "Naltrexone: A History and Future Directions," *Cerebrum* (September 1, 2018): cer-13-18, https://pubmed.ncbi.nlm.nih.gov/30746025/

6   A Benjamin Srivastava and Mark S Gold, "Naltrexone: A History and Future Directions," *Cerebrum* (September 1, 2018): cer-13-18, https://pubmed.ncbi.nlm.nih.gov/30746025/

7   Joseph Gal and Pedro Cintas, "Early History of the Recognition of Molecular Biochirality," *Topics in Current Chemistry* 333, (2013): 1-40, https://doi.org/10.1007/128_2012_406

8   Lien Ai Nguyen, Hua He and Chuong Pham-Huy, "Chiral Drugs: an Overview," *International Journal of Biomedical Science* 2, no. 2 (June 2006): 85-100, https://pubmed.ncbi.nlm.nih.gov/23674971/

9   Rachel Cant, Angus G Dalgleish and Rachel L Allen, "Naltrexone Inhibits IL-6 and TNFα Production in Human Immune Cell Subsets following Stimulation with Ligands for Intracellular Toll-Like Receptors," *Frontiers in Immunology* 8 (July 2017): 809, https://doi.org/10.3389/fimmu.2017.00809

10   Mark R Hutchinson et al., "Non-Stereoselective Reversal of Neuropathic Pain by Naloxone and Naltrexone: Involvement of Toll-Like Receptor 4 (TLR4)," *European Journal of Neuroscience* 28, no. 1 (July 2008): 20-9, https://doi.org/10.1111/j.1460-9568.2008.06321.x

11   Gemma Donovan et al., "Unlicensed Medicines Use: A UK Guideline Analysis Using AGREE II." *International Journal of Pharmacy Practice* 26, no. 6 (2018): 515–25, https://doi.org/10.1111/ijpp.12436

12   Alesha Wale et al., "Unlicensed "Special" Medicines: Understanding the Community Pharmacist Perspective," Integrated Pharmacy Research and Practice 9 (August 13, 2020): 93-104, https://doi.org/10.2147/IPRP. S263970

13   Gemma Donovan, Lindsay Parkin and Scott Wilkes, "Special Unlicensed Medicines: What We Do and Do Not Know About Them," *British Journal of General Practice* 65, no. 641 (December 2015): e861-e863, https://doi.org/10.3399/bjgp15X688033

Chapter Two

14   Eléonore Beurel, Marisa Toups and Charles B. Nemeroff, "The Bidirectional Relationship of Depression and Inflammation: Double Trouble," *Neuron* 107, no. 2 (July 2020): 234-56, https://doi. org/10.1016/j.neuron.2020.06.002

15   Eléonore Beurel, Marisa Toups and Charles B. Nemeroff, "The Bidirectional Relationship of Depression and Inflammation: Double Trouble," *Neuron* 107, no. 2 (July 2020): 234-56, https://doi. org/10.1016/j.neuron.2020.06.002

16   David Mischoulon, "S-Adenosylmethionine (SAMe) for Depression: What Does the Evidence Say?," *Natural Medications in Psychiatry* (September 6, 2018): https://psychopharmacologyinstitute.com/section/ s-adenosylmethionine-same-for-depression-what-does-the-evidence-say-2066-4181

17   S. R. Maxwell, "Coronary Artery Disease - Free Radical Damage, Antioxidant Protection and the Role of Homocysteine," *Basic Research in Cardiology* 95, Suppl 1 (2000): I65–I71, https://doi.org/10.1007/ s003950070012

18   Tengfei Luo et al., "De Novo Mutations in Folate-Related Genes Associated with Common Developmental Disorders," *Computational and Structural Biotechnology Journal* 19, (2021): 1414–22, https://doi. org/10.1016/j.csbj.2021.02.011

19   Eléonore Beurel, Marisa Toups and Charles B. Nemeroff, "The Bidirectional Relationship of Depression and Inflammation: Double Trouble," *Neuron* 107, no. 2 (July 2020): 234-56, https://doi. org/10.1016/j.neuron.2020.06.002

20   Benjamin E Deverman and Paul H Patterson, "Cytokines and CNS Development," *Neuron* 64, no.1, (2009 Oct 15): 61-78, https://doi. org/10.1016/j.neuron.2009.09.002

21 Eléonore Beurel, Marisa Toups and Charles B. Nemeroff, "The Bidirectional Relationship of Depression and Inflammation: Double Trouble," *Neuron* 107, no. 2 (July 2020): 234-56, https://doi.org/10.1016/j.neuron.2020.06.002

22 Eléonore Beurel, Marisa Toups and Charles B. Nemeroff, "The Bidirectional Relationship of Depression and Inflammation: Double Trouble," *Neuron* 107, no. 2 (July 2020): 234-56, https://doi.org/10.1016/j.neuron.2020.06.002

23 Samuel R Chamberlain et al., "Treatment-Resistant Depression and Peripheral C-Reactive Protein," *British Journal of Psychiatry* 214, no. 1 (January 2019): 11-19, https://doi.org/10.1192/bjp.2018.66

24 Gregory E. Miller and Steve W. Cole, "Clustering of Depression and Inflammation in Adolescents Previously Exposed to Childhood Adversity," *Biological Psychiatry* 72, no. 1 (July 2012): 34-40, https://doi.org/10.1016/j.biopsych.2012.02.034

25 L. Eugene Arnold, Nicholas Lofthouse, and Elizabeth Hurt, "Artificial Food Colors and Attention-Deficit/Hyperactivity Symptoms: Conclusions to Dye For," *Neurotherapeutics* 9, no. 3 (July 2012): 599–609, https://doi.org/10.1007/s13311-012-0133-x

26 Gregory E. Miller and Steve W. Cole, "Clustering of Depression and Inflammation in Adolescents Previously Exposed to Childhood Adversity," *Biological Psychiatry* 72, no. 1 (July 2012): 34-40, https://doi.org/10.1016/j.biopsych.2012.02.034

27 Gotthard G. Tribl, Thomas C. Wetter and Michael Schredl, "Dreaming Under Antidepressants: A Systematic Review on Evidence in Depressive Patients and Healthy Volunteers," *Sleep Medicine Reviews* 17, no. 2 (April 2013): 133-42, https://doi.org/10.1016/j.smrv.2012.05.001

28 Luciana Besedovsky, Tanja Lange, and Jan Born . "Sleep and Immune Function," *Pflügers Archiv - European Journal of Physiology* 463 (2012): 121–137, https://doi.org/10.1007/s00424-011-1044-0

29 Baland Jalal, "The Neuropharmacology of Sleep Paralysis Hallucinations: Serotonin 2A Activation and a Novel Therapeutic Drug," *Psychopharmacology* 235, no. 11 (Nov 2018): 3083-91, https://doi.org/10.1007/s00213-018-5042-1

30 Jon Johnson, Reviewed by Deborah Weatherspoon, "What to Know About Deep Sleep," *Medical news Today* (June 2019): https://www.medicalnewstoday.com/articles/325363#stage-two (11 Dec 2021)

31 Gebrehiwot Abraham, Roumen Milev and J. Stuart Lawson, "T3 Augmentation of SSRI Resistant Depression," *Journal of Affective Disorders* 91, no's 2-3 (April 2006): 211-5, https://doi.org/10.1016/j.jad.2006.01.013

32   Rena Cooper and Bernard Lerer, "The Use of Thyroid Hormones in the
      Treatment of Depression," *Harefuah* 149, no. 8 (August 2010): 529-34,
      549-50, https://pubmed.ncbi.nlm.nih.gov/21341434/

33   Qi Gao et al., "The Association Between Vitamin D eficiency and Sleep
      Disorders: A Systematic Review and Meta-Analysis," *Nutrients* 10, no.
      10 (October 2018): 1395, https://doi.org/10.3390/nu10101395

Chapter Three

34   Guang Zeng et al., "Infectivity of Severe Acute Respiratory Syndrome
      During its Incubation Period", *Biomedical and Environmental Sciences*
      22, no.6 (December 2009): 502-10, https://doi.org/10.1016/S0895-
      3988(10)60008-6

35   David S.C. Hui and Alimuddin Zumla, "Severe Acute Respiratory
      Syndrome: Historical, Epidemiologic, and Clinical Features," *Infectious
      Disease Clinics of North America* 33, no. 4, (December 2019): 869-89,
      https://doi.org/10.1016/j.idc.2019.07.001

36   Gregory Juckett, "Avian Influenza: Preparing for a Pandemic," *American
      Family Physician* 74, no. 5 (September 2006): 783-90, https://www.aafp.
      org/pubs/afp/issues/2006/0901/p783.html

37   Anita Patel et al., "Personal Protective Equipment Supply Chain:
      Lessons Learned from Recent Public Health Emergency Responses,"
      Health Security 15, no. 3 (June 2017): 244-52, https://doi.org/10.1089/
      hs.2016.0129

38   Eric Holderman, comment on "COVID-19: Not a Once-In-100-Years
      Event," *Disaster Zone, Government Technology*, posted 25 April 2020,
      https://www.govtech.com/em/emergency-blogs/disaster-zone/COVID19-
      not-a-once-in-100-years-event.html

39   Lawrence O Gostin and Jennifer B Nuzzo, "Twenty Years After the
      Anthrax Terrorist Attacks of 2001: Lessons Learned and Unlearned
      for the COVID-19 Response," *Georgetown Law Faculty Publications
      and Other Works, (October* 2021): 2417, https://doi.org/10.1001/
      jama.2021.19292

40   Gregory Juckett, "Avian Influenza: Preparing for a Pandemic," *American
      Family Physician* 74, no. 5 (September 2006): 783-90, https://www.aafp.
      org/pubs/afp/issues/2006/0901/p783.html

41   Hyunsuh Kim, Robert G. Webster, and Richard J. Webby, "Influenza
      Virus: Dealing with a Drifting and Shifting Pathogen," *Viral
      Immunology* 31, no. 2 (March 2018): 174-83, https://doi.org/10.1089/
      vim.2017.0141

42   George Santayana, "Reason in common sense." *Constable* 1, (1910).

43   Matthew Corbitt et al., "A Systematic Review of Cytokines in Chronic

Fatigue Syndrome/Myalgic Encephalomyelitis/Systemic Exertion Intolerance Disease (CFS/ME/SEID)," *BMC Neurology* 19, no. 207, (August 2019): https://doi.org/10.1186/s12883-019-1433-0

44 Tiansong Yang et al., "The Clinical Value of Cytokines in Chronic Fatigue Syndrome," *Journal of Translational Medicine* 17, no. 213, (June 2019): https://doi.org/10.1186/s12967-019-1948-6

45 Matthew Corbitt et al., "A Systematic Review of Cytokines in Chronic Fatigue Syndrome/Myalgic Encephalomyelitis/Systemic Exertion Intolerance Disease (CFS/ME/SEID)," *BMC Neurology* 19, no. 207 (2019): https://doi.org/10.1186/s12883-019-1433-0

46 Leslie A Hoffman and Joel A Vilensky, "Encephalitis Lethargica: 100 Years After the Epidemic," *Brain* 140, no. 8 (August 2017): 2246–51, https://doi.org/10.1093/brain/awx177

47 Leslie A Hoffman and Joel A Vilensky, "Encephalitis Lethargica: 100 Years After the Epidemic," *Brain* 140, no. 8 (August 2017): 2246–51, https://doi.org/10.1093/brain/awx177

48 Leslie A Hoffman and Joel A Vilensky, "Encephalitis Lethargica: 100 Years After the Epidemic," *Brain* 140, no. 8 (August 2017): 2246–51, https://doi.org/10.1093/brain/awx177

49 O.W. Sacks, "Postencephalitic Syndromes," In: Stern G, editor, Parkinson's Disease. Chapman & Hall, London, (1990): 415–28.

50 Leslie A Hoffman and Joel A Vilensky, "Encephalitis Lethargica: 100 Years After the Epidemic," *Brain* 140, no. 8 (August 2017): 2246–51, https://doi.org/10.1093/brain/awx177

51 Matthew Corbitt et al., "A Systematic Review of Cytokines in Chronic Fatigue Syndrome/Myalgic Encephalomyelitis/Systemic Exertion Intolerance Disease (CFS/ME/SEID)," *BMC Neurology* 19, no. 207 (2019): https://doi.org/10.1186/s12883-019-1433-0

52 Emily A Troyer, Jordan N Kohn and Suzi Hong, "Are We Facing a Crashing Wave of Neuropsychiatric Sequelae of COVID-19? Neuropsychiatric Symptoms and Potential Immunologic Mechanisms," *Brain, Behavior and Immunity* 87, (2020): 34-39, https://doi.org/10.1016/j.bbi.2020.04.027

53 Nicholas Kadar, Roberto Romero and Zoltán Papp, " Ignaz Semmelweis: The 'Savior Of Mothers': On The 200th Anniversary of His Birth," *American Journal of Obstetrics and Gynecology* 219, no. 6 (2018): 519–22, https://doi.org/10.1016/j.ajog.2018.10.036

54 Andreas Goebel et al., "Passive Transfer of Fibromyalgia Symptoms from Patients to Mice," *Journal of Clinical Investigation* 131, no. 13 (July 2021): e144201, https://doi.org/10.1172/JCI144201

55 Giusy Rita Maria La Rosa et al., "Association of Viral Infections

with Oral Cavity Lesions: Role of SARS-CoV-2 Infection," *Frontiers in Medicine* 7, (Jan 2021): 571214, https://doi.org/10.3389/fmed.2020.571214

56 Michael S.Nirenberg and María del Mar RuizHerrera, "Foot Manifestations in a Patient with COVID-19 and Epstein-Barr Virus: A Case Study," *The Foot* (Edinburgh, Scotland) 46, (2021): 101707, https://doi.org/10.1016/j.foot.2020.101707

57 Michael H. Hauer and Susan M. Gasser, "Chromatin and Nucleosome Dynamics in DNA Damage and Repair," *Genes & Development* 31, no. 22 (2017): 2204-21, https://doi.org/10.1101/gad.307702.117

58 Annamaria Hadnagy, Raymond Beaulieu and Danuta Balicki, "Histone Tail Modifications and Noncanonical Functions of Histones: Perspectives in Cancer Epigenetics," *Molecular Cancer Therapeutics* 7, no.4 (April 2008): 740-8, https://doi.org/10.1158/1535-7163.MCT-07-2284

59 Anna K. Serquiña, Joseph M. Ziegelbauer, "How Herpes Viruses Pass on their Genomes," *The Journal of Cell Biology* 216, no. 9 (2017): 2611-13, https://doi.org/10.1083/jcb.201708077

60 JingpingYangVictor G.Corces, "Chromatin Insulators: A Role in Nuclear Organization and Gene Expression," *Advances In Cancer Research* 110, (2011): 43-76, https://doi.org/10.1016/B978-0-12-386469-7.00003-7

61 Petros Kolovos et al., "Enhancers and Silencers: An Integrated and Simple Model for Their Function," *Epigenetics & Chromatin* 5, no. 1 (2012): https://doi.org/10.1186/1756-8935-5-1

62 Iain R. Konigsberg et al., "Host Methylation Predicts SARS-Cov-2 Infection and Clinical Outcome," *Communications Medicine* 1, no. 42 (2021): https://doi.org/10.1038/s43856-021-00042-y

63 Abeer M. Mahmoud and Mohamed M. Ali, "Methyl Donor Micronutrients that Modify DNA Methylation and Cancer Outcome," *Nutrients* 11, no. 3 (March 2019): 608, https://doi.org/10.3390/nu11030608

64 Ya-Fang Chiu et al., "Kaposi's sarcoma–associated herpesvirus stably clusters its genomes across generations to maintain itself extrachromosomally," *Journal of Cell Biology* 216, no. 9 (September 2017): 2745–58, https://doi.org/10.1083/jcb.201702013

65 R Sahaya Glingston et al., "Organelle Dynamics and Viral Infections: At Cross Roads," *Microbes and Infection* 21, no. 1 (2019): 20-32, https://doi.org/10.1016/j.micinf.2018.06.002

66 Jarred Younger, Luke Parkitny and David McLain, "The Use of Low-Dose Naltrexone (LDN) as a Novel Anti-Inflammatory Treatment for Chronic Pain," *Clinical Rheumatology* 33, no. 4 (April 2014): 451-9,

https://doi.org/10.1007/s10067-014-2517-2

67   Andreas Goebel et al., "Passive Transfer of Fibromyalgia Symptoms from Patients to Mice," *Journal of Clinical Investigation* 131, no. 13 (July 2021): e144201, https://doi.org/10.1172/JCI144201

68   Vincenzo Panichi et al., "Effects of Calcitriol on the Immune System: New Possibilities in the Treatment of Glomerulonephritis," *Clinical and Experimental Pharmacology & Physiology* 30, no. 11 (2003): 807-11, https://doi.org/10.1046/j.1440-1681.2003.03919.x

69   Joaquim Oristrell et al., "Association of Calcitriol Supplementation with Reduced COVID-19 Mortality in Patients with Chronic Kidney Disease: A Population-Based Study," *Biomedicines* 9, no. 5 (2021): 509, https://doi.org/10.3390/biomedicines9050509

70   Ravi Thadhani, "Is Calcitriol Life-Protective for Patients with Chronic Kidney Disease?" *Clinical Journal of the American Society of Nephrology* 20, no. 11 (November 2009): 2285-90, https://doi.org/10.1681/ASN.2009050494

71   Michal L. Melamed and Ravi I. Thadhani, "Vitamin D Therapy in Chronic Kidney Disease and End Stage Renal Disease," *Clinical Journal of the American Society of Nephrology* 7, no. 2 (2012): 358-65, https://doi.org/10.2215/CJN.04040411

72   Dominique Prié et al., "Plasma Fibroblast Growth Factor 23 Concentration is Increased and Predicts Mortality in Patients on the Liver-Transplant Waiting List," *PLoS ONE* 8, no.6 (June 2013): e66182, https://doi.org/10.1371/journal.pone.0066182

73   Maria L. Mace, Klaus Olgaard and Ewa Lewin, "New Aspects of the Kidney in the Regulation of Fibroblast Growth Factor 23 (FGF23) and Mineral Homeostasis," *International Journal of Molecular Sciences* 21, no. 22 (November 2020): 8810, https://doi.org/10.3390/ijms21228810

74   Boxiang Gui et al., "Effects of Calcitriol (1, 25-dihydroxy-vitamin D3) on the Inflammatory Response Induced by H9N2 Influenza Virus Infection in Human Lung A549 Epithelial Cells and in Mice," *Virology Journal* 14, no.10 (2017): https://doi.org/10.1186/s12985-017-0683-y

75   Stanislav R. Kurpe et al., "Antimicrobial and Amyloidogenic Activity of Peptides. Can Antimicrobial Peptides Be Used against SARS-CoV-2?" *International Journal of Molecular Sciences* 21, no. 24 (December 2020): 9552, https://doi.org/10.3390/ijms21249552

76   Carlos Antonio Amado Diago et al.,., "Calcitriol-Modulated Human Antibiotics: New Pathophysiological Aspects of Vitamin D," *Endocrinología y Nutrición* 63, no. 2 (March 2016): 87-94, https://doi.org/10.1016/j.endoen.2016.02.003

77   Danmei Su et al., "Vitamin D Signaling through Induction of Paneth Cell

Defensins Maintains Gut Microbiota and Improves Metabolic Disorders and Hepatic Steatosis in Animal Models," *Frontiers in Physiology* 7, no. 498 (November 2016): https://doi.org/10.3389/fphys.2016.00498

78   Yilan Zeng et al., "Vitamin D Signaling Maintains Intestinal Innate Immunity and Gut Microbiota: Potential Intervention for Metabolic Syndrome and NAFLD," *American Journal of Physiology. Gastrointestinal and Liver Physiology* 318, no. 3 (2020): G542-G553, https://doi.org/10.1152/ajpgi.00286.2019

79   Melissa Bersanelli, Alessandro Leonetti & Sebastiano Buti, "The Link Between Calcitriol and Anticancer Immunotherapy: Vitamin D as the Possible Balance Between Inflammation and Autoimmunity in the Immune-Checkpoint Blockade," *Immunotherapy* 9, no, 14 (2017):1127-31, https://doi.org/10.2217/imt-2017-0127

80   Masae Iwasaki et al., "Inflammation Triggered by SARS-CoV-2 and ACE2 Augment Drives Multiple Organ Failure of Severe COVID-19: Molecular Mechanisms and Implications," *Inflammation* 44, (2021): 13–34, https://doi.org/10.1007/s10753-020-01337-3

81   Shahanshah Khan et al., "SARS-CoV-2 Spike Protein Induces Inflammation via TLR2-Dependent Activation of the NF-κB Pathway," *bioRxiv* 3, no.16 (2021): 435700, https://doi.org/10.1101/2021.03.16.435700

82   Andrew J..Kwilasz et al., "Experimental Autoimmune Encephalopathy (EAE)-Induced Hippocampal Neuroinflammation and Memory Deficits are Prevented with the Non-Opioid TLR2/TLR4 Antagonist (+)-Naltrexone," *Behavioural Brain Research* 396, (2021): 112896, https://doi.org/10.1016/j.bbr.2020.112896

83   Linda Watkins, University of Colorado at Boulder, Boulder, CO, United States, 2021, "Targeting Toll Like Receptor 4 (TLR4) and TLR2 to Resolve EAE-Associated Paralysis, Pain and Cognitive Deficits: Efficacy of a Clinically-Relevant Blood Brain Permeable TLR4/TLR2 Antagonist,*"* 2016 NIH Grant Application.

84   Ganna Petruk et al., "SARS-CoV-2 Spike Protein Binds to Bacterial Lipopolysaccharide and Boosts Proinflammatory Activity," *Journal of Molecular Cell Biology* 12, no.12 (2020): 916-32, https://doi.org/10.1093/jmcb/mjaa067

85   Lize M. Grobbelaar et al., "SARS-CoV-2 Spike Protein S1 Induces Fibrin(Ogen) Resistant to Fibrinolysis: Implications for Microclot Formation in COVID-19," *medRxiv* (2021), https://doi.org/10.1101/2021.03.05.21252960

86   Mary Hongying Cheng et al., "Superantigenic Character of an Insert Unique to SARS-Cov-2 Spike Supported by Skewed TCR Repertoire

in Patients with Hyperinflammation," *Proceedings of the National Academy of Sciences* 117, no. 41 (October 2020): 25254-62, https://doi.org/10.1073/pnas.2010722117

87   Carlos A.Cañas et al., "Biomedical Applications of Snake Venom: From Basic Science to Autoimmunity and Rheumatology," *Journal of Translational Autoimmunity* 4, (2021): 100076, https://doi.org/10.1016/j.jtauto.2020.100076

88   Gayle J. Pageau et al., "The Disappearing Barr Body in Breast and Ovarian Cancers," *Nature Reviews Cancer* 7, (September 2007): 628-33, https://doi.org/10.1038/nrc2172

89   Manasi S. Apte andVictoria H. Meller, "Sex Differences in Drosophila Melanogaster Heterochromatin are Regulated by Non-Sex Specific Factors," *PLoS ONE* 10, no. 6 (June 2015): e0128114, https://doi.org/10.1371/journal.pone.0128114

90   Bo Hong et al., "Identification of an Autoimmune Serum Containing Antibodies Against the Barr Body," *Proceedings of the National Academy of Sciences* 98, no. 15 (July 2001): 8703-8, https://doi.org/10.1073/pnas.151259598

91   Jeffrey I. Cohen, "Herpes virus Latency," *Journal of Clinical Investigation* 130, no. 7 (May 2020): 3361-69, https://doi.org/10.1172/JCI136225 .

92   Jeffrey E. Gold et al., "Investigation of Long COVID Prevalence and Its Relationship to Epstein-Barr Virus Reactivation," *Pathogens* 10, no.6 (June 2021): 763, https://doi.org/10.3390/pathogens10060763

93   Jeffrey E. Gold et al., "Investigation of Long COVID Prevalence and its Relationship to Epstein-Barr Virus Reactivation," *Pathogens* 10, no.6 (June 2021): 763, https://doi.org/10.3390/pathogens10060763

94   Eleonora Forte et al., "Cytomegalovirus Latency and Reactivation: An Intricate Interplay With the Host Immune Response," *Frontiers in Cellular and Infection Microbiology*, (March 2020): https://doi.org/10.3389/fcimb.2020.00130

95   Francesco Drago et al., "Oral and Cutaneous Manifestations of Viral and Bacterial Infections: Not Only COVID-19 Disease," *Clinics in Dermatology* 39, no. 3 (2021): 384-404, https://doi.org/10.1016/j.clindermatol.2021.01.021

96   Jon B.Suzich and Anna R.Cliffe, "Strength in Diversity: Understanding the Pathways to Herpes Simplex Virus Reactivation," *Virology* 522 (September 2018): 81-91, https://doi.org/10.1016/j.virol.2018.07.011

97   David Kilpatrick and Abbas Vafai, "COVID-19 Infection Can Lead to the Reactivation of Varicella-Zoster Virus," *Viro Research*, (January 2, 2022): https://viroresearch.com/COVID-19-infection-can-lead-to-the-

reactivation-of-varicella-zoster-virus/

98   Kristina von Kietzell et al., "Antibody-Mediated Enhancement of Parvovirus B19 Uptake into Endothelial Cells Mediated by a Receptor for Complement Factor C1q," *Journal of Virology* 88, no. 14 (2014): 8102-15, https://doi.org/10.1128/JVI.00649-14

99   Francesco Drago et al., "Oral and Cutaneous Manifestations of Viral and Bacterial Infections: Not Only COVID-19 Disease," *Clinics in Dermatology* 39, no. 3 (2021): 384-404, https://doi.org/10.1016/j. clindermatol.2021.01.021

100 Francesco Drago et al., "Oral and Cutaneous Manifestations of Viral and Bacterial Infections: Not Only COVID-19 Disease," *Clinics in Dermatology* 39, no. 3 (2021): 384-404, https://doi.org/10.1016/j. clindermatol.2021.01.021

101 Anna K. Serquiña and Joseph M. Ziegelbauer, "How Herpes viruses Pass on their Genomes," *The Journal of Cell Biology* 216, no. 9 (2017): 2611-13, https://doi.org/10.1083/jcb.201708077

102 Jonathan R Kerr, "Epstein-Barr Virus (EBV) Reactivation and Therapeutic Inhibitors," *Journal of Clinical Pathology* 72, no. 10 (2019): 651-58, https://doi.org/10.1136/jclinpath-2019-205822

103 Julianna S. Deakyne et al., "Structural and Functional Basis for an EBNA1 Hexameric Ring in Epstein-Barr Virus Episome Maintenance," *Journal of Virology* 91, no. 19 (September 2017): https://doi. org/10.1128/JVI.01046-17

104 Stephanie A. Moquin et al., "The Epstein-Barr Virus Episome Maneuvers between Nuclear Chromatin Compartments during Reactivation," *Journal of Virology* 92, no. 3 (January 2018): https://doi. org/10.1128/JVI.01413-17

105 Jeffrey E. Gold et al., "Investigation of Long COVID Prevalence and Its Relationship to Epstein-Barr Virus Reactivation," *Pathogens (Basel, Switzerland)* 10, no.6 (June 2021): 763, https://doi.org/10.3390/ pathogens10060763

106 Guitao Zhang et al., "Enhanced IL-6/IL-6R Signaling Promotes Growth and Malignant Properties in EBV-Infected Premalignant and Cancerous Nasopharyngeal Epithelial Cells," *PLoS ONE* 8, no. 5 (May 2013): e62284, https://doi.org/10.1371/journal.pone.0062284

107 Georg Franz Lehner et al., "Correlation of Interleukin-6 With Epstein-Barr Virus Levels in COVID-19," *Critical Care (London, England)* 24, no. 657 (November 2020): https://doi.org/10.1186/s13054-020-03384-6

108 Paolo Antonio Ascierto, Binqing Fu and Haiming Wei, "IL-6 Modulation for COVID-19: The Right Patients at the Right Time?" *Journal for ImmunoTherapy of Cancer* 9, no. 4 (2021): e002285, https://doi.

org/10.1136/jitc-2020-002285

109 B Rostkowska-Nadolska et al. "Vitamin D Derivatives: Calcitriol and Tacalcitol Inhibits Interleukin-6 and Interleukin-8 Expression in Human Nasal Polyp Fibroblast Cultures," *Advances in Medical Sciences* 55, no. 1 (2010): 86-92, https://doi.org/10.2478/v10039-010-0012-9

110 Chun-Te Wu et al., "Effect of 1α,25-Dihydroxyvitamin D3 on the Radiation Response in Prostate Cancer: Association With IL-6 Signaling," *Frontiers in Oncology* 11, (May 2021): 619365, https://doi.org/10.3389/fonc.2021.619365

111 Ping-Tsung Chen et al., "1α,25-Dihydroxyvitamin D3 Inhibits Esophageal Squamous Cell Carcinoma Progression by Reducing IL6 Signaling," *Molecular Cancer Therapeutics* 14, no. 6 (June 2015):1365-1375, https://doi.org/10.1158/1535-7163.MCT-14-0952

112 Xavier Nogues et al., "Calcifediol Treatment and COVID-19-Related Outcomes," *The Journal of Clinical Endocrinology and Metabolism* 106, no. 10 (October 2021): e4017-e4027, https://doi.org/10.1210/clinem/dgab405

113 Carlos Loucera et al., "Real world evidence of calcifediol or vitamin D prescription and mortality rate of COVID-19 in a retrospective cohort of hospitalized Andalusian patients," *Scientific Reports* 11, no. 23380 (December 2021): https://doi.org/10.1038/s41598-021-02701-5

114 Philipp Koehler et al., "Defining and Managing COVID-19-Associated Pulmonary Aspergillosis: The 2020 ECMM/ISHAM Consensus Criteria for Research and Clinical Guidance," *The Lancet Infectious Diseases* 21, no. 6 (December 2020): E149-E162, HTTPS://DOI.ORG/10.1016/S1473-3099(20)30847-1

115 Sanjay Kalra, Atul Kalhan and Zhanay A Akanov, "COVID-and Endocrinology – A Bidirectional Relationship," *Touch Endocrinology* (March 30, 2020): https://www.touchendocrinology.com/insight/COVID-19-and-endocrinology-a-bidirectional-relationship/

116 Li Hi Shing S. et al. "Post-polio Syndrome: More Than Just a Lower Motor Neuron Disease," *Frontiers in Neurology* 10, no. 773 (July 2019): https://doi.org/10.3389/fneur.2019.00773

117 Jung, H.E., Lee, H.K., "Current Understanding of the Innate Control of Toll-like Receptors in Response to SARS-CoV-2 Infection," Viruses 13, no. 11 (October 2021): 2132, https://doi.org/10.3390/v13112132

118 Yingchi Zhao et al., "SARS-Cov-2 Spike Protein Interacts with and Activates TLR4," *Cell Research* 31, (2021): 818–20, https://doi.org/10.1038/s41422-021-00495-9

119 Glassman, P.M., Muzykantov V.R., "Pharmacokinetic and Pharmacodynamic Properties of Drug Delivery Systems," *The Journal*

of Pharmacology and Experimental Therapeutics 370, no.3 (September 2019): 570-80, https://doi.org/10.1124/jpet.119.257113

120 Jatta Huotari and Ari Helenius, "Endosome Maturation," *The EMBO Journal* 30, (August 2011): 3481-500, https://doi.org/10.1038/emboj.2011.286

121 Bruce K. Patterson et al., "Persistence of SARS CoV-2 S1 Protein in CD16+ Monocytes in Post-Acute Sequelae of COVID-19 (PASC) Up to 15 Months Post-Infection," *bioRxiv* 6, no. 25 (June 2021): 449905, https://doi.org/10.1101/2021.06.25.449905

122 Bruce K. Patterson et al., "Persistence of SARS CoV-2 S1 Protein in CD16+ Monocytes in Post-Acute Sequelae of COVID-19 (PASC) Up to 15 Months Post-Infection," *bioRxiv* 6, no. 25 (June 2021): 449905, https://doi.org/10.1101/2021.06.25.449905

123 SF Yanuck et al., "Evidence Supporting a Phased Immuno-physiological Approach to COVID-19 From Prevention Through Recovery," *Integrative medicine (Encinitas)* 19, Suppl no.1 (May 2020): 8-35, https://pubmed.ncbi.nlm.nih.gov/32425712/

124 R.Miller, A.R.Wentzel and G.A.Richards, "COVID-19: NAD^+ Deficiency May Predispose the Aged, Obese and Type2 Diabetics to Mortality Through its Effect on SIRT1 Activity," *Medical Hypotheses* 144, (November 2020): 110044, https://doi.org/10.1016/j.mehy.2020.110044

125 Undurti N.Das, "Bioactive Lipids in COVID-19-Further Evidence," *Archives of Medical Research* 52, no.1 (2021): 107-20, https://doi.org/10.1016/j.arcmed.2020.09.006

126 Yanuck, S.F. et al., "Evidence Supporting a Phased Immuno-physiological Approach to COVID-19 From Prevention Through Recovery," *Integrative Medicine (Encinitas)* 19, Suppl no.1 (2020): 8-35, https://pubmed.ncbi.nlm.nih.gov/32425712/

127 Yanuck, S.F. et al., "Evidence Supporting a Phased Immuno-physiological Approach to COVID-19 From Prevention Through Recovery," *Integrative medicine (Encinitas)* 19, Suppl no.1 (2020): 8-35, https://pubmed.ncbi.nlm.nih.gov/32425712/

128 Yanuck, S.F. et al., "Evidence Supporting a Phased Immuno-physiological Approach to COVID-19 From Prevention Through Recovery," *Integrative medicine (Encinitas)* 19, Suppl no.1 (2020): 8-35, https://pubmed.ncbi.nlm.nih.gov/32425712/

129 Yanuck, S.F. et al., "Evidence Supporting a Phased Immuno-physiological Approach to COVID-19 From Prevention Through Recovery," *Integrative medicine (Encinitas)* 19, Suppl no.1 (2020): 8-35, https://pubmed.ncbi.nlm.nih.gov/32425712/

130 Jonathan R Kerr, "Epstein-Barr Virus (EBV) Reactivation and Therapeutic inhibitors," *Journal of Clinical Pathology* 72, no. 10 (2019): 651-58, https://doi.org/10.1136/jclinpath-2019-205822

131 Jonathan R Kerr, "Epstein-Barr Virus (EBV) Reactivation and Therapeutic Inhibitors," *Journal of Clinical Pathology* 72, no. 10 (2019): 651-58, https://doi.org/10.1136/jclinpath-2019-205822

Chapter Four

132 Megan Gannon, "China's First Emperor Ordered Official Search for Immortality Elixir," *Live Science,* (December 27, 2017): https://www.livescience.com/61286-first-chinese-emperor-sought-immortality.html

133 Dave Asprey, "Super Human: The Bulletproof Plan to Age Backward and Maybe Even Live Forever," *Harper Wave* (October 1, 2019): Bulletproof, 5

134 Emily Willingham, "Humans Could Live up to 150 Years, New Research Suggests," *Scientific American*, December 18, 2021, https://www.scientificamerican.com/article/humans-could-live-up-to-150-years-new-research-suggests/

135 Elie Dolgin, "There's No Limit to Longevity, Says Study That Revives Human Lifespan Debate," *Nature 559, (2018):* 14–15, https://doi.org/10.1038/d41586-018-05582-3

136 Jennifer Welsh, "Extending Life: 7 Ways to Live Past 100," *Livescience,* (December 06, 2011): https://www.livescience.com/17314-tips-live-longer-longevity.html

137 Philip Hunter, "The Inflammation Theory of Disease," *EMBO Reports* 13, no. 11, (November 1, 2012): 968–70, https://doi.org/10.1038/embor.2012.142

138 Denham Harman, "Aging: A Theory Based on Free Radical and Radiation Chemistry," *Journal of Gerontology* 11, no. 3 (July 1956): 298-300, https://doi.org/10.1093/geronj/11.3.298

139 Ward Dean, "Neuroendocrine Theory Of Aging," *Anti-Aging and Life Extension Medicine*, Chapter 1, (Accessed January 9, 2021): https://warddeanmd.com/articles/neuroendocrine-theory-of-aging-chapter-1/

140 Denham Harman, "Aging: A Theory Based on Free Radical and Radiation Chemistry," *Journal of Gerontology* 11, no. 3 (July 1956): 298-300, https://doi.org/10.1093/geronj/11.3.298

141 Yichen Dai et al., "Steroid Hormone 20-Hydroxyecdysone Induces the Transcription and Complex Assembly of V-Atpases to Facilitate Autophagy in Bombyx Mori," *Insect Biochemistry and Molecular Biology* 116 (January 2020*):* 103255*,* https://doi.org/10.1016/j.ibmb.2019.103255

142 ZS- NAGY, "The Membrane Hypothesis of Aging," *International Antiaging Systems (IAS)*, Article, https://www.antiaging-systems.com/articles/the-membrane-hypothesis-of-aging/

143 Leonard Hayflick, "Theories of Biological Aging," *Experimental Gerontology 20, no's* 3–4, (1985): 145–59, https://doi.org/10.1016/0531-5565(85)90032-4

144 E S Epel et al., "Meditation and Vacation Effects Have an Impact on Disease-Associated Molecular Phenotypes," *Translational Psychiatry* 6, (2016): e880, https://doi.org/10.1038/tp.2016.164

145 David Zelman, "Inflammation," *Medical Review of Inflammation* by WebMD, October 15, 2020, https://www.webmd.com/arthritis/about-inflammation

146 Joel Zindel and Paul Kubes, "DAMPs, PAMPs, and LAMPs in Immunity and Sterile Inflammation," *Annual Review of Pathology* 15, (January 2020): 493–518, https://doi.org/10.1146/annurev-pathmechdis-012419-032847

147 Rachel Cant, Angus G. Dalgleish and Rachel L. Allen, "Naltrexone Inhibits IL-6 and TNFα Production in Human Immune Cell Subsets following Stimulation with Ligands for Intracellular Toll-Like Receptors," *Frontiers in Immunology* 8, no. 809 (July 11, 2017): https://doi.org/10.3389/fimmu.2017.00809

148 Luke Parkitny and Jarred Younger, "Reduced Pro-Inflammatory Cytokines After Eight Weeks of Low-Dose Naltrexone for Fibromyalgia," *Biomedicines* 5, no. 2 (April 18, 2017): 16, https://doi.org/10.3390/biomedicines5020016

149 Ricardo David Couto and Bruno Jose Dumêt Fernandes, "Low Doses Naltrexone: The Potential Benefit Effects for its Use in Patients with Cancer," *Current Drug Research Reviews* 13, no. 2 (January 26, 2021): 86–89, https://doi.org/10.2174/2589977513666210127094222

150 Elaine A Moore and Samantha Wilkinson, "The Promise of Low Dose Naltrexone Therapy: Potential Benefits in Cancer, Autoimmune, Neurological and Infectious Disorders*,"* Jefferson, N.C. McFarland, 2009, ISBN: 0786437154 9780786437153

151 XinWen and Daniel J.Klionsky, "At A Glance: A History of Autophagy and Cancer," *Seminars in Cancer Biology* 66 (November 2020): 3–11, https://doi.org/10.1016/j.semcancer.2019.11.005

152 S. M. Mir et al., "Shelterin Complex at Telomeres: Implications in Ageing," *Clinical Interventions in Aging* 15, (June 3, 2020): 827–39, https://doi.org/10.2147/CIA.S256425

153 Anna Marrone, Amanda Walne and Inderjeet Dokal, "Dyskeratosis Congenita: Telomerase, Telomeres and Anticipation," *Current Opinion*

in Genetics & Development 15, no. 3 (June 2005): 249-57, https://doi.org/10.1016/j.gde.2005.04.004

154 J Carrillo et al., "High Resolution Melting Analysis for the Identification of Novel Mutations in DKC1 and TERT Genes in Patients with Dyskeratosis Congenita," *Blood Cells Molecules and Diseases* 49, no. 3-4 (December 2012): 140-6. https://doi.org/10.1016/j.bcmd.2012.05.008

155 Chi-Hau Chen and Ruey-Jien Chen, "Prevalence of Telomerase Activity in Human Cancer," *Journal of the Formosan Medical Association* 110, no. 5 (May 2011): 275-89, https://doi.org/10.1016/S0929-6646(11)60043-0

156 Wai M. Liu et al., "Naltrexone at Low Doses Upregulates a Unique Gene Expression Not Seen with Normal Doses: Implications for its Use in Cancer Therapy," *International Journal of Oncology* 49, no. 2 (August 2016): 793-802, https://doi.org/10.3892/ijo.2016.3567

157 Dongmei Sun et al., "Exosomes Are Endogenous Nanoparticles That Can Deliver Biological Information Between Cells," *Advanced Drug Delivery Reviews* 65, no. 3 (March 2013): 342–347, https://doi.org/10.1016/j.addr.2012.07.002

158 Xin Luan et al., "Engineering Exosomes as Refined Biological Nanoplatforms for Drug Delivery," *Acta Pharmacologica Sinica* 38, no. 6 (April 10, 2017): 754–763, https://doi.org/10.1038/aps.2017.12

159 Yousra Hamdan, Loubna Mazini and Gabriel Malka, "Exosomes and Micro-Rnas in Aging Process," *Biomedicines* 9, no. 8 (August 6, 2021): 968, https://doi.org/10.3390/biomedicines9080968

160 Bao Zhu et al., "Stem Cell-Derived Exosomes Prevent Aging-Induced Cardiac Dysfunction Through a Novel Exosome/Lncrna MALAT1/NF-Kb/TNF-A Signaling Pathway," *Oxidative Medicine and Cellular Longevity* 2019, 9739258 (April 8, 2019): https://doi.org/10.1155/2019/9739258

161 DijanaBalenovic et al., "Inhibition of Methyldigoxin-Induced Arrhythmias by Pentadecapeptide BPC 157: A Relation With NO-System," *Regulatory Peptides* 156, no. 1–3 (August 2009): 83–89, https://doi.org/10.1016/j.regpep.2009.05.008

162 Khavinson peptides - History and Mission of Khavinson Peptides Foundation, (n.d.). Khavinson-Peptides.Com. Retrieved December 18, 2021, from https://khavinson-peptides.com/history

163 Xin Xu et al., "Protective Effect of Scorpion Venom Heat-Resistant Synthetic Peptide Against PM2.5-Induced Microglial Polarization Via TLR4-Mediated Autophagy Activating PI3K/AKT/NF-Kb Signaling Pathway," *Journal of Neuroimmunology* 355, 57756 (June 15, 2021):

https://doi.org/10.1016/j.jneuroim.2021.577567

164   YichenDai et al,. "Steroid Hormone 20-Hydroxyecdysone Induces
       the Transcription and Complex Assembly of V-Atpases to Facilitate
       Autophagy in Bombyx Mori," *Insect Biochemistry and Molecular
       Biology* 116, 103255 (January 2020): https://doi.org/10.1016/j.
       ibmb.2019.103255

165   Izabela Sadowska-Bartosz and Grzegorz Bartosz, "Effect of
       Antioxidants Supplementation on Aging and Longevity," *BioMed
       Research International* 2014, Article 404680 (March 25, 2014): https://
       doi.org/10.1155/2014/404680

166   Cheng Peng et al., "Biology of Ageing and Role of Dietary
       Antioxidants," *BioMed Research International* 214 (2014): Article
       831841, https://doi.org/10.1155/2014/831841

167   Jamshid Faraji and Gerlinde A.S Metz, "Aging, Social Distancing,
       and COVID-19 Risk: Who is more Vulnerable and Why?" *Aging
       and Disease* 12, no. 7 (2021): 1624–43, https://doi.org/10.14336/
       AD.2021.0319

168   David Mischoulon et al., "Randomized, Proof-Of-Concept Trial of
       Low Dose Naltrexone for Patients with Breakthrough Symptoms of
       Major Depressive Disorder on Antidepressants," *Journal of Affective
       Disorders* 208 (January 15, 2017): 6–14, https://doi.org/10.1016/j.
       jad.2016.08.029

169   Steven C. Moore et al., "Leisure Time Physical Activity of Moderate
       to Vigorous Intensity and Mortality: A Large Pooled Cohort
       Analysis," *PLoS Medicine* 9, no. 11 (November 6, 2012): e1001335,
       https://doi.org/10.1371/journal.pmed.1001335

170   Vincent Gremeaux et al., "Exercise and Longevity." *Maturitas* 73,
       no. 4 (October 1, 2012): 312–17, https://doi.org/10.1016/j.
       maturitas.2012.09.012

171   Daniel G. Blackmore et al., "An Exercise "Sweet Spot" Reverses
       Cognitive Deficits of Aging by Growth-Hormone-Induced
       Neurogenesis," *iScience* 24, no. 11 (October 14, 2021): 103275, https://
       doi.org/10.1016/j.isci.2021.103275

172   Diego Robles Mazzotti et al., "Human Longevity is Associated
       with Regular Sleep Patterns, Maintenance of Slow Wave Sleep, and
       Favorable Lipid Profile," *Frontiers in Aging Neuroscience* 6, no. 134
       (June 24, 2014): https://doi.org/10.3389/fnagi.2014.00134

173   Francesco P. Cappuccio et al., "Sleep Duration and All-Cause Mortality: A
       Systematic Review and Meta-Analysis of Prospective Studies," *Sleep 33,
       no. 5 (May* 2010): 585–92, https://doi.org/10.1093/sleep/33.5.585

174   Jarred Younger, Luke Parkitny and David McLain, "The use of low-dose

naltrexone (LDN) as a novel anti-inflammatory treatment for chronic pain," *Clinical Rheumatology* 33, no. 4 (April 2014): 451-9, https://doi.org/10.1007/s10067-014-2517-2

175 Madhuri Tolahunase, Rajesh Sagar and Rima Dada, "Impact of Yoga and Meditation on Cellular Aging in Apparently Healthy Individuals: A Prospective, Open-Label Single-Arm Exploratory Study," *Oxidative Medicine and Cell Longevity* (September 24, 2017): Article 7928981, https://doi.org/10.1155/2017/7928981

176 William C. Bushell, "Longevity: Potential Life Span and Health Span Enhancement Through Practice of the Basic Yoga Meditation Regimen," *Annals of the New York Academy of Sciences* 1172, no. 1 (August 2009): 20–7, https://doi.org/10.1111/j.1749-6632.2009.04538.x

177 Fabien Pifferi et al., "Caloric Restriction Increases Lifespan but Affects Brain Integrity in Grey Mouse Lemur Primates," *Communications Biology* 1, no. 30 (April 5, 2018): https://doi.org/10.1038/s42003-018-0024-8

178 David A. Sinclair and Lenny Guarente, "Unlocking the Secrets of Longevity Genes," *Scientific American* 294, no. 3 (March 2006): 48-51, 54-7, https://doi.org/10.1038/scientificamerican1206-68sp

179 Genetic variation in CETP and human longevity, *Senescence.Info*, Retrieved December 18, 2021, from https://genomics.senescence.info/longevity/gene.php?id=CETP

180 Jian-Kang Yang et al., "Association Study of Promoter Polymorphisms in The CETP Gene with Longevity in the Han Chinese Population," *Molecular Biology Reports* 41, no. 1 (2014): 325–9, https://doi.org/10.1007/s11033-013-2865-z

181 B. J. Morris et al.,."FOXO3: A Major Gene for Human Longevity--A Mini-Review," *Gerontology* 61, no. 6 (October 2015): 515–25. https://doi.org/10.1159/000375235

Chapter Five

182 Binita Sapkota and Yasir Al Khalili, "Mixed Connective Tissue Disease." PubMed, Treasure Island (FL), StatPearls Publishing, (2020): https://www.ncbi.nlm.nih.gov/books/NBK542198/

183 Vito Racanelli et al., "Autoantibodies to Intracellular Antigens: Generation and Pathogenesis Role," *Autoimmunity Reviews* 10, no. 8 (June 2011): 503-8, https://doi.org/10.1016/j.autrev.2011.03.001

184 Vito Racanelli et al., "Autoantibodies to Intracellular Antigens: Generation and Pathogenesis Role," *Autoimmunity Reviews* 10, no. 8 (June 2011): 503-8, https://doi.org/10.1016/j.autrev.2011.03.001

185 Elena Carnero-Montoro et al., "Epigenome-Wide Comparative Study

Reveals Key Differences Between Mixed Connective Tissue Disease and Related Systemic Autoimmune Diseases," *Frontiers in Immunology* 10 (August 7, 2019): 1880, https://doi.org/10.3389/fimmu.2019.01880

186   Barbara Stypińska et al., "Association Study Between Immune-Related MiRNAs and Mixed Connective Tissue Disease," *Arthritis Research & Therapy* 23, no. 1 (January 11, 2021): 19, https://doi.org/10.1186/s13075-020-02403-9

187   Alastair Crisp et al., "Expression of Multiple Horizontally Acquired Genes is a Hallmark of Both Vertebrate and Invertebrate Genomes," *Genome Biology* 16 (2015): 50, https://doi.org/10.1186/s13059-015-0607-3

188   Alastair Crisp et al., "Expression of Multiple Horizontally Acquired Genes is a Hallmark of Both Vertebrate and Invertebrate Genomes," *Genome Biology* 16 (2015): 50, https://doi.org/10.1186/s13059-015-0607-3

189   Rossella Talotta et al., "The Microbiome in Connective Tissue Diseases and Vasculitides: An Updated Narrative Review," *Journal of Immunology Research* 3 (August 2017): 1-11, https://doi.org/10.1155/2017/6836498

190   Elena Carnero-Montoro et al., "Epigenome-Wide Comparative Study Reveals Key Differences Between Mixed Connective Tissue Disease and Related Systemic Autoimmune Diseases," *Frontiers in Immunology* 10 (August 7, 2019): 1880, https://doi.org/10.3389/fimmu.2019.01880

191   M E Mercer and M D Holder, "Food Cravings, Endogenous Opioid Peptides, and Food Intake: A Review," *Appetite* 29, no. 3 (December 1997): 325-52, https://doi.org/10.1006/appe.1997.0100

192   Natalia Kučić et al., "Immunometabolic Modulatory Role of Naltrexone in BV-2 Microglia Cells," *International Journal of Molecular Sciences* 22, no. 16 (August 5, 2021): 8429, https://doi.org/10.3390/ijms22168429

193   Edited By Robert E. Faith et al., "Cytokines: Stress and Immunity," Second Edition (Page 362), CRC Press (September 19, 2019): 362.

194   Robert W McMurray and Warren May, "Sex Hormones and Systemic Lupus Erythematosus: Review and Meta-Analysis," *Arthritis and Rheumatism* 48, no. 8 (August 2003): 2100-10, https://doi.org/10.1002/art.11105

195   Svetlana Trifunovic et al., "The Function of the Hypothalamic-Pituitary-Adrenal Axis During Experimental Autoimmune Encephalomyelitis: Involvement of Oxidative Stress Mediators," *Frontiers in Neuroscience* 15 (June 17, 2021): 649485, https://doi.org/10.3389/fnins.2021.649485

196   "Toxic Chemicals Released by Industries – Worldometers," *Worldometers.info* (2019): https://www.worldometers.info/view/

toxchem/

197 David Goldstein, "Eye on the Environment - Tracking Toxins and Talking Transitions," *Ventura County Public Works Agency* (October 28, 2020), https://www.vcpublicworks.org/2020/10/28/toxins/

198 "National Report on Human Exposure to Environmental Chemicals | CDC," (2020): https://www.cdc.gov/exposurereport/

199 Nazzareno Ballatori, "Transport of Toxic Metals by Molecular Mimicry," *Environmental Health Perspectives* 110, Suppl 5 (October 2002): 689–694, https://doi.org/10.1289/ehp.02110s5689

200 SA Ahmed, "The Immune System as a Potential Target for Environmental Estrogens (Endocrine Disrupters): A New Emerging Field," *Toxicology* 150, no. 1-3 (September 7, 2000): 191–206, https://doi.org/10.1016/s0300-483x(00)00259-6

201 Jeffrey M Smith, "Genetic Roulette -The Gamble of Our Lives," *Institute for Responsible Technology* (2012): https://geneticroulettemovie.com/

202 Bruce Richardson, "Primer: Epigenetics of Autoimmunity," *Nature Clinical Practice Rheumatology* 3, no. 9 (September 2007): 521-7, https://doi.org/10.1038/ncprheum0573

203 Svetlana Trifunovic et al., "The Function of the Hypothalamic-Pituitary-Adrenal Axis During Experimental Autoimmune Encephalomyelitis: Involvement of Oxidative Stress Mediators," *Frontiers in Neuroscience* 15 (June 17, 2021): 649485, https://doi.org/10.3389/fnins.2021.649485

204 M E Mercer and M D Holder, "Food Cravings, Endogenous Opioid Peptides, and Food Intake: A Review," *Appetite* 29, no. 3 (December 1997): 325-52, https://doi.org/10.1006/appe.1997.0100

205 Kayoko Urashima et al., "The Prevalence of Insomnia and Restless Legs Syndrome Among Japanese Outpatients with Rheumatic Disease: A Cross-Sectional Study," *PLoS ONE* 15, no. 3 (March 20, 2020): e0230273, https://doi.org/10.1371/journal.pone.0230273

206 Rene Cortese, "Epigenetics of Sleep Disorders: An Emerging Field in Diagnosis and Therapeutics," *Diagnostics (Basel)* 11, no. 5 (May 10, 2021): 851, https://doi.org/10.3390/diagnostics11050851

207 Alexandru-Dan Costache et al., "Beyond the Finish Line: The Impact and Dynamics of Biomarkers in Physical Exercise-A Narrative Review," *Journal of Clinical Medicine* 10, no. 21 (27 October, 2021): 4978, https://doi.org/10.3390/jcm10214978

208 Brietta Gerrard et al., "Chronic Mild Stress Exacerbates Severity of Experimental Autoimmune Encephalomyelitis in Association with Altered Non-coding RNA and Metabolic Biomarkers," *Neuroscience* 359 (July 2017): https://doi.org/10.1016/j.neuroscience.2017.07.033

209 Kim Penberthy et al., "Mindfulness Based Therapies for Autoimmune Diseases and Related Symptoms," *OBM Integrative and Complementary Medicine* 3, no. 4 (December 28, 2018): https://doi.org/10.21926/obm.icm.1804039

Chapter Six

210 Ritchie Shoemaker, http://SurvivingMold.com

211 Patti Schmidt, Ritchie C. Shoemaker and James L. Schaller, Mold Warriors: Fighting America's Hidden Health Threat," Gateway Press 2005, ISBN-10 0966553535

212 Hermina Drah, "21 Critical Mold Statistics We Have to Be Aware of in 2022," *ComfyLiving*, (January 20, 2022), https://comfyliving.net/mold-statistics/

213 J Carahan, "How EMFs Could Be Making Your Mold Illness Symptoms Worse." (October 16, 2021): https://www.jillcarnahan.com/2021/10/16/struggling-with-mold-illness-how-emfs-could-be-making-your-symptoms-worse/

214 "EMR Induces Mold and Yeast Growth: The Evidence." *World-News* (June 18, 2008): https://omeganews.wordpress.com/2008/06/18/emr-induces-mold-and-yeast-growth-the-evidence/

215 Lloyd Burrell, "EMFs And Indoor Mold – The Connection," (August 17, 2003): https://www.electricsense.com/emfs-indoor-mold-connection/

216 J Carahan, "How EMFs Could Be Making Your Mold Illness Symptoms Worse." (October 16, 2021): https://www.jillcarnahan.com/2021/10/16/struggling-with-mold-illness-how-emfs-could-be-making-your-symptoms-worse/

217 "EMR Induces Mold and Yeast Growth: The Evidence." *World-News* (June 18, 2008): https://omeganews.wordpress.com/2008/06/18/emr-induces-mold-and-yeast-growth-the-evidence/

218 Lloyd Burrell, "EMFs And Indoor Mold – The Connection," (August 17, 2003): https://www.electricsense.com/emfs-indoor-mold-connection/

219 Ritchie Shoemaker, http://SurvivingMold.com

220 Patti Schmidt, Ritchie C Shoemaker and James L Schaller, "Mold Warriors: Fighting America's Hidden Health Threat," Gateway Press 2005, ISBN-10 0966553535

221 Patti Schmidt, Ritchie C Shoemaker and James L Schaller, "Mold Warriors: Fighting America's Hidden Health Threat," Gateway Press 2005, ISBN-10 0966553535

222 Ritchie Shoemaker, "Use of Visual Contrast Sensitivity and Cholestyramine in Diagnosis and Treatment of Indoor Aquired, Chronic, Neurotoxin-Mediated Illness," n.d., https://www.survivingmold.com/

docs/Use_of_visual_contrast_sensitivity.PDF

223 Ritchie Shoemaker, "Linkage disequilibrium in alleles of HLA DR: differential association with susceptibility to chronic illness following exposure to biologically produced neurotoxins," *American Society of Microbiology* 2003. (conference peer review), https://www.survivingmold.com/docs/Linkage_disequilibrium_in_alleles_of_HLA_DR.PDF

224 E John Wherry and Makoto Kurachi, "Molecular and Cellular Insight into T Cell Exhaustion," *Nature Reviews: Immunology* 15, no. 8 (2015): 486-99, https://doi.org/10.1038/nri3862

225 John S Yi, Maureen A Cox and Allan J Zajac, "T-Cell Exhaustion: Characteristics, Causes and Conversion," *Immunology* 129, no. 4 (April 2015): 474-81, https://doi.org/10.1111/j.1365-2567.2010.03255.x

226 E A Ojo-Amaize, E J Conley and J B Peter, "Decreased Natural Killer Cell Activity is Associated with Severity of Chronic Fatigue Immune Dysfunction Syndrome," *Clinical Infectious Diseases* 18, Suppl 1 (January 1994): S157-9, https://doi.org/10.1093/clinids/18.supplement_1.s157

227 E John Wherry and Makoto Kurachi, "Molecular and Cellular Insight into T Cell Exhaustion," Nature Reviews: *Immunology* 15, no. 8 (2015): 486-99, https://doi.org/10.1038/nri3862

228 John S Yi, Maureen A Cox and Allan J Zajac, "T-Cell Exhaustion: Characteristics, Causes and Conversion," *Immunology* 129, no. 4 (April 2015): 474-81, https://doi.org/10.1111/j.1365-2567.2010.03255.x

229 E A Ojo-Amaize, E J Conley and J B Peter, "Decreased Natural Killer Cell Activity is Associated with Severity of Chronic Fatigue Immune Dysfunction Syndrome," *Clinical Infectious Diseases* 18, Suppl 1 (January 1994): S157-9, https://doi.org/10.1093/clinids/18.supplement_1.s157

230 John S Yi, Maureen A Cox and Allan J Zajac, "T-Cell Exhaustion: Characteristics, Causes and Conversion," *Immunology* 129, no. 4 (April 2015): 474-81, https://doi.org/10.1111/j.1365-2567.2010.03255.x

231 E John Wherry and Makoto Kurachi, "Molecular and Cellular Insight into T Cell Exhaustion," Nature Reviews: *Immunology* 15, no. 8 (2015): 486-99, https://doi.org/10.1038/nri3862

232 John S Yi, Maureen A Cox and Allan J Zajac, "T-Cell Exhaustion: Characteristics, Causes and Conversion," *Immunology* 129, no. 4 (April 2015): 474-81, https://doi.org/10.1111/j.1365-2567.2010.03255.x

233 R B Stricker et al., "Complement Split Products C3A and C4A in Chronic Lyme Disease," *Scandinavian Journal of Clinical Immunology* 69, no. 1 (January 2009): 64-9, https://doi.org/10.1111/j.1365-3083.2008.02191.x

234   E A Ojo-Amaize, E J Conley and J B Peter, "Decreased Natural
      Killer Cell Activity is Associated with Severity of Chronic Fatigue
      Immune Dysfunction Syndrome," *Clinical Infectious Diseases* 18,
      Suppl 1 (January 1994): S157-9, https://doi.org/10.1093/clinids/18.
      supplement_1.s157

235   Eduardo Candelario-Jalil et al., "Matrix Metalloproteinases are
      Associated with Increased Blood-Brain Barrier Opening in Vascular
      Cognitive Impairment," *Stroke* 42, no. 5 (May 2011): 1345-50, https://
      doi.org/10.1161/STROKEAHA.110.600825

236   Kent Holtorf, "Peripheral Thyroid Hormone Conversion and its Impact
      on TSH and Metabolic Activity," *Journal of Restorative Medicine* 3, no.
      1 (April 2014): 30-51

237   Ritchie C. Shoemaker, James Schaller and Patti Schmidt,"Mold
      Warriors: Fighting America's Hidden Health Threat, Biotoxin Related
      Illness Treatment Pathway-A Warriors," Gateway Health 2005, ISBN
      13: 9780966553536

238   Aaron Hartman, "A New Paradigm for Chronic Disease. Part IV: CIRS
      Treatment Pathway - A Guide to Biotoxin Related Illness Treatment,"
      Richmond Integrative & Functional Medicine (February 2019): https://
      richmondfunctionalmedicine.com/mold-related-biotoxin-illness-part4/

239   Gabriele Siciliano et al., "Human Mitochondrial Transcription Factor a
      Reduction and Mitochondrial Dysfunction in Hashimoto's Hypothyroid
      Myopathy," *Molecular Medicine* 8, no. 6 (June 2002): 326-33

240   Predrag Sikiric et al., "Brain-gut Axis and Pentadecapeptide BPC 157:
      Theoretical and Practical Implications," *Current Neuropharmacology*
      14, no. 8 (November 2016): 857-865, https://doi.org/10.2174/157015
      9x13666160502153022

241   Predrag Sikiric et al., "Brain-gut Axis and Pentadecapeptide BPC 157:
      Theoretical and Practical Implications," *Current Neuropharmacology*
      14, no. 8 (November 2016): 857-865, https://doi.org/10.2174/157015
      9x13666160502153022

242   R M Jones, J W Mercante and A S Neish, "Reactive Oxygen Production
      Induced by the Gut Microbiota: Pharmacotherapeutic Implications,"
      Current Medicinal Chemistry 19, no. 10 (April 2012): 1519-29, https://
      doi.org/10.2174/092986712799828283

243   Predrag Sikiric et al., "Brain-gut Axis and Pentadecapeptide BPC 157:
      Theoretical and Practical Implications," *Current Neuropharmacology*
      14, no. 8 (November 2016): 857-865, https://doi.org/10.2174/157015
      9x13666160502153022

244   Predrag Sikiric et al., "Stable Gastric Pentadecapeptide BPC 157: Novel
      Therapy in Gastrointestinal Tract," *Current Pharmaceutical Design* 17,

no. 16 (2011): 1612-32, https://doi.org/10.2174/138161211796196954

245   Predrag Sikiric et al., "Stress in Gastrointestinal Tract and Stable Gastric Pentadecapeptide BPC 157. Finally, Do We Have a Solution?," *Current Pharmaceutical Design* 23, no. 27 (August 2017): 4012-28, https://doi.or g/10.2174/1381612823666170220163219

246   Anna Catania et al., "The Melanocortin System in Control of Inflammation," *The Scientific World Journal* 10 (September 2010): 1840-53, https://doi.org/10.1100/tsw.2010.173

247   Madhuri Singh and Kasturi Mukhopadhyay, "Alpha-Melanocyte Stimulating Hormone: An Emerging Anti-Inflammatory Antimicrobial Peptide," *BioMed Research International* 2014 (July 2014): 874610, https://doi.org/10.1155/2014/874610

248   Balazs Varga et al., "Protective Effect of Alpha-Melanocyte-Stimulating Hormone (-α MSH) on the Recovery of Ischemia/Reperfusion (I/R)-Induced Retinal Damage in a Rat Model," *Journal of Molecular Neuroscience* 50, no. 3 (July 2013): 558–70, https://doi.org/10.1007/s12031-013-9998-3

249   M Cutuli et al., "Antimicrobial Effects of Alpha-MSH Peptides," *Journal of Leukocyte Biology* 67, no. 2 (February 2000): 233-9, https://doi.org/10.1002/jlb.67.2.233

250   Madhuri Singh and Kasturi Mukhopadhyay, "Alpha-Melanocyte Stimulating Hormone: An Emerging Anti-Inflammatory Antimicrobial Peptide," *BioMed Research International* 2014 (July 2014): 874610, https://doi.org/10.1155/2014/874610

251   Anna Catania et al., "The Melanocortin System in Control of Inflammation," *The Scientific World Journal* 10 (September 2010): 1840-53, https://doi.org/10.1100/tsw.2010.173

252   Anna Catania et al., "The Melanocortin System in Control of Inflammation," *The Scientific World Journal* 10 (September 2010): 1840-53, https://doi.org/10.1100/tsw.2010.173

253   Aaron Hartman, "A New Paradigm for Chronic Disease. Part IV: CIRS Treatment Protocol — A Guide to Biotoxin Related Illness Treatment," *Richmond Integrative & Functional Medicine* (21 February 2019), https://richmondfunctionalmedicine.com/mold-related-biotoxin-illness-part4/

254   Yvonne Berry, "A physician's Guide to Understanding and Treating Biotoxin Illness (Based on the work of Ritchie Shoemaker, M.D," *SurvivingMold.com* (April 3, 2014), https://www.survivingmold.com/legal-resources/works-citing-dr.-shoemaker/a-physicians-guide-to-biotoxin-illness

255   Kent Holtorf, "Diagnosis and Treatment of Hypothalamic-Pituitary-

Adrenal (HPA) Axis Dysfunction in Patients with Chronic Fatigue Syndrome (CFS) and Fibromyalgia (FM)," *Journal of Chronic Fatigue Syndrome* 14, no. 3 (January 2008): 59-88, https://doi.org/10.1300/J092v14n03_06

256   Aaron Hartman, "A New Paradigm for Chronic Disease. Part IV: CIRS Treatment Protocol — A Guide to Biotoxin Related Illness Treatment*,"* *Richmond Integrative & Functional Medicine* (21 February 2019), https://richmondfunctionalmedicine.com/mold-related-biotoxin-illness-part4/

257   Yvonne Berry, "A physician's Guide to Understanding and Treating Biotoxin Illness (Based on the work of Ritchie Shoemaker, M.D," *SurvivingMold.com* (April 3, 2014), https://www.survivingmold.com/legal-resources/works-citing-dr.-shoemaker/a-physicians-guide-to-biotoxin-illness

258   Natasha Thomas, "Understanding Chronic Inflammatory Response Syndrome (CIRS)," *Survivingmold.com* (n.d.) https://www.survivingmold.com/docs/UNDERSTANDING_CIRS_EDITV2A.PDF

259   C E Crist, D E Berg and H H Harrison, "Does Borreliosis (Lyme Disease) Activate the Coagulation System and is a Coagulation Regulatory Protein Defect Predispositional?," *Infectious Diseases Society of America* (Oct 2003), https://idsa.confex.com/idsa/2003/webprogram/Paper18421.html

260   Mahesh Yadav and Edward J Goetzl, "Vasoactive Intestinal Peptide-Mediated Th17 Differentiation," *Annals of the New York Acadamy of Sciences* 1144 (November 2008): 83-9, https://doi.org/10.1196/annals.1418.020

261   R Newman et al., "Vasoactive Intestinal Peptide Impairs Leucocyte Migration but Fails to Modify Experimental Murine Colitis," *Clinical and Experimental Immunology* 139, no. 3 (March 2005): 411–20, https://doi.org/10.1111/j.1365-2249.2005.02673.x

262   Aaron Hartman, "A New Paradigm for Chronic Disease. Part IV: CIRS Treatment Protocol — A Guide to Biotoxin Related Illness Treatment," *Richmond Integrative & Functional Medicine* (21 February 2019), https://richmondfunctionalmedicine.com/mold-related-biotoxin-illness-part4/

263   Ritchie C. Shoemaker, James Louis Schaller and Patti Schmidt, "Mold Warriors: Fighting America's Hidden Health Threat," Gateway Press (2005)

264   Ritchie C. Shoemaker, James Louis Schaller and Patti Schmidt, "Mold Warriors: Fighting America's Hidden Health Threat," Gateway Press (2005)

265 Aaron Hartman, "A New Paradigm for Chronic Disease. Part IV: CIRS Treatment Protocol — A Guide to Biotoxin Related Illness Treatment," *Richmond Integrative & Functional Medicine* (21 February 2019), https://richmondfunctionalmedicine.com/mold-related-biotoxin-illness-part4/

266 Mahesh Yadav and Edward J Goetzl, "Vasoactive Intestinal Peptide-Mediated Th17 Differentiation," *Annals of the New York Academy of Sciences* 1144 (November 2008): 83-9, https://doi.org/10.1196/annals.1418.020

267 John S Yi, Maureen A Cox and Allan J Zajac, "T-Cell Exhaustion: Characteristics, Causes and Conversion," *Immunology* 129, no. 4 (April 2010): 474-81, https://doi.org/10.1111/j.1365-2567.2010.03255.x

268 Mahesh Yadav, Jennifer Rosenbaum and Edward J. Goetzl , "Cutting Edge: Vasoactive Intestinal Peptide (VIP) Induces Differentiation of Th17 Cells with a Distinctive Cytokine Profile," *Journal of Immunology* 180, no. 5 (March 1, 2008): 27772-6, https://doi.org/10.4049/jimmunol.180.5.2772

269 Mahesh Yadav and Edward J Goetzl, "Vasoactive Intestinal Peptide-Mediated Th17 Differentiation," *Annals of the New York Acadamy of Sciences* 1144 (November 2008): 83-9, https://doi.org/10.1196/annals.1418.020

270 Mahesh Yadav, Jennifer Rosenbaum and Edward J. Goetzl , "Cutting Edge: Vasoactive Intestinal Peptide (VIP) Induces Differentiation of Th17 Cells with a Distinctive Cytokine Profile," *Journal of Immunology* 180, no. 5 (March 1, 2008): 27772-6, https://doi.org/10.4049/jimmunol.180.5.2772

271 Ritchie C. Shoemaker, James Louis Schaller and Patti Schmidt, "Mold Warriors: Fighting America's Hidden Health Threat," Gateway Press (2005)

272 Mahesh Yadav, Jennifer Rosenbaum and Edward J. Goetzl , "Cutting Edge: Vasoactive Intestinal Peptide (VIP) Induces Differentiation of Th17 Cells with a Distinctive Cytokine Profile," *Journal of Immunology* 180, no. 5 (March 1, 2008): 27772-6, https://doi.org/10.4049/jimmunol.180.5.2772

273 Mahesh Yadav, Jennifer Rosenbaum and Edward J. Goetzl , "Cutting Edge: Vasoactive Intestinal Peptide (VIP) Induces Differentiation of Th17 Cells with a Distinctive Cytokine Profile," *Journal of Immunology* 180, no. 5 (March 1, 2008): 27772-6, https://doi.org/10.4049/jimmunol.180.5.2772

274 T Chalastras et al., "Expression of Substance P, Vasoactive Intestinal Peptide and Heat Shock Protein 70 in Nasal Mucosal Smears of Patients

with Allergic Rhinitis: Investigation Using a Liquid-Based Method,"
Journal of Laryngology & Otology 122, no. 7 (July 2008): 700-6, https://
doi.org/10.1017/S0022215107001454

275   Mahesh Yadav, Jennifer Rosenbaum and Edward J. Goetzl , "Cutting
      Edge: Vasoactive Intestinal Peptide (VIP) Induces Differentiation of
      Th17 Cells with a Distinctive Cytokine Profile," *Journal of Immunology*
      180, no. 5 (March 1, 2008): 27772-6, https://doi.org/10.4049/
      jimmunol.180.5.2772

276   Mahesh Yadav, Jennifer Rosenbaum and Edward J. Goetzl , "Cutting
      Edge: Vasoactive Intestinal Peptide (VIP) Induces Differentiation of
      Th17 Cells with a Distinctive Cytokine Profile," *Journal of Immunology*
      180, no. 5 (March 1, 2008): 27772-6, https://doi.org/10.4049/
      jimmunol.180.5.2772

277   T Chalastras et al., "Expression of Substance P, Vasoactive Intestinal
      Peptide and Heat Shock Protein 70 in Nasal Mucosal Smears of Patients
      with Allergic Rhinitis: Investigation Using a Liquid-Based Method,"
      Journal of Laryngology & Otology 122, no. 7 (July 2008): 700-6, https://
      doi.org/10.1017/S0022215107001454

278   Global Burden of Disease Study 2013 Collaborators, "Global, Regional,
      and National Incidence, Prevalence, and Years Lived with Disability for
      301 Acute and Chronic Diseases and Injuries in 188 Countries, 1990–
      2013: A Systematic Analysis for the Global Burden of Disease Study
      2013," *The Lancet* 386, no. 9995 (August 2015): 743-800, https://doi.
      org/10.1016/S0140-6736(15)60692-4

279   Robin Osborn et al., "Older Americans Were Sicker and Faced
      More Financial Barriers to Health Care Than Counterparts in Other
      Countries," *Health Affairs* 36, no. 12 (15 November 2017): https://doi.
      org/10.1377/hlthaff.2017.1048

280   Aristo Vojdani et al., "Saliva Secretory IgA Antibodies Against
      Molds and Mycotoxins in Patients Exposed to Toxigenic Fungi,"
      Immunopharmacology and Immunotoxicology 25, no. 4 (November
      2003): 595-614, https://doi.org/10.1081/iph-120026444

281   Aristo Vojdani et al., "Antibodies Against Molds and Mycotoxins
      Following Exposure to Toxigenic Fungi in a Water-Damaged Building,"
      Archives of Environmental Health 58, no. 6 (June 2003): 324-36, https://
      pubmed.ncbi.nlm.nih.gov/14992307/

282   Andrew W Campbell et al., "Mold, and Mycotoxins: Effects on the
      Neurological and Immune Systems in Humans," *Advances in Applied
      Microbiology* 55 (2004): 373-406, https://doi.org/10.1016/S0065-
      2164(04)55015-3

283   Andrew W Campbell et al., "Neural Autoantibodies and

Neurophysiologic Abnormalities in Patients Exposed to Molds in Water-Damaged Buildings," *Archives of Environmental Health* 58, no. 8 (August 2003): 464-74, https://doi.org/10.3200/AEOH.58.8.464-474

284 Andrew W Campbell et al., "Mold, and Mycotoxins: Effects on the Neurological and Immune Systems in Humans," *Advances in Applied Microbiology* 55 (2004): 373-406, https://doi.org/10.1016/S0065-2164(04)55015-3

285 Andrew W Campbell et al., "Neural Autoantibodies and Neurophysiologic Abnormalities in Patients Exposed to Molds in Water-Damaged Buildings," *Archives of Environmental Health* 58, no. 8 (August 2003): 464-74, https://doi.org/10.3200/AEOH.58.8.464-474

286 Stephanie Kraft, Lisa Buchenauer and Tobias Polte, "Mold, Mycotoxins, and a Dysregulated Immune System: A Combination of Concern?," *International Journal of Molecular Sciences* 22, no. 22 (November 2021): 12269, https://doi.org/10.3390/ijms222212269

287 John S Yi, Maureen A Cox and Allan J Zajac, "T-cell Exhaustion: Characteristics, Causes, and Conversion," *Immunology* 129, no. 4 (April 2010): 474-81, https://doi.org/10.1111/j.1365-2567.2010.03255.x

288 E John Wherry, "T Cell Exhaustion," *Nature Immunology* 12, no. 6 (June 2011): 492-99, https://doi.org/10.1038/ni.2035

289 Ebere Anyanwu et al., "The Neurological Significance of Abnormal Natural Killer Cell Activity in Chronic Toxigenic Mold Exposures," *Scientific World Journal* 3 (November2003): 1128-37, https://doi.org/10.1100/tsw.2003.98

290 Andrew W Campbell et al., "Mold and Mycotoxins: Effects on the Neurological and Immune Systems in Humans," *Advances in Applied Microbiology* 55 (2004): 375-406, https://doi.org/10.1016/S0065-2164(04)55015-3

291 Stephanie Kraft, Lisa Buchenauer and Tobias Polte, "Mold, Mycotoxins and a Dysregulated Immune System: A Combination of Concern?," *International Journal of Molecular Sciences* 22, no. 22 (November 2021): 12269, https://doi.org/10.3390/ijms222212269

292 E A Ojo-Amaize, E J Conley and J B Peter, "Decreased Natural Killer Cell Activity is Associated with the Severity of Chronic Fatigue Immune Dysfunction Syndrome," *Clinical Infectious Diseases* 18, no. 1 (January 1994): S157-9, https://doi.org/10.1093/clinids/18.supplement_1.s157

293 Michael R Gray et al., "Mixed Mold Mycotoxicosis: Immunological Changes in Humans following Exposure in Water-Damaged Buildings," *Archives of Environmental Health* 58, no.7 (July 2003): 410-420, https://doi.org/10.1080/00039896.2003.11879142

294 Andrew W Campbell et al., "Mold and Mycotoxins: Effects on the

Neurological and Immune Systems in Humans," *Advances in Applied Microbiology* 55 (2004): 375-406, https://doi.org/10.1016/S0065-2164(04)55015-3

295   Ebere Anyanwu et al., "The Neurological Significance of Abnormal Natural Killer Cell Activity in Chronic Toxigenic Mold Exposures," *Scientific World Journal* 3 (November 2003): 1128–37, https://doi.org/10.1100/tsw.2003.98

296   Andrew W Campbell et al., "Mold and Mycotoxins: Effects on the Neurological and Immune Systems in Humans," *Advances in Applied Microbiology* 55 (2004): 375-406, https://doi.org/10.1016/S0065-2164(04)55015-3

297   Ebere Anyanwu et al., "The Neurological Significance of Abnormal Natural Killer Cell Activity in Chronic Toxigenic Mold Exposures," *Scientific World Journal* 3 (November 2003): 1128–37, https://doi.org/10.1100/tsw.2003.98

298   Stephanie Kraft, Lisa Buchenauer and Tobias Polte, "Mold, Mycotoxins and a Dysregulated Immune System: A Combination of Concern?," *International Journal of Molecular Sciences* 22, no. 22 (November 2021): 12269, https://doi.org/10.3390/ijms222212269

299   Ebere Anyanwu et al., "The Neurological Significance of Abnormal Natural Killer Cell Activity in Chronic Toxigenic Mold Exposures," *Scientific World Journal* 3 (November2003): 1128-37, https://doi.org/10.1100/tsw.2003.98

300   Stephanie Kraft, Lisa Buchenauer and Tobias Polte, "Mold, Mycotoxins and a Dysregulated Immune System: A Combination of Concern?," *International Journal of Molecular Sciences* 22, no. 22 (November 2021): 12269, https://doi.org/10.3390/ijms222212269

301   Ebere Anyanwu et al., "The Neurological Significance of Abnormal Natural Killer Cell Activity in Chronic Toxigenic Mold Exposures," *Scientific World Journal* 3 (November2003): 1128-37, https://doi.org/10.1100/tsw.2003.98

302   E A Ojo-Amaize, E J Conley and J B Peter, "Decreased Natural Killer Cell Activity is Associated with the Severity of Chronic Fatigue Immune Dysfunction Syndrome," *Clinical Infectious Diseases* 18, no. 1 (January 1994): S157-9, https://doi.org/10.1093/clinids/18.supplement_1.s157

303   Stephanie Kraft, Lisa Buchenauer and Tobias Polte, "Mold, Mycotoxins and a Dysregulated Immune System: A Combination of Concern?," *International Journal of Molecular Sciences* 22, no. 22 (November 2021): 12269, https://doi.org/10.3390/ijms222212269

304   Ebere Anyanwu et al., "The Neurological Significance of Abnormal Natural Killer Cell Activity in Chronic Toxigenic Mold Exposures,"

Scientific World Journal 3 (November2003): 1128-37, https://doi. org/10.1100/tsw.2003.98

305 Stephanie Kraft, Lisa Buchenauer and Tobias Polte, "Mold, Mycotoxins and a Dysregulated Immune System: A Combination of Concern?," *International Journal of Molecular Sciences* 22, no. 22 (November 2021): 12269, https://doi.org/10.3390/ijms222212269

306 Ebere Anyanwu et al., "The Neurological Significance of Abnormal Natural Killer Cell Activity in Chronic Toxigenic Mold Exposures," *Scientific World Journal* 3 (November2003): 1128-37, https://doi. org/10.1100/tsw.2003.98

307 Stephanie Kraft, Lisa Buchenauer and Tobias Polte, "Mold, Mycotoxins and a Dysregulated Immune System: A Combination of Concern?," *International Journal of Molecular Sciences* 22, no. 22 (November 2021): 12269, https://doi.org/10.3390/ijms222212269

308 Ebere Anyanwu et al., "The Neurological Significance of Abnormal Natural Killer Cell Activity in Chronic Toxigenic Mold Exposures," *Scientific World Journal* 3 (November2003): 1128-37, https://doi. org/10.1100/tsw.2003.98

309 Stephanie Kraft, Lisa Buchenauer and Tobias Polte, "Mold, Mycotoxins and a Dysregulated Immune System: A Combination of Concern?," *International Journal of Molecular Sciences* 22, no. 22 (November 2021): 12269, https://doi.org/10.3390/ijms222212269

310 Jarred Younger and Sean Mackey, "Fibromyalgia Symptoms are Reduced by Low-Dose Naltrexone: A Pilot Study," *Pain Medicine* 10, no. 4 (June 2009): 663–72, https://doi.org/10.1111/j.1526-4637.2009.00613.x

311 V G Morozov and V K Khavinson, "Natural and Synthetic Thymic Peptides as Therapeutics for Immune Dysfunction," *International Journal of Immunopharmacology* 19, no. 9-10 (October 1997): 501-5, https://doi.org/10.1016/S0192-0561(97)00058-1

312 Laura J Cobb et al., "Naturally Occurring Mitochondrial-Derived Peptides Are Age-Dependent Regulators of Apoptosis, Insulin Sensitivity, and Inflammatory Markers," *Aging* 8, no. 4 (April 2016): 796-808, https://doi.org/10.18632/aging.100943

313 Andrew W Campbell et al., "Mold and Mycotoxins: Effects on the Neurological and Immune Systems in Humans," *Advances in Applied Microbiology* 55 (2004): 375-406, https://doi.org/10.1016/S0065-2164(04)55015-3

314 Stephanie Kraft, Lisa Buchenauer and Tobias Polte, "Mold, Mycotoxins and a Dysregulated Immune System: A Combination of Concern?," *International Journal of Molecular Sciences* 22, no. 22 (November

2021): 12269, https://doi.org/10.3390/ijms222212269

315 Ebere Anyanwu et al., "The Neurological Significance of Abnormal Natural Killer Cell Activity in Chronic Toxigenic Mold Exposures," *Scientific World Journal* 3 (November2003): 1128-37, https://doi.org/10.1100/tsw.2003.98

316 E John Wherry and Makoto Kurachi, "Molecular and Cellular Insight into T Cell Exhaustion," *Nature Reviews: Immunology* 15, no. 8 (August 2015): 486-99, https://doi.org/10.1038/nri3862

317 E John Wherry and Makoto Kurachi, "Molecular and Cellular Insight into T Cell Exhaustion," *Nature Reviews: Immunology* 15, no. 8 (August 2015): 486-99, https://doi.org/10.1038/nri3862

318 John S Yi, Maureen A Cox and Allan J Zajac, "T-Cell Exhaustion: Characteristics, Causes, and Conversion," *Immunology* 129, no. 4 (April 2010): 474-81, https://doi.org/10.1111/j.1365-2567.2010.03255.x

319 E A Ojo-Amaize, E J Conley and J B Peter, "Decreased Natural Killer Cell Activity is Associated with the Severity of Chronic Fatigue Immune Dysfunction Syndrome," *Clinical Infectious Diseases* 18, no. 1 (January 1994): S157-9, https://doi.org/10.1093/clinids/18.supplement_1.s157

320 John S Yi, Maureen A Cox and Allan J Zajac, "T-Cell Exhaustion: Characteristics, Causes, and Conversion," *Immunology* 129, no. 4 (April 2010): 474-81, https://doi.org/10.1111/j.1365-2567.2010.03255.x

321 E John Wherry, "T Cell Exhaustion," *Nature Immunology* 12, no. 6 (June 2011): 492-9, https://doi.org/10.1038/ni.2035

322 E John Wherry and Makoto Kurachi, "Molecular and Cellular Insight into T Cell Exhaustion," *Nature Reviews: Immunology* 15, no. 8 (August 2015): 486-99, https://doi.org/10.1038/nri3862

323 John S Yi, Maureen A Cox and Allan J Zajac, "T-Cell Exhaustion: Characteristics, Causes, and Conversion," *Immunology* 129, no. 4 (April 2010): 474-81, https://doi.org/10.1111/j.1365-2567.2010.03255.x

324 Xiao-Hua Luo et al., "T Cell Immunobiology and Cytokine Storm of COVID-19," *Scandinavian Journal of Immunology* 93, no. 3 (March 2021): e12989, https://doi.org/10.1111/sji.12989

325 Sara De Biasi et al., "Marked T Cell Activation, Senescence, Exhaustion and Skewing Towards Th17 in Patients with COVID-19 Pneumonia," *Nature Communications* 11, no. 3434 (July 2020): https://doi.org/10.1038/s41467-020-17292-4

326 Bo Diao et al., "Reduction and Functional Exhaustion of T Cells in Patients with Coronavirus Disease," *Frontiers in Immunology* 11 (May 2020): 827, https://doi.org/10.3389/fimmu.2020.00827

327 Jeffrey E. Gold et al., "Investigation of Long COVID Prevalence and its

Relationship to Epstein-Barr Virus Reactivation," *Pathogens* 10, no. 6 (June 2021): 763, https://doi.org/10.3390/pathogens10060763

328   Jeffrey E. Gold et al., "Investigation of Long COVID Prevalence and its Relationship to Epstein-Barr Virus Reactivation," *Pathogens* 10, no. 6 (June 2021): 763, https://doi.org/10.3390/pathogens10060763

329   Daniel Kinderlehrer, "What Can Chronic Lyme Disease Teach Us About Long COVID?," *Lymedisease.org Focus-Opinions and Features* (January 24, 2022), https://www.lymedisease.org/kinderlehrer-lyme-long-COVID/

330   R Consolini et al., "Distribution of Age-Related Thymulin Titres in Normal Subjects Through the Course of Life," *Clinical and Experimental Immunology* 121, no. 3 (September 2000): 444-7, https://doi.org/10.1046/j.1365-2249.2000.01315.x

331   Jingang Gui et al., "Thymus Size and Age-related Thymic Involution: Early Programming, Sexual Dimorphism, Progenitors and Stroma," *Aging and Disease* 3, no. 3 (June 2012): 280-90, https://pubmed.ncbi.nlm.nih.gov/22724086/

332   Stephanie Kraft, Lisa Buchenauer and Tobias Polte, "Mold, Mycotoxins, and a Dysregulated Immune System: A Combination of Concern?," *International Journal of Molecular Sciences* 22, no. 22 (November 2021): 12269, https://doi.org/10.3390/ijms222212269

333   E A Ojo-Amaize, E J Conley and J B Peter, "Decreased Natural Killer Cell Activity is Associated with the Severity of Chronic Fatigue Immune Dysfunction Syndrome," *Clinical Infectious Diseases* 18, no. 1 (January 1994): S157-9, https://doi.org/10.1093/clinids/18.supplement_1.s157

334   Jarred Younger and Sean Mackey, "Fibromyalgia Symptoms are Reduced by Low-Dose Naltrexone: A Pilot Study," *Pain Medicine* 10, no. 4 (June 2009): 663–72, https://doi.org/10.1111/j.1526-4637.2009.00613.x

335   V G Morozov and V K Khavinson, "Natural and Synthetic Thymic Peptides as Therapeutics for Immune Dysfunction," *International Journal of Immunopharmacology* 19, no. 9-10 (October 1997): 501-5, https://doi.org/10.1016/S0192-0561(97)00058-1

336   V G Morozov and V K Khavinson, "Natural and Synthetic Thymic Peptides as Therapeutics for Immune Dysfunction," *International Journal of Immunopharmacology* 19, no. 9-10 (October 1997): 501-5, https://doi.org/10.1016/S0192-0561(97)00058-1

337   R Consolini et al., "Distribution of Age-Related Thymulin Titres in Normal Subjects Through the Course of Life," *Clinical and Experimental Immunology* 121, no. 3 (September 2000): 444-7, https://doi.org/10.1046/j.1365-2249.2000.01315.x

338 Jingang Gui et al., "Thymus Size and Age-related Thymic Involution: Early Programming, Sexual Dimorphism, Progenitors and Stroma," *Aging and Disease* 3, no. 3 (June 2012): 280-90, https://pubmed.ncbi.nlm.nih.gov/22724086/

339 R Consolini et al., "Distribution of Age-Related Thymulin Titres in Normal Subjects Through the Course of Life," *Clinical and Experimental Immunology* 121, no. 3 (September 2000): 444-7, https://doi.org/10.1046/j.1365-2249.2000.01315.x

340 Jingang Gui et al., "Thymus Size and Age-related Thymic Involution: Early Programming, Sexual Dimorphism, Progenitors and Stroma," *Aging and Disease* 3, no. 3 (June 2012): 280-90, https://pubmed.ncbi.nlm.nih.gov/22724086/

341 Yehezqel Elyahu and Alon Monsonego, "Thymus Involution Sets the Clock of Declined Immunity and Repair with Aging," *Aging Research Reviews* 65 (November 2020): 101231, https://doi.org/10.1016/j.arr.2020.101231

342 H Hancı et al., "Can Prenatal Exposure to a 900 Mhz Electromagnetic Field Affect the Morphology of the Spleen and Thymus, and Alter Biomarkers of Oxidative Damage in 21-Day-Old Male Rats?," *Biotechnic and Histochemistry* 90, no. 7 (2015): 535-43, https://doi.org/10.3109/10520295.2015.1042051

343 Laura J Cobb et al., "Naturally Occurring Mitochondrial-Derived Peptides are Age-Dependent Regulators of Apoptosis, Insulin Sensitivity, and Inflammatory Markers," *Aging* 8, no. 4 (April 2016): 796-808, https://doi.org/10.18632/aging.100943

344 V G Morozov and V K Khavinson, "Natural and Synthetic Thymic Peptides as Therapeutics for Immune Dysfunction," *International Journal of Immunopharmacology* 19, no. 9-10 (October 1997): 501-5, https://doi.org/10.1016/S0192-0561(97)00058-1

345 M Cutuli et al., "Antimicrobial Effects of Alpha-MSH Peptides," *Journal of Leukocyte Biology* 67, no. 2 (February 2000): 233-9, https://doi.org/10.1002/jlb.67.2.233

346 Pablo Nakagawa et al., "Ac-SDKP Decreases Mortality and Cardiac Rupture After Acute Myocardial Infarction," *PLoS ONE* 13, no. 1 (January 2018): e0190300, https://doi.org/10.1371/journal.pone.0190300

347 N A Gavrisheva et al., "Effect of Peptide Vilon on the Content of Transforming Growth Factor-B and Permeability of Microvessels During Experimental Chronic Renal Failure," *Bulletin of Experimental Biology and Medicine* 139, no. 1 (January 2005): 24-6 https://doi.org/10.1007/s10517-005-0202-9

348 V N Anisimov et al., "The Effect of the Synthetic Immunomodulator

Thymogen on Radiation-Induced Carcinogenesis in Rats," *Voprosy Onkologii* 38, no. 4 (1992): 451-8, PMID: 1300740

349   Predrag Sikiric et al., "Stable Gastric Pentadecapeptide BPC 157: Novel Therapy in Gastrointestinal Tract," *Current Pharmaceutical Design* 17, no. 16 (2011): 1612-32, https://doi.org/10.2174/138161211796196954

350   Dennis Ruff et al., "A Randomized, Placebo-Controlled, Single and Multiple-Dose Study of Intravenous Thymosin Beta4 in Healthy Volunteers," *Annals of New York Academy of Sciences* 1194 (April 2010): 223-9, https://doi.org/10.1111/j.1749-6632.2010.05474.x

351   Jarred Younger and Sean Mackey, "Fibromyalgia Symptoms are Reduced by Low-Dose Naltrexone: A Pilot Study," *Pain Medicine* 10, no. 4 (June 2009): 663–72, https://doi.org/10.1111/j.1526-4637.2009.00613.x

352   Jarred Younger et al., "Low-Dose Naltrexone for the Treatment of Fibromyalgia: Findings of a Small, Randomized, Double-Blind, Placebo-Controlled, Counterbalanced, Crossover Trial Assessing Daily Pain Levels," *Arthritis & Rheumatism* 65, no. 2 (February 2013): 529-38, https://doi.org/10.1002/art.37734

353   V G Morozov and V K Khavinson, "Natural and Synthetic Thymic Peptides as Therapeutics for Immune Dysfunction," *International Journal of Immunopharmacology* 19, no. 9-10 (October 1997): 501-5, https://doi.org/10.1016/S0192-0561(97)00058-1

354   Laura J Cobb et al., "Naturally Occurring Mitochondrial-Derived Peptides Are Age-Dependent Regulators of Apoptosis, Insulin Sensitivity, and Inflammatory Markers," *Aging* 8, no. 4 (April 2016): 796-808, https://doi.org/10.18632/aging.100943

355   Cynthia Tuthill, Israel Rios and Randy McBeath, "Thymosin Alpha 1: Past Clinical Experience and Future Promise," *Annals of the New York Academy of Sciences* 1194 (April 2010); 130-5, https://doi.org/10.1111/j.1749-6632.2010.05482.x

356   Jarred Younger and Sean Mackey, "Fibromyalgia Symptoms are Reduced by Low-Dose Naltrexone: A Pilot Study," *Pain Medicine* 10, no. 4 (June 2009): 663–72, https://doi.org/10.1111/j.1526-4637.2009.00613.x

357   E John Wherry and Makoto Kurachi, "Molecular and Cellular Insight into T Cell Exhaustion," *Nature Reviews: Immunology* 15, no. 8 (August 2015): 486-99, https://doi.org/10.1038/nri3862

358   E John Wherry, "T Cell Exhaustion," *Nature Immunology* 12, no. 6 (June 2011): 492-9, https://doi.org/10.1038/ni.2035

359   Juan Li, Chun Hui Liu and Feng Shan Wang, "Thymosin Alpha 1: Biological Activities, Applications and Genetic Engineering

Production," *Peptides* 31, no. 11 (November 2010): 2151-8, https://doi.org/10.1016/j.peptides.2010.07.026

360   Jing Zhang et al., "Thymosin Beta4 Promotes Oligodendrogenesis in the Demyelinating Central Nervous System," *Neurobiology of Disease* 88 (April 2016): 85-95, https://doi.org/10.1016/j.nbd.2016.01.010

361   Predrag Sikiric et al., "Stable Gastric Pentadecapeptide BPC 157: Novel Therapy in Gastrointestinal Tract," *Current Pharmaceutical Design* 17, no. 16 (2011): 1612-32, https://doi.org/10.2174/138161211796196954

362   Jianfeng Zhang et al., "Function of Thymosin Beta-4 in Ethanol Induced Microglial Activation," *Cellular Physiology and Biochemistry* 38, no. 6 (2016): 2230-8, https://doi.org/10.1159/000445578

363   Kyoko Nitta et al., "Oral Administration of N-Acetyl-Seryl-Aspartyl-Lysyl-Proline Ameliorates Kidney Disease in Both Type 1 and Type II Diabetic Mice Via a Therapeutic Regimen," *BioMed Research International* 9172157 (2016): 1-11, https://doi.org/10.1155/2016/9172157

364   Pablo Nakagawa et al., "Ac-SDKP Decreases Mortality and Cardiac Rupture After Acute Myocardial Infarction," *PLoS ONE* 13, no. 1 (January 2018): e0190300, https://doi.org/10.1371/journal.pone.0190300

365   Megumi Kanasaki et al., "Elevation of the Antifibrotic Peptide N-Acetyl-Seryl-Aspartyl-Lysyl-Proline: A Blood Pressure-Independent Beneficial Effect of Angiotensin I-Converting Enzyme Inhibitors," *Fibrogenesis & Tissue Repair* 4, no. 1 (November 2011): 25, https://doi.org/10.1186/1755-1536-4-25

366   V G Morozov and V K Khavinson, "Natural and Synthetic Thymic Peptides as Therapeutics for Immune Dysfunction," *International Journal of Immunopharacology* 19, no. 9-10 (October 1997): 501-5, https://doi.org/10.1016/S0192-0561(97)00058-1

367   E V Koplik et al., "Effect of Dipeptide Vilon on Emotional Stress Resistance in Rats," *Rossiiskii Fiziologicheskii Zhurnal Imeni I.M. Sechenova* 88, no. 11 (November 2002): 1440-52, PMID: 12587272

368   Vladimir Kh Khavinson and Vyacheslav G Morozov, "Peptides of Pineal Gland and Thymus Prolong Human Life," *Neuro Endocrinology Letters* 24, no. 3-4 (August 2003): 233-40, PMID: 14523363

369   V N Anisimov, V K Khavinson and V G Morozov, "Immunomodulatory Synthetic Dipeptide L-Glu-L-Trp Slows Down Aging and Inhibits Spontaneous Carcinogenesis in Rats," *Biogerontology* 1, no. 1 (2000): 55-9, https://doi.org/10.1023/A:1010042008969

370   D H Kim et al., "Peptide Fragment of Thymosin ß4 Increases Hippocampal Neurogenesis and Facilitates Spatial Memory," *Neuroscience* 310 (December 2015): 51-62, https://doi.org/10.1016/j.

neuroscience.2015.09.017

371   Deborah Philp and Hynda K Kleinman, "Animal Studies with Thymosin B4, a Multifunctional Tissue Repair and Regeneration Peptide," *Annals of the New York Academy of Sciences* 1194 (April 2010): 81-6, https://doi.org/10.1111/j.1749-6632.2010.05479.x

372   V G Morozov and V K Khavinson, "Natural and Synthetic Thymic Peptides as Therapeutics for Immune Dysfunction*," International Journal of Immunopharacology* 19, no. 9-10 (October 1997): 501-5, https://doi.org/10.1016/S0192-0561(97)00058-1

373   L S Kogosova et al., "The Effect of Vilozen on the Immune Status of Bronchial Asthma Patients," *Vrachebnoe Delo* 10 (October 1990): 48-50, PMID: 2080579

374   Giovanna Castoldi et al., "Prevention of Myocardial Fibrosis by N-Acetyl-Seryl-Aspartyl-Lysyl-Proline in Diabetic Rats," *Clinical science* 118, no. 3 (October 2009): 211-20, https://doi.org/10.1042/cs20090234

375   Kyoko Nitta et al., "Oral Administration of N-Acetyl-Seryl-Aspartyl-Lysyl-Proline Ameliorates Kidney Disease in Both Type 1 and Type II Diabetic Mice Via a Therapeutic Regimen," *BioMed Research International* 9172157 (2016): 1-11, https://doi.org/10.1155/2016/9172157

376   Megumi Kanasaki et al., "Elevation of the Antifibrotic Peptide N-Acetyl-Seryl-Aspartyl-Lysyl-Proline: A Blood Pressure-Independent Beneficial Effect of Angiotensin I-Converting Enzyme Inhibitors," *Fibrogenesis & Tissue Repair* 4, no. 1 (November 2011): 25, https://doi.org/10.1186/1755-1536-4-25

377   T A Kudriavtseva et al., "Effect of Vilon on the Neuroendocrine Status and Sexual Function of old Male Rats," *Advances in Gerontology* 19 (2006): 97-101, PMID: 17152729

378   E V Koplik et al., "Effect of Dipeptide Vilon on Emotional Stress Resistance in Rats," *Rossiiskii Fiziologicheskii Zhurnal Imeni I.M. Sechenova* 88, no. 11 (November 2002): 1440-52, PMID: 12587272

379   O P Barykina et al., "Combined Effect of Vilon and Cyclophosphane on Tumor Transplants and Lymphoid Tissue Explants in Mice and Rats of Various Age," *Advances in Gerontology* 12 (2003): 128-31, PMID: 14743610

380   G B Pliss et al., "Inhibitory Effect of Peptide Vilon on the Development of Induced Rate Urinary Bladder Tumors in Rats," *Bulletin of Experimental Biology and Medicine* 131, no. 6 (June 2001): 558-64, https://doi.org/10.1023/a:1012354603132

381   V K Khavinson et al., "Effect of Vilon on Biological Age and Lifespan

in Mice," *Bulletin of Experimental Biology and Medicine* 130, no. 7 (July 2000): 88-91, https://doi.org/10.1007/BF02682106

382   B I Kuznik et al., "Effect of Vilon on the Immunity Status and Coagulation Hemostasis in Patients of Different Age with Diabetes Mellitus," *Advances in Gerontology* 20, no, 2 (2007): 106-15, PMID: 18306698

383   B I Kuznik et al., "Effect of Vilon on the Immunity Status and Coagulation Hemostasis in Patients of Different Age with Diabetes Mellitus," *Advances in Gerontology* 20, no, 2 (2007): 106-15, PMID: 18306698

384   L. S, Kozina et al., "Regulatory Peptides Protect Brain Neurons from Hypoxia in Vivo," *Doklady Biological Sciences* 418, no. 1 (February 2008): 7-10, https://doi.org/10.1134/S0012496608010031

385   Rita Rezzani et al., "Thymus-Pineal Gland Axis: Revisiting its Role in Human Life and Ageing," *International Journal of Molecular Sciences* 21, no. 22 (November 20, 2020): 8806, https://doi.org/10.3390/ijms21228806

386   B. I. Kuznik et al., "The Effect of Lys–Glu–Asp–Gly and Ala–Glu–Asp–Gly Peptides on Hormone Activity and the Thyroid Structure in Sexually Mature and Old Hypophysectomized Birds," *Advances in Gerontology* 1, no. 4 (2011): 340-5, https://doi.org/10.1134/s2079057011040072

387   V Kh Khavinson et al., "Short Peptides and Telomere Length Regulator Hormone Irisin," *Bulletin of Experimental Biology and Medicine* 160, no. 3 (January 2016): 347-9, https://doi.org/10.1007/s10517-016-3167-y

388   Vladimir N Anisimov et al., "Inhibitory Effect of the Peptide Epitalon on the Development of Spontaneous Mammary Tumors in HER-2/Neu Transgenic Mice," *International Journal of Cancer* 101, no. 1 (September 1, 2002): 7-10, https://doi.org/10.1002/ijc.10570

389   V Kh Khavinson et al., "Short Peptides and Telomere Length Regulator Hormone Irisin," *Bulletin of Experimental Biology and Medicine* 160, no. 3 (January 2016): 347-9, https://doi.org/10.1007/s10517-016-3167-y

390   R Sandyk and G I Awerbuch, "Pineal Calcification and its Relationship to the Fatigue of Multiple Sclerosis," *International Journal of Neuroscience* 74, no. 1-4 (February 1994): 95-103, https://doi.org/10.3109/00207459408987233

391   Vladimir Kh Khavinson and Vyacheslav G Morozov, "Peptides of Pineal Gland and Thymus Prolong Human Life," *Neuro Endocrinology Letters* 24, no. 3-4 (August 2003): 233-40, PMID: 14523363

392   Vladimir Kh Khavinson and Vyacheslav G Morozov, "Peptides of Pineal Gland and Thymus Prolong Human Life," *Neuro Endocrinology Letters* 24, no. 3-4 (August 2003): 233-40, PMID: 14523363

393 V N Anisimov, A V Arutjunyan and V K Khavinson, "Effects of Pineal Peptide Preparation Epitalon on Free-Radical Processes in Humans and Animals," *Neuroendocrinology Letters* 22, no. 1 (2001): 9–18, PMID: 11335874

394 S V Anisimov et al., "Studies of the Effects of Vilon and Epithalon on Gene Expression in Mouse Heart Using DNA-Microarray Technology," *Bulletin of Experimental Biology and Medicine* 133, no. 3 (March 2002): 293-9, https://doi.org/10.1023/A:1015859322630

395 Predrag Sikiric et al., "Stable Gastric Pentadecapeptide BPC 157: Novel Therapy in Gastrointestinal Tract," *Current Pharmaceutical Design* 17, no. 16 (2011): 1612-32, https://doi.org/10.2174/138161211796196954

396 Chung-Hsun Chang et al., "The Promoting Effect of Pentadecapeptide BPC 157 on Tendon Healing Involves Tendon Outgrowth, Cell Survival, and Cell Migration," *Journal of Applied Physiology* 110, no. 3 (March 2011): 774-80, https://doi.org/10.1152/japplphysiol.00945.2010

397 Alenka Boban-Blagaic et al., "The Influence of Gastric Pentadecapeptide BPC 157 on Acute and Chronic Ethanol Administration in Mice. The Effect of N (G)-Nitro-L-Arginine Methyl Ester and L-Arginine," *Medical Science Monitor* 12, no. 1 (January 2006): BR36-45, PMID: 16369461

398 Tonglie Huang et al., "Body Protective Compound-157 Enhances alkali-Burn Wound Healing in Vivo and Promotes Proliferation, Migration, and Angiogenesis in Vitro," *Drug Design, Development and Therapy* 9 (April 2015): 2485-99, https://doi.org/10.2147/DDDT.S82030

399 Predrag Sikiric et al., "Stress in Gastrointestinal Tract and Stable Gastric Pentadecapeptide BPC 157. Finally, Do we Have a Solution?." *Current Pharmaceutical Design* 23, no. 27 (2017): 4012-28, https://doi.org/10.21 74/1381612823666170220163219

400 Predrag Sikiric et al., "Revised Robert's Cytoprotection and Adaptive Cytoprotection and Stable Gastric Pentadecapeptide BPC 157. Possible Significance and Implications for a Novel Mediator," *Current Pharmaceutical Design* 16, no. 10 (2010): 1224–34, https://doi. org/10.2174/138161210790945977

401 Nermin Lojo et al., "Effects of Diclofenac, L-NAME, L-Arginine, and Pentadecapeptide BPC 157 on Gastrointestinal, Liver, and Brain Lesions, Failed Anastomosis, and Intestinal Adaptation Deterioration in 24 Hour-Short-Bowel Rats," *PLoS ONE* 11, no. 9 (September 14, 2016): e0162590, https://doi.org/10.1371/journal.pone.0162590

402 P Sikiric et al., "The Antidepressant Effect of an Antiulcer Pentadecapeptide BPC 157 in Porsolt's Test and Chronic Unpredictable Stress in Rats. A Comparison with Antidepressants," *Journal of*

Physiology-Paris 94, no. 2 (March-April 2009): 99-104, https://doi.org/10.1016/s0928-4257(00)00148-0

403   Sanja Masnec et al., "Perforating Corneal Injury in Rat and Pentadecapeptide BPC 157," *Experimental Eye Research* 136 (July 2015): 9-15, https://doi.org/10.1016/j.exer.2015.04.016

404   Annika Roth et al., "LL-37 fights SARS-CoV-2: The vitamin D-Inducible Peptide LL-37 Inhibits Binding of SARS-COV-2 Spike Protein to its Cellular Receptor Angiotensin-Converting Enzyme 2 in Vitro," *BioRxiv Preprint* (December 2, 2020): https://doi.org/10.1101/2020.12.02.408153

405   Hanlin Zhang et al., "Preliminary Evaluation of the Safety and Efficacy of Oral Human Antimicrobial Peptide LL-37 in the Treatment of Patients of COVID-19, A Small-Scale, Single-Arm, Exploratory Safety Study," *MedRxiv Preprint* (May 15, 2020): https://doi.org/10.1101/2020.05.11.20064584

406   Predrag Sikiric et al., "Stable Gastric Pentadecapeptide BPC 157: Novel Therapy in Gastrointestinal Tract," *Current Pharmaceutical Design* 17, no. 16 (2011): 1612-32, https://doi.org/10.2174/138161211796196954

407   Ben Greenfiled, "How to Reverse the Damage from Cell Phone Radiation, Hidden Sources of EMF, the Best Way to Measure your EMF Exposure & Much More with Dr. Joseph Mercola," (2019): Podcast, https://bengreenfieldlife.com/podcast/lifestyle-podcasts/dr-mercola-emf-recommendations/

408   Dimitris J. Panagopoulos, Olle Johansson and George L. Carlo, "Polarization: a Key Difference Between Man-made and Natural Electromagnetic Fields, in Regard to Biological Activity," *Scientific Reports* 5 (October 12, 2015): 14914, https://doi.org/10.1038/srep14914

409   J L Phillips, N P Singh and H Lai, "Electromagnetic Fields and DNA Damage," *Pathophysiology* 16, no. 2-3 (August 2009): 79–88, https://doi.org/10.1016/j.pathophys.2008.11.005

410   Carl Blackman, "Cell Phone Radiation: Evidence From ELF and RF Studies Supporting More Inclusive Risk Identification and Assessment," *Pathophysiology* 16, no. 2-3 (August 2009): 205–16, https://doi.org/10.1016/j.pathophys.2009.02.001

411   Vini G Khurana et al., "Cell Phones and Brain Tumors: A Review Including the Long-Term Epidemiologic Data," *Surgical Neurology* 72, no. 3 (September 2009): 205–14, https://doi.org/10.1016/j.surneu.2009.01.019

412   Dimitris J. Panagopoulos, "Analyzing the Health Impacts of Modern Telecommunications Microwaves", L. V. Berhardt (Ed), *Advances in Medicine and Biology* 17 (September 2011): 1-55, Nova Science

Publishers, Inc., New York, USA.

413   Dimitris J Panagopoulos, Evangelia D Chavdoula and Lukas H Margaritis, "Bioeffects of Mobile Telephony Radiation in Relation to its Intensity or Distance from the Antenna," *International Journal of Radiation Biology* 86, no. 5 (May 2010): 345–57, https://doi.org/10.3109/09553000903567961

414   H Hancı et al., "Can Prenatal Exposure to a 900 MHz Electromagnetic Field Affect the Morphology of the Spleen and Thymus, and Alter Biomarkers of Oxidative Damage in 21-day-old Male Rats?," *Biotechnic and Histochemistry* 90, no. 7 (2015): 1-9, https://doi.org/10.3109/10520295.2015.1042051

415   H Hancı et al., "Can Prenatal Exposure to a 900 MHz Electromagnetic Field Affect the Morphology of the Spleen and Thymus, and Alter Biomarkers of Oxidative Damage in 21-day-old Male Rats?," *Biotechnic and Histochemistry* 90, no. 7 (2015): 1-9, https://doi.org/10.3109/10520295.2015.1042051

416   M R Duchen, "Topical Review: Mitochondria and Calcium: from Cell Signaling to Cell Death," *Journal of Physiology* 529, no. 1 (November 2000): 57-68, https://doi.org/10.1111/j.1469-7793.2000.00057.x

417   Robert K Naviaux, "Metabolic Features and Regulation of the Healing Cycle—A New Model For Chronic Disease Pathogenesis and Treatment," *Mitochondrion* 46 (May 2019): 278-97, https://doi.org/10.1016/j.mito.2018.08.001

418   Veronica Eisner et al., "Mitochondria Fine-Tune the Slow Ca2+ Transients Induced by Electrical Stimulation of Skeletal Myotubes," *Cell Calcium* 48, no. 6 (December 2010): 358-70, https://doi.org/10.1016/j.ceca.2010.11.001

419   Magda Havas, "Radiation From Wireless Technology Affects the Blood, the Heart, and the Autonomic Nervous System," *Reviews on Environmental Health* 28, no. 2-3 (2013): 75-84, https://doi.org/10.1515/reveh-2013-0004

420   H Hancı et al., "Can Prenatal Exposure to a 900 MHz Electromagnetic Field Affect the Morphology of the Spleen and Thymus, and Alter Biomarkers of Oxidative Damage in 21-day-old Male Rats?," *Biotechnic and Histochemistry* 90, no. 7 (2015): 1-9, https://doi.org/10.3109/10520295.2015.1042051

421   L LloydMorgan, Santosh Kesari and Devra Lee Davis, "Why Children Absorb More Microwave Radiation Than Adults: The Consequences," *Journal of Microscopy and Ultrastructure* 2, no. 4 (December 2014): 197–204, https://doi.org/10.1016/j.jmau.2014.06.005

422   Tamir S Aldad et al., "Fetal Radiofrequency Radiation Exposure from

800-1900 Mhz-Rated Cellular Telephones Affects Neurodevelopment and Behavior in Mice," *Science Reports* 2, (2012): 312, https://doi.org/10.1038/srep00312

423   Jun Tang et al., "Exposure to 900mhz Electromagnetic Fields Activates the Mkp-1/ERK Pathway and Causes Blood-Brain Barrier Damage and Cognitive Impairment in Rats," *Brain Research* 1601 (March 19, 2015): 92-101, https://doi.org/10.1016/j.brainres.2015.01.019

424   Nidhi Saikhedkar et al., "Effects of Mobile Phone Radiation (900mhz Radiofrequency) on Structure and Functions of Rat Brain," *Neurological Research* 36, no. 12 (December 2014): 1072– 9, https://doi.org/10.1179/1743132814Y.0000000392

425   Ayşe İkinci Keleş et al., "The Effects of a Continuous 1-H a Day 900-Mhz Electromagnetic Field Applied Throughout Early and Mid-Adolescence on Hippocampus Morphology and Learning Behavior in Late Adolescent Male Rats," *Journal of Chemical Neuroanatomy* 94 (December 2018): 46–53, https://doi.org/10.1016/j.jchemneu.2018.08.006

426   Ayşe İkinci Keleş et al., "The Effects of a Continuous 1-H a Day 900-Mhz Electromagnetic Field Applied Throughout Early and Mid-Adolescence on Hippocampus Morphology and Learning Behavior in Late Adolescent Male Rats," *Journal of Chemical Neuroanatomy* 94 (December 2018): 46–53, https://doi.org/10.1016/j.jchemneu.2018.08.006

427   Jun-Ping Zhang et al., "Effects of 1.8 Ghz Radiofrequency Fields on the Emotional Behavior and Spatial Memory of Adolescent Mice," *International Journal of Environmental Research and Public Health* 14, no. 11 (November 2017): 1344, https://doi.org/10.3390/ijerph14111344

428   Vladimir Kh Khavinson and Vyacheslav G Morozov, "Peptides of Pineal Gland and Thymus Prolong Human Life," *Neuro Endocrinology Letters* 24, no. 3-4 (August 2003): 233-40, PMID: 14523363

429   Vladimir Kh. Khavinson et al., "Experimental Studies of the Pineal Gland Preparation Epithalamin," *The Pineal Gland and Cancer: Neuroimmunoendocrine Mechanisms in Malignancy* (2001): 294-306, https://doi.org/10.1007/978-3-642-59512-7_14

430   Vladimir Kh Khavinson and Vyacheslav G Morozov, "Peptides of Pineal Gland and Thymus Prolong Human Life," *Neuro Endocrinology Letters* 24, no. 3-4 (August 2003): 233-40, PMID: 14523363

431   L S Kogosova et al., "The Effect of Vilozen on the Immune Status of Bronchial Asthma Patients," *Vrachebnoe Delo* 10 (October 1990): 48-50, PMID: 2080579

432   V G Morozov and V K Khavinson, "Natural and Synthetic Thymic

Peptides as Therapeutics for Immune Dysfunction," *International Journal of Immunopharmacology* 19, no. 9-10 (October 1997): 501-5, https://doi.org/10.1016/S0192-0561(97)00058-1

433 V. K. Khavinson and V. V. Malinin, "Gerontological Aspects of Genome Peptide Regulation," *Karger* (2005): https://doi.org/10.1159/isbn.978-3-318-01193-7

434 E A Ojo-Amaize, E J Conley and J B Peter, "Decreased Natural Killer Cell Activity is Associated with the Severity of Chronic Fatigue Immune Dysfunction Syndrome," *Clinical Infectious Diseases* 18, no. 1 (January 1994): 1:S157-9, https://www.jstor.org/stable/4457628

435 Keizo Kanasaki et al., "N-Acetyl-Seryl-Aspartyl-Lysyl-Proline Inhibits TGF-β–Mediated Plasminogen Activator Inhibitor-1 Expression via Inhibition of Smad Pathway in Human Mesangial Cells," *Journal of the American Society of Nephrology* 14, no. 4 (April 2003): 863-72, https://10.1097/01.asn.0000057544.95569.ec

436 Kent Holtorf, "Peripheral Thyroid Hormone Conversion and its Impact on TSH and Metabolic Activity," *Journal of Restorative Medicine* 3, no. 1 (April 2014): 30-51, https://doi.org/10.14200/jrm.2014.3.0103

437 Kent Holtorf, "Peripheral Thyroid Hormone Conversion and its Impact on TSH and Metabolic Activity," *Journal of Restorative Medicine* 3, no. 1 (April 2014): 30-51, https://doi.org/10.14200/jrm.2014.3.0103

438 Kent Holtorf, "Diagnosis and Treatment of Hypothalamic-Pituitary-Adrenal (HPA) Axis Dysfunction in Patients with Chronic Fatigue Syndrome (CFS) and Fibromyalgia (FM)," *Journal of Chronic Fatigue Syndrome* 14, no. 3 (January 2008): 59-88, https://doi.org/10.1300/J092v14n03_06

439 Keizo Kanasaki et al., "N-Acetyl-Seryl-Aspartyl-Lysyl-Proline Inhibits TGF-β–Mediated Plasminogen Activator Inhibitor-1 Expression via Inhibition of Smad Pathway in Human Mesangial Cells," *Journal of American Society of Nephrology* 14, no. 4 (April 2003): 863-872, https://doi.org/10.1097/01.ASN.0000057544.95569.EC

440 Kent Holtorf, "Peripheral Thyroid Hormone Conversion and its Impact on TSH and Metabolic Activity," *Journal of Restorative Medicine* 3, no. 1 (April 2014): 30-51, https://doi.org/10.14200/jrm.2014.3.0103

441 Erika T. Schwartz and Kent Holtorf, "Hormones in Wellness and Disease Prevention: Common Practices, Current State of the Evidence, and Questions for the Future," *Primary Care: Clinics in Office Practice* 35, no. 4 (December 1, 2008): 669–705, https://doi.org/10.1016/j.pop.2008.07.015

442 Kent Holtorf, "Thyroid Hormone Transport into Cellular Tissue," *Journal of Restorative Medicine* 3, no. 1 (April 1, 2014): 53-68, https://

doi.org/10.14200/jrm.2014.3.0104

443   Kent Holtorf, "Peripheral Thyroid Hormone Conversion and its Impact
      on TSH and Metabolic Activity," *Journal of Restorative Medicine* 3, no.
      1 (April 2014): 30-51, https://doi.org/10.14200/jrm.2014.3.0103

444   Erika Schwartz, Vincent Morelli and Kent Holtorf, "Hormone
      Replacement Therapy in the Geriatric Patient: Current State of the
      Evidence and Questions for the Future: Estrogen, Progesterone,
      Testosterone, Growth Hormone and Thyroid Hormone Augmentation
      in the Geriatric Clinical Practice: Part 2," *Clinics in Geriatric Medicine*
      27, no. 4 (November 2011): 561-75, https://doi.org/10.1016/j.
      cger.2011.07.004

445   Kent Holtorf, "Diagnosis and Treatment of Hypothalamic-Pituitary-
      Adrenal (HPA) Axis Dysfunction in Patients with Chronic Fatigue
      Syndrome (CFS) and Fibromyalgia (FM)," *Journal of Chronic Fatigue
      Syndrome* 14, no. 3 (January 2008): 59-88, https://doi.org/10.1300/
      J092v14n03_06

446   Kent Holtorf, "Diagnosis and Treatment of Hypothalamic-Pituitary-
      Adrenal (HPA) Axis Dysfunction in Patients with Chronic Fatigue
      Syndrome (CFS) and Fibromyalgia (FM)," *Journal of Chronic Fatigue
      Syndrome* 14, no. 3 (January 2008): 59-88, https://doi.org/10.1300/
      J092v14n03_06

447   Kent Holtorf, "Diagnosis and Treatment of Hypothalamic-Pituitary-
      Adrenal (HPA) Axis Dysfunction in Patients with Chronic Fatigue
      Syndrome (CFS) and Fibromyalgia (FM)," *Journal of Chronic Fatigue
      Syndrome* 14, no. 3 (January 2008): 59-88, https://doi.org/10.1300/
      J092v14n03_06

448   M Cutuli et al., "Antimicrobial Effects of Alpha-MSH Peptides,"
      Journal of Leukocyte Biology 67, no. 2 (February 2000): 233-9, https://
      doi.org/10.1002/jlb.67.2.233

449   Madhuri Singh and Kasturi Mukhopadhyay, "Alpha-Melanocyte
      Stimulating Hormone: An Emerging Anti-Inflammatory Antimicrobial
      Peptide," *BioMed Research International* 2014 (July 2014): 874610,
      https://doi.org/10.1155/2014/874610

450   Anna Catania et al., "The Melanocortin System in Control of
      Inflammation," *The Scientific World Journal* 10 (September 2010):
      1840-53, https://doi.org/10.1100/tsw.2010.173

451   M Cutuli et al., "Antimicrobial Effects of Alpha-MSH Peptides,"
      Journal of Leukocyte Biology 67, no. 2 (February 2000): 233-9, https://
      doi.org/10.1002/jlb.67.2.233

452   Balazs Varga et al., "Protective Effect of Alpha-Melanocyte-Stimulating
      Hormone (-α MSH) on the Recovery of Ischemia/Reperfusion (I/R)-

Induced Retinal Damage in a Rat Model," *Journal of Molecular Neuroscience* 50, no. 3 (July 2013): 558–70, https://doi.org/10.1007/s12031-013-9998-3

453 M Cutuli et al., "Antimicrobial Effects of Alpha-MSH Peptides," *Journal of Leukocyte Biology* 67, no. 2 (February 2000): 233-9, https://doi.org/10.1002/jlb.67.2.233

454 Madhuri Singh and Kasturi Mukhopadhyay, "Alpha-Melanocyte Stimulating Hormone: An Emerging Anti-Inflammatory Antimicrobial Peptide," *BioMed Research International* 2014 (July 2014): 874610, https://doi.org/10.1155/2014/874610

455 Madhuri Singh and Kasturi Mukhopadhyay, "Alpha-Melanocyte Stimulating Hormone: An Emerging Anti-Inflammatory Antimicrobial Peptide," *BioMed Research International* 2014 (July 2014): 874610, https://doi.org/10.1155/2014/874610

456 Evelien T M Berends et al., "Bacteria Under Stress by Complement and Coagulation," *FEMS Microbiology Reviews* 38, no. 6 (November 2014): 1146-71, https://doi.org/10.1111/1574-6976.12080

457 C E Crist, D E Berg and H. H. Harrison, "Does Borreliosis (Lyme Disease) Activate the Coagulation System and is a Coagulation Regulatory Protein Defect Predispositional?," *Infectious Diseases Society of America* (Oct 2003), https://idsa.confex.com/idsa/2003/webprogram/Paper18421.html

458 Evelien T M Berends et al., "Bacteria Under Stress by Complement and Coagulation," *FEMS Microbiology Reviews* 38, no. 6 (November 2014): 1146-71, https://doi.org/10.1111/1574-6976.12080

459 Sabine Bork et al., "Growth-inhibitory Effect of Heparin on Babesia Parasites," *Antimicrobial Agents and Chemotherapy* 48, no. 1 (January 2004): 236-41, https://doi.org/10.1128/AAC.48.1.236-241.2004

460 C E Crist, D E Berg and H. H. Harrison, "Does Borreliosis (Lyme Disease) Activate the Coagulation System and is a Coagulation Regulatory Protein Defect Predispositional?," *Infectious Diseases Society of America* (Oct 2003), https://idsa.confex.com/idsa/2003/webprogram/Paper18421.html

461 Neil A Zakai et al., "Activated Partial Thromboplastin Time and Risk of Future Venous Thromboembolism," *American Journal of Medicine* 121, no. 3 (March 2008): 231-8, https://doi.org/10.1016/j.amjmed.2007.10.025

462 Sabine Bork et al., "Growth-inhibitory Effect of Heparin on Babesia Parasites," *Antimicrobial Agents and Chemotherapy* 48, no. 1 (January 2004): 236-41, https://doi.org/10.1128/AAC.48.1.236-241.2004

463 Karin C A A Wildhagen et al., "Nonanticoagulant Heparin Prevents Histone-Mediated Cytotoxicity in Vitro and Improves Survival in Sepsis," *Blood* 123, no. 7 (February 2014) 1098-1101, https://doi.org/10.1182/blood-2013-07-514984

464 Masaharu Hatakeyama et al., "Heparin Inhibits IFN-Gamma-Induced Fractalkine/CX3CL1 Expression in Human Endothelial Cells," *Inflammation* 28, no. 1 (February 2004): 7-13, https://doi.org/10.1023/b:ifla.0000014706.49598.78

465 Petra H Wirtz et al., "Oral Melatonin Reduces Blood Coagulation Activity: A Placebo-Controlled Study in Healthy Young Men," *Journal of Pineal Research* 44, no. 2 (March 2008): 127-33, https://doi.org/10.1111/j.1600-079X.2007.00499.x

466 Mirjana Stupnisek et al., "Pentadecapeptide BPC-157 Reduces Bleeding Time and Thrombocytopenia after Amputation in Rats Treated with Heparin, Warfarin or Aspirin," *Thrombosis Research* 129, no. 5 (May 2012): 652-9, https://doi.org/10.1016/j.thromres.2011.07.035

467 Sabine Bork et al., "Growth-inhibitory Effect of Heparin on Babesia Parasites," *Antimicrobial Agents and Chemotherapy* 48, no. 1 (January 2004): 236-41, https://doi.org/10.1128/AAC.48.1.236-241.2004

468 Mahesh Yadav, Jennifer Rosenbaum and Edward J. Goetzl , "Cutting Edge: Vasoactive Intestinal Peptide (VIP) Induces Differentiation of Th17 Cells with a Distinctive Cytokine Profile," *Journal of immunology* 180, no. 5 (March 1, 2008): 27772-6, https://doi.org/10.4049/jimmunol.180.5.2772

469 Catalina Abad et al., "Vasoactive Intestinal Peptide Loss Leads to Impaired CNS Parenchymal T-Cell Infiltration and Resistance to Experimental Autoimmune Encephalomyelitis," *Proceedings of the National Academy of Sciences of the United States of America* 107, no. 45 (November 2010): 19555-60, https://doi.org/10.1073/pnas.1007622107

470 Mahesh Yadav and Edward J Goetzl, "Vasoactive Intestinal Peptide-Mediated Th17 Differentiation," *Annals of the New York Acadamy of Sciences* 1144 (November 2008): 83-9, https://doi.org/10.1196/annals.1418.020

471 Mahesh Yadav, Jennifer Rosenbaum and Edward J. Goetzl , "Cutting Edge: Vasoactive Intestinal Peptide (VIP) Induces Differentiation of Th17 Cells with a Distinctive Cytokine Profile," *Journal of Immunology* 180, no. 5 (March 1, 2008): 27772-6, https://doi.org/10.4049/jimmunol.180.5.2772

472 Catalina Abad et al., "Vasoactive Intestinal Peptide Loss Leads to Impaired CNS Parenchymal T-Cell Infiltration and Resistance to

Experimental Autoimmune Encephalomyelitis," *Proceedings of the National Academy of Sciences of the United States of America* 107, no. 45 (November 2010): 19555-60, https://doi.org/10.1073/pnas.1007622107

473 Per Anderson and Elena Gonzalez-Rey, "Vasoactive Intestinal Peptide Induces Cell Cycle Arrest and Regulatory Functions in Human T Cells at Multiple Levels," *Molecular and Cellular Biology* 30, no. 10 (May 2010): 2537-51, https://doi.org/10.1128/MCB.01282-09

474 John S Yi, Maureen A Cox and Allan J Zajac, "T-cell exhaustion: characteristics, causes and conversion," *Immunology* 129, no. 4 (April 2010): 474-81, https://doi.org/10.1111/j.1365-2567.2010.03255.x

475 Per Anderson and Elena Gonzalez-Rey, "Vasoactive Intestinal Peptide Induces Cell Cycle Arrest and Regulatory Functions in Human T Cells at Multiple Levels," *Molecular and Cellular Biology* 30, no. 10 (May 2010): 2537-51, https://doi.org/10.1128/MCB.01282-09

476 John S Yi, Maureen A Cox and Allan J Zajac, "T-cell exhaustion: characteristics, causes and conversion," *Immunology* 129, no. 4 (April 2010): 474-81, https://doi.org/10.1111/j.1365-2567.2010.03255.x

477 E John Wherry, "T Cell Exhaustion," *Nature Immunology* 12, no. 6 (June 2011): 492-9, https://doi.org/10.1038/ni.2035

478 M Delgado et al., "Vasoactive Intestinal Peptide and Pituitary Adenylate Cyclase-Activating Polypeptide Stimulate the Induction of Th2 Responses by Up-Regulating B7.2 Expression," *Journal of Immunology* 163, no. 7 (October 1999): 3629-35, https://pubmed.ncbi.nlm.nih.gov/10490956/

479 Giovanna Castoldi et al., "Prevention of Myocardial Fibrosis By N-Acetyl-Seryl-Aspartyl-Lysyl-Proline in Diabetic Rats," *Clinical Science* 118, no.3 (October 2009): 211-20, https://doi.org/10.1042/cs20090234

480 N A Gavrisheva et al., "Effect of Peptide Vilon on the Content of Transforming Growth Factor-Beta and Permeability of Microvessels During Experimental Chronic Renal Failure," *Bulletin of Experimental Biology and Medicine* 139, no. 1 (January 2005): 24–6, https://doi.org/10.1007/s10517-005-0202-9

481 Keizo Kanasaki et al., "N-Acetyl-Seryl-Aspartyl-Lysyl-Proline Inhibits TGF-Beta-Mediated Plasminogen Activator Inhibitor-1 Expression Via Inhibition of Smad Pathway in Human Mesangial Cells*," Journal of the American Society of Nephrology* 14, no. 4 (April 2003): 863-72, https://doi.org/10.1097/01.asn.0000057544.95569.ec

482 Mahesh Yadav and Edward J Goetzl, "Vasoactive Intestinal Peptide-Mediated Th17 Differentiation," *Annals of the New York Acadamy*

of Sciences 1144 (November 2008): 83-9, https://doi.org/10.1196/annals.1418.020

483   Catalina Abad et al., "Vasoactive Intestinal Peptide Loss Leads to Impaired CNS Parenchymal T-Cell Infiltration and Resistance to Experimental Autoimmune Encephalomyelitis," *Proceedings of the National Academy of Sciences of the United States of America* 107, no. 45 (November 2010): 19555-60, https://doi.org/10.1073/pnas.1007622107

484   E John Wherry and Makoto Kurachi, "Molecular and Cellular Insight into T Cell Exhaustion," *Nature Reviews: Immunology* 15, no. 8 (August 2015): 486-99, https://doi.org/10.1038/nri3862

485   Kent Holtorf, "Peripheral Thyroid Hormone Conversion and its Impact on TSH and Metabolic Activity," *Journal of Restorative Medicine* 3, no. 1 (April 2014): 30-51, https://doi.org/10.14200/jrm.2014.3.0103

486   Kent Holtorf, "A Confounding Condition: Treating chronic fatigue syndrome and fibromyalgia requires addressing the underlying problems," *Healthy Aging* (Nov/Dec) 2008, http://truemedmd.com/wp-content/uploads/2013/03/Treating_Chronic_Fatigue_Syndrome_Kent_Holtorf_Womens_Health.pdf

487   Ming-Jer Hsieh et al., "Therapeutic Potential of Pro-Angiogenic BPC157 is Associated with VEGFR2 Activation and Up-Regulation," *Journal of Molecular Medicine* 95, no. 3 (March 2017): 323–33, https://doi.org/10.1007/s00109-016-1488-y

488   Tonglie Huang et al., "Body Protective Compound-157 Enhancesalkali-Burn Wound Healing in Vivo and Promotes Proliferation, Migration, and Angiogenesis in Vitro," *Drug Design, Development and Therapy* 9 (April 2015): 2485-99, https://doi.org/10.2147/DDDT.S82030

Chapter Seven

489   "World Report on Vision," *World Health Organization*, License: CC BY-NC-SA 3.0 IGO https://apps.who.int/iris/bitstream/handle/10665/328717/9789241516570-eng.pdf?sequence=18&isAllowed=y

490   Gray's Anatomy, 42nd Edition, "The Anatomical Basis of Clinical Practice," Editor-in-Chief : Susan Standring, Hardcover ISBN: 9780702077050

491   Caleb L. Shumway, Mahsaw Motlagh and Matthew Wade, "Anatomy, Head and Neck, Eye Conjunctiva," *StatPearls [Internet]*, Treasure Island (FL): StatPearls Publishing (January 2022), PMID: 30137787, [Updated Jul 26, 2021]

492   Ru Zhou and Rachel R Caspi, "Ocular Immune Privilege," *F1000 Biology Reports* (January 18, 2010): 2:3, https://doi.org/10.3410/B2-3

493   Bruce Alberts et al., "Molecular Biology of the Cell, 4th edition," New York: *Garland Science* (2002): Chapter 24, The Adaptive Immune System, ISBN-10: 0-8153-3218-1

494   Fu-Shin X Yu and Linda D Hazlett, "Toll-like Receptors and the Eye," *Investigative Ophthalmology & Visual Science* 47, no. 4 (April 2006): 1255-1263, https://doi.org/10.1167/iovs.05-0956

495   Bruce Alberts et al., "Molecular Biology of the Cell, 4th edition," New York: *Garland Science* (2002): Chapter 24, The Adaptive Immune System, ISBN-10: 0-8153-3218-1

496   Andreea E. Bodoki et al., "Perspectives of Molecularly Imprinted Polymer-Based Drug Delivery Systems in Ocular Therapy," *Polymers (Basel)* 13, no. 21 (November 2021): 3649, https://doi.org/10.3390/polym13213649

497   Keith M Meek and Carlo Knupp, "Corneal Structure and Transparency," *Progress in Retinal and Eye Research* 49 (November 2015): 1-16, https://doi.org/10.1016/j.preteyeres.2015.07.001

498   E K Akpek and J D Gottsch, "Immune Defense at the Ocular Surface," *Eye* 17, no. 8 (November 2003): 949–956, https://doi.org/10.1038/sj.eye.6700617

499   M A Lemp and H J Blackman, "Ocular Surface Defense Mechanisms," *Annals Ophthalmology* 13, no. 1 (January 1981): 61-3, https://pubmed.ncbi.nlm.nih.gov/7247160/

500   U. Pleyer and H. Baatz, "Antibacterial Protection of the Ocular Surface," *Ophthalmologica* 211, Suppl 1 (1997): 2-8, https://doi.org/10.1159/000310878

501   Charles A Dinarello, "Overview of the IL-1 Family in Innate Inflammation and Acquired Immunity," *Immunological Reviews* 281, no. 1 (January 2018): 8-27, https://doi.org/10.1111/imr.12621

502   Bruce Alberts et al., "Molecular Biology of the Cell, 4th edition," New York: *Garland Science* (2002): Chapter 24, The Adaptive Immune System, ISBN-10: 0-8153-3218-1

503   Charles A Dinarello, "Overview of the IL-1 Family in Innate Inflammation and Acquired Immunity," *Immunological Reviews* 281, no. 1 (January 2018): 8-27, https://doi.org/10.1111/imr.12621

504   Judith A West-Mays and Dhruva J Dwivedi, "The Keratocyte: Corneal Stromal Cell with Variable Repair Phenotypes," *The International Journal of Biochemistry & Cell Biology* 38, no. 10 (2006): 1625-1631, https://doi.org/10.1016/j.biocel.2006.03.010

505   Ian A Parish et al., "Tissue Destruction Caused by Cytotoxic T Lymphocytes Induces Deletional Tolerance," *Proceedings of the National Academy of Sciences of the United States of America* 106, no.

10 (March 10,2009): 3901-6, https://doi.org/10.1073/pnas.0810427106

506   Eric Vivier et al., "Functions of Natural Killer Cells," *Nature Immunology* 9, (2008): 503–10, https://doi.org/10.1038/ni1582

507   Teruo Nishida, "Commanding Roles of Keratocytes in Health and Disease," *Cornea* 29, Suppl 1 (November 2010): S3-6, https://doi.org/10.1097/ICO.0b013e3181f2d578

508   Haitham T. Idriss and James H. Naismith, "TNF Alpha and the TNF Receptor Superfamily: Structure-Function Relationship(s)," *Microscopy Research and Technique* 50, no. 3 (July 6, 2000): 184-95, https://doi.org/10.1002/1097-0029(20000801)50:3<184::AID-JEMT2>3.0.CO;2-H

509   Erin T Livingston, Md Huzzatul Mursalin and Michelle C Callegan, "A Pyrrhic Victory: The PMN Response to Ocular Bacterial Infections," *Microorganisms* 7, no. 11 (November 7, 2019): 537, https://doi.org/10.3390/microorganisms7110537

510   Beatriz E Brito et al., "Toll-Like Receptor 4 and CD14 Expression in Human Ciliary Body and TLR-4 in Human Iris Endothelial Cells," *Experimental Eye Research* 79, no. 2 (August 2004): 203-8, https://doi.org/ 10.1016/j.exer.2004.03.012. PMID: 15325567

511   Matam Vijay Kumar et al., "Innate Immunity: Toll-Like Receptor (TLR) Signaling in Human Retinal Pigment Epithelial Cells," *Journal of Neuroimmunology* 153, no. 1-2 (August 2004): 7-15, https://doi.org/10.1016/j.jneuroim.2004.04.018

512   Sascha K R Spencer, Ian C Francis and Minas T Coroneo, "Spontaneous Face- and Eye-Touching: Infection Risk Versus Potential Microbiome Gain," *The Ocular Surface* 21 (July 2021): 64-65, https://doi.org/10.1016/j.jtos.2021.04.008

513   Qiong Liu et al., "NK Cells Modulate the Inflammatory Response to Corneal Epithelial Abrasion and Thereby Support Wound Healing," *American Journal of Pathology* 181, no. 2 (August 2012): 452-62, https://doi.org/10.1016/j.ajpath.2012.04.010

514   Davis Willmann, Lanxing Fu and Scott W. Melanson, "Corneal Injury," *StatPearls [Internet]*, Treasure Island (FL): StatPearls Publishing; (January 2022): https://www.ncbi.nlm.nih.gov/books/NBK459283/

515   Scott M. Whitcup, "The Double-Edged Ocular Immune Response - The Cogan Lecture," *Investigative Ophthalmology & Visual Science* 41, no. 11 (November 2000): 3243-8, https://pubmed.ncbi.nlm.nih.gov/11006209/

516   Mary Ann Stepp and A. Sue Menko, "Immune Responses to Injury and Their Links to Eye Disease," *Translational Research* 236 (October 1, 2021): 52-71, https://doi.org/10.1016/j.trsl.2021.05.005

517   Manuel J. Amador-Patarroyo, Alba Cristina Peñaranda and María Teresa

Bernal, "Autoimmune Uveitis,". *Autoimmunity: From Bench to Bedside* 37, (July 18, 2013): El Rosario University Press. https://www.ncbi.nlm.nih.gov/books/NBK459445/

518 S. Sharma, "Keratitis," *Bioscience Reports* 21, no. 4 (August 2001): 419–44, https://doi.org/10.1023/a:1017939725776

519 Maarten P. Rozing, et al., "Age-Related Macular Degeneration: A Two-Level Model Hypothesis," *Progress in Retinal and Eye Research* 76 (May 2020): 100825, https://doi.org/10.1016/j.preteyeres.2019.100825

520 "Age-Related Macular Degeneration," *National Eye Institute*, Nih.gov. 2019, https://www.nei.nih.gov/learn-about-eye-health/eye-conditions-and-diseases/age-related-macular-degeneration

521 Philip Hunter, "The Inflammation Theory of Disease, The Growing Realization That Chronic Inflammation is Crucial in Many Diseases Opens New Avenues For Treatment," *EMBO Reports* 13, no. 11 (November 6, 2012): 968-70, https://doi.org/10.1038/embor.2012.142

522 Qingdong Guan et al., "Cytokines in Autoimmune Disease," *Mediators of Inflammation* 2017 (July 11, 2017): 5089815, https://doi.org/10.1155/2017/5089815

523 Erwan Mortier et al., "Modulating Cytokines as Treatment for Autoimmune Diseases and Cancer," *Frontiers in Immunology* 11 (2020): 608636, https://doi.org/10.3389/fimmu.2020.608636

524 Judy H. Cho and Peter K. Gregersen, "Genomics and the Multifactorial Nature of Human Autoimmune Disease," *New England Journal of Medicine* 365, no. 17 (October 27, 2011): 1612-23, https://doi.org/10.1056/NEJMra1100030

525 Akbar Mohammad Hosseini et al., "Toll-Like Receptors in the Pathogenesis of Autoimmune Diseases," *Advanced Pharmaceutical Bulletin* 5, no. 1 (December 2015): 605–14, https://doi.org/10.15171/apb.2015.082

526 Kelly Mai et al., "Role of toll-like receptors in human iris pigment epithelial cells and their response to pathogen-associated molecular patterns," *Journal of Inflammation* 11, no. 20 (July 16, 2014): https://doi.org/10.1186/1476-9255-11-20

527 Henry J. Kaplan, Deming Sun and Hui Shao, "Damage-Associated Molecular Patterns in Clinical and Animal Models of Uveitis," *Ocular Immunology and Inflammation* (September 3, 2021): 1 – 7, https://doi.org/10.1080/09273948.2021.1954203

528 Jing Wang et al., "The Effect of Toll-Like Receptor 4 in the Aqueous Humor of Endotoxin-Induced Uveitis," *International Journal of Molecular Sciences* 13, no. 2 (2012): 2110-8, https://doi.org/10.3390/ijms13022110

529   Jian-Ying Zhou et al., "Association Study of Toll-Like Receptors 4
      Polymorphisms and The Risk of Age-Related Macular Degeneration: A
      Meta-Analysis," *Ophthalmic Genetics* 41, no. 6 (December 2020): 579-
      84, https://doi.org/10.1080/13816810.2020.1814348

530   Alexa Klettner and Johann Roider, "Retinal Pigment Epithelium
      Expressed Toll-like Receptors and Their Potential Role in Age-Related
      Macular Degeneration," *International Journal of Molecular Sciences* 22,
      no. 16 (August 4, 2021): 8387, https://doi.org/10.3390/ijms22168387

531   Amandeep Kaur et al., "Toll-Like Receptor-Associated Keratitis and
      Strategies for its Management," *3 Biotech* 5, no. 5 (October 2015): 611-
      19, https://doi.org/10.1007/s13205-015-0280-y

532   Rachel L Redfern et al., "Dry Eye Modulates the Expression of Toll-
      Like Receptors on the Ocular Surface," *Experimental Eye Research* 134
      (May 2015): 80-9, https://doi.org/10.1016/j.exer.2015.03.018

533   Jeremy Kiripolsky and Jill M Kramer, "Current and Emerging Evidence
      for Toll-Like Receptor Activation in Sjögren's Syndrome," *Journal of
      Immunology Research* 2018 (December 20, 2018): 1246818, https://doi.
      org/10.1155/2018/1246818

534   Michael E Stern, Chris S Schaumburg and Stephen C Pflugfelder, "Dry
      Eye as a Mucosal Autoimmune Disease," *International Reviews of
      Immunology* 32, no. 1 (February 2013): 19-41, https://doi.org/10.3109/0
      8830185.2012.748052

535   Hui Lin and Samuel C Yiu, "Dry Eye Disease: A Review of Diagnostic
      Approaches and Treatments," *Saudi Journal of Ophthalmology* 28, no. 3
      (July 2014): 173-181, https://doi.org/10.1016/j.sjopt.2014.06.002

536   Rajeev K Pandey, Fu-Shin Yu and Ashok Kumar, "Targeting Toll-Like
      Receptor Signaling as a Novel Approach to Prevent Ocular Infectious
      Diseases," *Indian Journal of Medical Research* 138, no. 5 (November
      2013): 609-19, https://pubmed.ncbi.nlm.nih.gov/24434316/

537   Robert J. Barry et al., "Pharmacotherapy for Uveitis: Current
      Management and Emerging Therapy," *Clinical Ophthalmology* 8 (2014):
      1891-1911, https://doi.org/10.2147/OPTH.S47778

538   Sapna Gangaputra et al., "Methotrexate For Ocular Inflammatory
      Diseases," *Ophthalmology* 116, no. 11 (November 2009): 2188-98.e1,
      https://di:10.1016/j.ophtha.2009.04.020

539   Stefano Bonini et al., "Phase II Randomized, Double-Masked, Vehicle-
      Controlled Trial of Recombinant Human Nerve Growth Factor for
      Neurotrophic Keratitis," *Ophthalmology* 125, no. 9 (September 2018):
      1332–43, https://doi.org/10.1016/j.ophtha.2018.02.022

540   Stephen C Pflugfelder et al., "Topical Recombinant Human Nerve
      Growth Factor (Cenergermin) For Neurotrophic Keratopathy:

A Multicenter Randomized Vehicle-Controlled Pivotal Trial," *Ophthalmology* 127, no. 1 (January 2020): 14–26, https://doi.org/10.1016/j.ophtha.2019.08.020

541 Xiaohong Cen, Shuwen Liu and Kui Cheng, "The Role of Toll-Like Receptor in Inflammation and Tumor Immunity," *Frontiers in Pharmacology* 9, no. 878 (August 6, 2018): https://doi.org/10.3389/fphar.2018.00878

542 Carisa K Petris and Arghavan Almony, "Ophthalmic Manifestations of Rheumatologic Disease: Diagnosis and Management," *Missouri Medicine* 109, no. 1 (February 2012): 53-58, https://pubmed.ncbi.nlm.nih.gov/22428448/

543 Alfred Yu Ting Chia et al., "Managing Psoriatic Arthritis with Inflammatory Bowel Disease and/or Uveitis," *Frontiers in Medicine (Lausanne)* 8 (September 16, 2021): 737256 https://doi.org/10.3389/fmed.2021.737256

544 Elvis Hysa et al., "Immunopathophysiology and Clinical Impact of Uveitis in Inflammatory Rheumatic Diseases: An Update," *European Journal of Clinical Investigation* 51, no. 8 (April 13, 2021): e13572, https://doi.org/10.1111/eci.13572

545 Ruchi Shah et al., "Systemic Diseases and the Cornea," *Experimental Eye Research* 204 (March 2021): 108455, https://doi.org/10.1016/j.exer.2021.108455

546 Thomas Boehm, "Evolution of Vertebrate Immunity," *Current Biology* 22, no. 17 (September 11, 2012): R722-R732, https://doi.org/10.1016/j.cub.2012.07.003

547 Jared C. Roach et al., "The Evolution of Vertebrate Toll-Like Receptors," *Proceedings of the National Academy of Sciences* 102, no. 27 (July 5, 2005): 9577-82, https://doi.org/10.1073/pnas.0502272102

548 Teva Canada Limited, "Revia Product Monograph," (April 14, 2015): https://pdf.hres.ca/dpd_pm/00030323.PDF accessed Nov 2020.

549 Brandon R. Selfridge et al., "Structure-Activity Relationships of (+)-Naltrexone-Inspired Toll-like Receptor 4 (TLR4) Antagonists," *Journal of Medicinal Chemistry* 58, no. 12 (May 26, 2015): 38-52, https://doi.org/10.1021/acs.jmedchem.5b00426

550 Xiaozheng Zhang et al., "Dissecting the Innate Immune Recognition of Opioid Inactive Isomer (+)-Naltrexone Derived Toll-like Receptor 4 (TLR4) Antagonists," *Journal of Chemical Information and Modeling* 58, no. 4 (March 8, 2018): 816-25, https://doi.org/10.1021/acs.jcim.7b00717

551 Rachel Cant, Angus G Dalgleish and Rachel L Allen, "Naltrexone Inhibits IL-6 and TNFα Production in Human Immune Cell Subsets following Stimulation with Ligands for Intracellular Toll-Like

Receptors," *Frontiers in Immunology* 8, no. 809 (July 11, 2017): https://doi.org/10.3389/fimmu.2017.00809

552   L. Charles Murrin, "[Leu]enkephalin," *xPharm: The Comprehensive Pharmacology Reference* (2007): 1-6, https://doi.org/10.1016/B978-008055232-3.61077-3

553   JianFei Wang et al., "Toll-like Receptors Expressed by Dermal Fibroblasts Contribute to Hypertrophic Scarring," *Journal of Cell Physiology* 226, no. 5 (May 2011): 1265-73, https://doi.org/10.1002/jcp.22454

554   Ian S Zagon, Michael F Verderame and Patricia J McLaughlin, "The Biology of the Opioid Growth Factor Receptor (OGFr)," *Brain Research. Brain Research Reviews* 38, no. 3 (February 2002): 351-76, https://doi.org/10.1016/s0165-0173(01)00160-6

555   Ian S Zagon, Michael F Verderame and Patricia J McLaughlin, "The Biology of the Opioid Growth Factor Receptor (OGFr)," *Brain Research. Brain Research Reviews* 38, no. 3 (February 2002): 351-76, https://doi.org/10.1016/s0165-0173(01)00160-6

556   Patricia J. McLaughlin, J W Sassani and Ian S Zagon, "Dysregulation of the OGF-OGFr Pathway and Associated Diabetic Complications," *Journal of Diabetes and Clinical Research* 3, no. 3 (July 19, 2021): 64-7, https://www.scientificarchives.com/article/dysregulation-of-the-ogf-ogfr-pathway-and-associated-diabetic-complications

557   Nancy P Kren, Ian S Zagon and Patricia J McLaughlin, "Mutations in the Opioid Growth Factor Receptor in Human Cancers Alter Receptor Function," *International Journal of Molecular Medicine* 36, no. 1 (July 2015): 289-93, https://doi.org/10.3892/ijmm.2015.2221

558   Patricia J. McLaughlin et al., "Diabetic Keratopathy and Treatment by Modulation of the Opioid Growth Factor (OGF)–OGF Receptor (Ogfr) Axis With Naltrexone: A Review," *Brain Research Bulletin* 81, no. 2-3 (February 15,2010): 236–247, https://doi.org/10.1016/j.brainresbull.2009.08.008

559   Jessica A Immonen, Ian S Zagon and Patricia J McLaughlin, "Selective Blockade of the OGF-Ogfr Pathway by Naltrexone Accelerates Fibroblast Proliferation and Wound Healing," *Experimental Biology and Medicine* 239, no. 10 (July 16, 2014): 1300-09, https://doi.org/10.1177/1535370214543061

560   Ning Liu, et al., "Low-Dose Naltrexone Inhibits the Epithelial-Mesenchymal Transition of Cervical Cancer Cells in Vitro and Effects Indirectly on Tumor-Associated Macrophages in Vivo," *International Immunopharmacology* 86 (September 2020): 106718, https://doi.org/10.1016/j.intimp.2020.106718

561 Matthew S Klocek et al., "Topically Applied Naltrexone Restores Corneal Reepithelialization in Diabetic Rats," *Journal of Ocular Pharmacology and Therapeutics* 23, no. 2 (April 2007): 89-102, https://doi.org/10.1089/jop.2006.0111

562 Hanane Chajra, "Cutaneous Opioid Receptors and Stress Responses: Molecular Interactions and Opportunities for Therapeutic Intervention," *Skin Stress Response Pathways* (August 23, 2016): 265-280, https://doi.org/10.1007/978-3-319-43157-4_13

563 Luke Parkitny and Jarred Younger, "Reduced Pro-Inflammatory Cytokines after Eight Weeks of Low-Dose Naltrexone for Fibromyalgia," *Biomedicines* 5, no. 2 (April 18, 2017): 16, https://doi.org/10.3390/biomedicines5020016

564 D Wakefield and A Lloyd, "The Role of Cytokines in the Pathogenesis of Inflammatory Eye Disease," *Cytokine* 4, no. 1 (January 1992): 1-5, https://doi.org/10.1016/1043-4666(92)90028-P

565 Alessandro Lambiase et al., "Toll-Like Receptors in Ocular Surface Diseases: Overview and New Findings," *Clinical Science* 120, no. 10 (May 2011): 441-50, https://doi.org/10.1042/CS20100425

566 Hyun Soo Lee et al., "Expression of Toll-Like Receptor 4 Contributes to Corneal Inflammation in Experimental Dry Eye Disease," *Investigative Ophthalmology and Visual Science* 53, no. 9 (August 17, 2012): 5632-40, https://doi.org/10.1167/iovs.12-9547

567 I S Zagon et al., "Topical Application of Naltrexone Facilitates Reepithelialization of the Cornea in Diabetic Rabbits," *Brain Research Bulletin* 81, no. 2-3 (February 15, 2010): 248-55, https://doi.org/10.1016/j.brainresbull.2009.10.009

568 Monica Bolton et al., "Serious Adverse Events Reported in Placebo Randomized Controlled Trials of Oral Naltrexone: A Systematic Review and Meta-Analysis," *BMC Medicine* 17, no. 1 (January 15, 2019): 10, https://doi.org/10.1186/s12916-018-1242-0

569 David Liang et al., "Topical Application of Naltrexone to the Ocular Surface of Healthy Volunteers: A Tolerability Study," *Journal of Ocular Pharmacology and Therapeutics* 32, no. 2 (March 2016): 127-32, https://doi.org/10.1089/jop.2015.0070

570 P J McLaughlin et al., "Efficacy and Safety of a Novel Naltrexone Treatment for Dry Eye in Type 1 Diabetes," *BMC Ophthalmology* 19, no. 35 (2019): https://doi.org/10.1186/s12886-019-1044-y

571 MG Maguire, "Age-related Macular Degeneration," *The Aging Retina* 1. No. 3 (December 2006): http://www.focus-ed.net/AMD_AR%20v1n3.pdf

572 Maarten P. Rozing, et al., "Age-Related Macular Degeneration: A Two-

Level Model Hypothesis," *Progress in Retinal and Eye Research* 76 (May 2020): 100825, https://doi.org/10.1016/j.preteyeres.2019.100825

573 S Zashin, "Sjogren's Syndrome and Clinical Benefits of Low-Dose Naltrexone Therapy: Additional Case Reports," *Cureus* 12, no. 7 (July 1, 2020): e8948, https://doi.org/10.7759/cureus.8948

574 Gabriela Dieckmann et al., "Low-Dose Naltrexone is Effective and Well-Tolerated for Modulating Symptoms in Patients with Neuropathic Corneal Pain," *The Ocular Surface* 20 (April 2021): 33-8, https://doi.org/10.1016/j.jtos.2020.12.003

575 Fabiana Mallone et al., "Understanding Drivers of Ocular Fibrosis: Current and Future Therapeutic Perspectives," *International Journal of Molecular Sciences* 22, no. 21 (October 27, 2021): 11748, https://doi.org/10.3390/ijms222111748

576 Ashaben Patel et al., "Ocular Drug Delivery Systems: An Overview," *World Journal of Pharmacology* 2, no. 2 (2013): 47-64, https://doi.org/10.5497/wjp.v2.i2.47

577 "USP 795," Draft 2021, www.usp.org. https://www.usp.org/compounding/general-chapter-795

578 NAPRA, "Model Standards for Pharmacy Compounding of Non-hazardous Sterile Preparations," (March 28, 2018): https://www.napra.ca/general-practice-resources/model-standards-pharmacy-compounding-non-sterile-preparations

579 MHRA Guidance for Specials Manufacturers, Manufacture of Sterile Medicinal Products, Revision 2 (January 2021): 13, https://assets.publishing.service.gov.uk/government/uploads/system/uploads/attachment_data/file/964017/QA_Version_3_-_Aseptic_manip_updates.pdf

580 "Pharmacy Board of Australia - Codes, Guidelines and Policies." *Pharmacyboard.gov.au,* 2017: https://www.pharmacyboard.gov.au/codes-guidelines.aspx.

Chapter Eight

581 European Centre for Disease Prevention and Control. COVID-19 situation update worldwide, as of week 52, updated 5 January 2022. Accessed: 6 January 2022. https://www.ecdc.europa.eu/en/geographical-distribution-2019-ncov-cases

582 Markus Hoffmann et al., "SARS-CoV-2 Cell Entry Depends on ACE2 and TMPRSS2 and is Blocked by a Clinically Proven Protease Inhibitor", *Cell* 181, no. 2 (April 16, 2020): 270-80, https://doi.org/10.1016/j.cell.2020.02.052

583 I Hamming et al., "Tissue Distribution of ACE2 Protein, The Functional

Receptor for SARS Coronavirus. A First Step in Understanding SARS Pathogenesis," *Journal of Pathology* 203, no. 2 (June 2004): 631-7, https://doi.org/10.1002/path.1570

584   Centers for Disease Control and Prevention, Symptoms of COVID-19, Updated: 22 February 2021, Accessed: 6 January 2022, https://www.cdc.gov/coronavirus/2019-ncov/symptoms-testing/symptoms.html

585   NICE guideline [NG188] Published: 18 December 2020 Last updated: 11 November 2021 https://app.magicapp.org/#/guideline/EQpzKn/section/n3vwoL

586   Elena Ortona and Walter Malorni, "Long COVID: To Investigate Immunological Mechanisms and Sex/Gender Related Aspects as Fundamental Steps for a Tailored Therapy," *European Respiratory Journal* 2102245 (16 September 2021): https://doi.org/10.1183/13993003.02245-2021

587   H. Cook et al., "Long COVID—mechanisms, risk factors, and management," *British Medical Journal* 374 (July 2021): https://doi.org/10.1136/bmj.n1648

588   J. M. Arthur et al., "Development of ACE2 Autoantibodies After SARS-CoV-2 Infection," *PLoS ONE* 16, no. 9 (September 3, 2021): e0257016, https://doi.org/10.1371/journal.pone.0257016

589   "Prevalence of Long COVID Symptoms and COVID-19 Complications - Office for National Statistics," *www.ons.gov.uk* (December 16, 2020): https://www.ons.gov.uk/peoplepopulationandcommunity/healthandsocialcare/healthandlifeexpectancies/datasets/prevalenceoflongCOVIDsymptomsandCOVID19complications.

590   Nicholas S Hopkinson, Gisli Jenkins and Nicholas Hart, "COVID-19 and What Comes After?" *Thorax* 76, (February 15, 2021): 324-5, http://dx.doi.org/10.1136/thoraxjnl-2020-216226

591   Swapna Mandal et al., "Long-COVID': a Cross-Sectional Study of Persisting Symptoms, Biomarker and Imaging Abnormalities Following Hospitalisation for COVID-19," *Thorax* 76, no. 4 (March 15, 2021): 396-8, https://thorax.bmj.com/content/76/4/396

592   David T Arnold et al., "Patient Outcomes After Hospitalisation with COVID-19 and Implications for Follow-Up: Results From a Prospective UK Cohort," *Thorax* 76, no. 4 (March 15, 2021): 399-401, https://thorax.bmj.com/content/76/4/399

593   Vineet Chopra et al., "Sixty-Day Outcomes Among Patients Hospitalized with COVID-19," *Annals of Internal Medicine* 174, no. 4 (November 11, 2020): 576-8, https://doi.org/10.7326/M20-5661

594   Ani Nalbandian et al., "Post-acute COVID-19 Syndrome," *Nature Medicine* 27, no. 4 (March 22, 2021): 601-15, https://doi.org/10.1038/

s41591-021-01283-z

595   Laura A Huppert, Michael A Matthay and Lorraine B Ware,
       "Pathogenesis of Acute Respiratory Distress Syndrome," *Seminars in
       Respiratory and Critical Care Medicine* 40, no. 1 (February 2019): 31-9,
       https://doi.org/10.1055/s-0039-1683996.

596   Dane Parker and Alice Prince, "Innate Immunity in the Respiratory
       Epithelium," *The American Journal of Respiratory Cell and Molecular
       Biology* 45, no. 2 (August 2011): 189-201, https://doi.org/10.1165/
       rcmb.2011-0011RT

597   Toshio Tanaka, Masashi Narazaki and Tadamitsu Kishimoto, "IL-
       6 in Inflammation, Immunity, And Disease," *Cold Spring Harbor
       Perspectives in Biology* 6, no. 10 (September 4, 2014): a016295, https://
       doi.org/10.1101/cshperspect.a016295

598   J D Gillmore et al., "Amyloid Load and Clinical Outcome in AA
       Amyloidosis in Relation to Circulating Concentration of Serum Amyloid
       A Protein," *Lancet (London, England)* 358, no. 9275 (July 7, 2001): 24-
       9, https://doi.org/10.1016/S0140-6736(00)05252-1

599   Luca Carsana et al., "Pulmonary Post-Mortem Findings in a Series
       of COVID-19 Cases from Northern Italy: A Two-Centre Descriptive
       Study," *The Lancet, Infectious Diseases* 20, no. 10 (October 2020):
       1135-40, https://doi.org/10.1016/S1473-3099(20)30434-5

600   "Updated Estimates of the Prevalence of Long COVID Symptoms -
       Office for National Statistics." n.d. Www.ons.gov.uk. Accessed January
       6, 2022. https://www.ons.gov.uk/peoplepopulationandcommunity/
       healthandsocialcare/healthandlifeexpectancies/
       adhocs/12788updatedestimatesoftheprevalenceoflongCOVIDsymptoms

601   Carolina X Sandler et al., "Long COVID and Post-infective Fatigue
       Syndrome: A Review," *Open Forum Infectious Diseases* 8, no. 10
       (September 8, 2021): ofab440, https://doi.org/10.1093/ofid/ofab440

602   Melanie Newman, "Chronic Fatigue Syndrome and Long COVID:
       Moving Beyond the Controversy," *British Medical Journal* 373 (June
       24, 2021): n1559, https://doi.org/10.1136/bmj.n1559

603   Angelo Carfì, Roberto Bernabei and Francesco Landi, "Persistent
       Symptoms in Patients After Acute COVID-19," *JAMA* 324, no. 6
       (August 11, 2020): 603-5, https://doi.org/10.1001/jama.2020.12603

604   Alexandra H Mandarano et al., "Myalgic Encephalomyelitis/Chronic
       Fatigue Syndrome Patients Exhibit Altered T Cell Metabolism and
       Cytokine Associations," *Journal of Clinical Investigation* 130, no. 3
       (March 2, 2020): 1491-1505, https://doi.org/10.1172/JCI132185

605   Liam Townsend et al., "Persistent Fatigue Following SARS-Cov-2
       Infection is Common and Independent of Severity of Initial Infection,"

PLoS ONE 15, no. 11 (November 9, 2020): e0240784, https://doi.org/10.1371/journal.pone.0240784

606   Kieron South et al., "Preceding Infection and Risk of Stroke: An Old Concept Revived by The COVID-19 Pandemic," *International Journal of Stroke* 15, no. 7 (October 2020): 722-32, https://doi.org/10.1177/1747493020943815

607   Bindu D. Paul et al., "Redox Imbalance Links COVID-19 and Myalgic Encephalomyelitis/Chronic Fatigue Syndrome," *Proceedings of the National Academy of Sciences* 118, no. 34 (August 24, 2021): e2024358118, https://doi.org/10.1073/pnas.2024358118

608   Mady Hornig et al., "Distinct Plasma Immune Signatures in ME/CFS are Present Early in the Course of Illness," *Science Advances* 1, no. 1 (February 2015): e1400121, https://doi.org/10.1126/sciadv.1400121

609   Marta Curriu et al., "Screening NK-, B- and T-cell Phenotype and Function in Patients Suffering from Chronic Fatigue Syndrome," *Journal of Translational Medicine* 11, no.68 (March 20, 2013): https://doi.org/10.1186/1479-5876-11-68

610   Anna Schurich et al., "Distinct Metabolic Requirements of Exhausted and Functional Virus-Specific CD8 T Cells in the Same Host," *Cell Reports* 16, no. 5 (August 2, 2016): 1243-52, https://doi.org/10.1016/j.celrep.2016.06.078

611   Luke Parkitny and Jarred Younger, "Reduced Pro-Inflammatory Cytokines after Eight Weeks of Low-Dose Naltrexone for Fibromyalgia," *Biomedicines* 5, no. 2 (April 18, 2017): 16, https://doi.org/10.3390/biomedicines5020016

612   Lisanne Mirja Plein and Heike L Rittner, "Opioids and the Immune System - Friend or Foe," *British Journal of Pharmacology* 175, no. 14 (July 2018): 2717-25, https://doi.org/10.1111/bph.13750

613   J M Bidlack, "Detection and Function of Opioid Receptors on Cells from the Immune System," *Clinical and Diagnostic Laboratory Immunology* 7, no. 5 (September 2000): 719-23, https://doi.org/10.1128/CDLI.7.5.719-723.2000

614   Toby K Eisenstein, "The Role of Opioid Receptors in Immune System Function," *Frontiers in Immunology* 10 (December 20, 2019): 2904, https://doi.org/10.3389/fimmu.2019.02904

615   M. J. Bolton, B. P. Chapman and H. Van Marwijk, "Low-Dose Naltrexone as a Treatment For Chronic Fatigue Syndrome," *BMJ Case Reports* 13, no. 1 (January 6, 2020): e232502, https://casereports.bmj.com/content/13/1/e232502

616   Rachel Cant, Angus G Dalgleish and Rachel L Allen, "Naltrexone Inhibits IL-6 and TNFα Production in Human Immune Cell Subsets

following Stimulation with Ligands for Intracellular Toll-Like
Receptors," *Frontiers in Immunology* 8 (July 11, 2017): 809, https://doi.
org/10.3389/fimmu.2017.008

617 Birger Sørensen, Andres Susrud and Angus G Dalgleish, "Biovacc-19:
A Candidate Vaccine for COVID-19 (SARS-CoV-2) Developed from
Analysis of its General Method of Action for Infectivity," Published
online by Cambridge University Press, *QRB Discovery* 1 (June 2, 2020):
e6 https://doi.org/10.1017/qrd.2020.8

618 David H Brann et al., "Non-Neuronal Expression of SARS-Cov-2
Entry Genes in the Olfactory System Suggests Mechanisms Underlying
COVID-19-Associated Anosmia," *Science Advances* 6, no. 31 (July 31,
2020): eabc5801, https://doi.org/10.1126/sciadv.abc5801

619 Alexander P Bye et al., "Aberrant Glycosylation of Anti-SARS-Cov-2
Spike Igg is a Prothrombotic Stimulus for Platelets," *Blood* 138, no. 16
(October 21, 2021): 1481-89, https://doi.org/10.1182/blood.2021011871

620 B Joseph Elmunzer et al., "Digestive Manifestations in Patients
Hospitalized with Coronavirus Disease 2019," *Clinical Gastroenterology
and Hepatology* 19, no. 7 (July 2021): 1355-65.e4, https://doi.
org/10.1016/j.cgh.2020.09.041

621 Helene Cabanas et al., "Potential Therapeutic Benefit of Low Dose
Naltrexone in Myalgic Encephalomyelitis/Chronic Fatigue Syndrome:
Role of Transient Receptor Potential Melastatin 3 Ion Channels in
Pathophysiology and Treatment," *Frontiers in Immunology* 12 (July 13,
2021): 687806, https://doi.org/10.3389/fimmu.2021.687806

622 M J Bolton, B P Chapman and H Van Marwijk, "Low-Dose Naltrexone
as a Treatment for Chronic Fatigue Syndrome," *BMJ Case Report* 13,
no. 1 (January 6, 2020): e232502, https://doi.org/10.1136/bcr-2019-
232502

623 Helene Cabanas et al., "Potential Therapeutic Benefit of Low Dose
Naltrexone in Myalgic Encephalomyelitis/Chronic Fatigue Syndrome:
Role of Transient Receptor Potential Melastatin 3 Ion Channels in
Pathophysiology and Treatment," *Frontiers in Immunology* 12 (July 13,
2021): 687806, https://doi.org/10.3389/fimmu.2021.687806

624 Helene Cabanas et al., "Potential Therapeutic Benefit of Low Dose
Naltrexone in Myalgic Encephalomyelitis/Chronic Fatigue Syndrome:
Role of Transient Receptor Potential Melastatin 3 Ion Channels in
Pathophysiology and Treatment," *Frontiers in Immunology* 12 (July 13,
2021): 687806, https://doi.org/10.3389/fimmu.2021.687806

625 "WHO Recommends Life-Saving Interleukin-6 Receptor Blockers for
COVID-19 and Urges Producers to Join Efforts to Rapidly Increase
Access." www.who.int., Published: 6 July 2021. Accessed: 6 January

2022 https://www.who.int/news/item/06-07-2021-who-recommends-life-saving-interleukin-6-receptor-blockers-for-COVID-19-and-urges-producers-to-join-efforts-to-rapidly-increase-access

Chapter Nine

626 Angus G Dalgleish and Ken J O'Byrne, "Chronic Immune Activation and Inflammation in the Pathogenesis of AIDS and Cancer," *Advances in Cancer Research* 84 (2002): 231-76, https://doi.org/10.1016/s0065-230x(02)84008-8

627 P Arbuthnot and M Kew, "Hepatitis B Virus and Hepatocellular Carcinoma," *International Journal of Experimental Pathology* 82, no. 2 (April 2001): 77-100, https://doi.org/10.1111/j.1365-2613.2001.iep0082-0077-x

628 Janos Terzić et al., "Inflammation and Colon Cancer," *Gastroenterology* 138, no. 6 (June 2010):2101-14.e5, https://doi.org/10.1053/j.gastro.2010.01.058

629 Tonya Walser et al., "Smoking and Lung Cancer," *Proceedings of the American Thoracic Society* 5, no. 8 (December 2008): 811-15, https://doi.org/10.1513/pats.200809-100TH

630 Emanuela Ricciotti, Kirk J. Wangensteen and Garret A. FitzGerald, "Aspirin in Hepatocellular Carcinoma," *Cancer Research* 81, no. 14 (July 15, 2021): 3751-61, https://doi.org/10.1158/0008-5472.CAN-21-0758

631 Wai M Liu and Angus G Dalgleish, "Naltrexone at Low Doses (LDN) and its Relevance to Cancer Therapy," *Expert Review of Anticancer Therapy* 22, no. 3 (March 2022): 269-74, https://doi.org/10.1080/14737140.2022.2037426

632 Angus G. Dalgleish et al., "Long-Term Benefit from Immune Modulation and Anti-Inflammatory Treatment in Metastatic Mesothelioma," *Respiratory Medicine Case Reports* 29 (2020): 100971, https://doi.org/10.1016/j.rmcr.2019.100971

633 Akbar Khan, "Long-Term Remission of Adenoid Cystic Tongue Carcinoma with Low Dose Naltrexone and Vitamin D3--A Case Report," *Oral Health and Dental Management* 13, no. 3 (September 2014): 721-4, PMID: 25284545

634 Angus G Dalgleish et al., "Randomised, Open-Label, Phase II Study of Gemcitabine with and without IMM-101 For Advanced Pancreatic Cancer," *British Journal of Cancer* 115, no. 7 (September 2016): 789-96, https://doi.org/10.1038/bjc.2016.271

635 Karen S Sfanos and Angelo M De Marzo, "Prostate Cancer and Inflammation: The Evidence," *Histopathology* 60, no.1 (January 2012):

199-215, https://doi.org/10.1111/j.1365-2559.2011.04033.x

636   Jeffrey A Miskoff and Moiuz Chaudhri, "Low Dose Naltrexone and
       Lung Cancer: A Case Report and Discussion," *Cureus* 10, no. 7 (July
       2018): e2924, https://doi.org/10.7759/cureus.2924

637   Burton M Berkson and Francisco Calvo Riera, "The Long-Term
       Survival of a Patient with Stage IV Renal Cell Carcinoma Following
       an Integrative Treatment Approach Including the Intravenous
       α-Lipoic Acid/Low-Dose Naltrexone Protocol," *Integrative Cancer
       Therapies* 17, no. 3 (September 2018): 986-993, https://doi.
       org/10.1177/1534735417747984

638   Moshe Rogosnitzky et al., "Opioid Growth Factor (OGF) for
       Hepatoblastoma: a Novel Non-Toxic Treatment," *Investigational New
       Drugs* 31, no. 4 (August 2013): 1066-70, https://doi.org/10.1007/
       s10637-012-9918-3

639   Burton M Berkson, Daniel M Rubin and Arthur J Berkson, "Revisiting
       the ALA/N (Alpha-Lipoic Acid/Low-Dose Naltrexone) Protocol for
       People with Metastatic and Nonmetastatic Pancreatic Cancer: A Report
       of 3 New Cases," *Integrative Cancer Therapies* 8, no. 4 (December
       2009): 416-22, https://doi.org/10.1177/1534735409352082

640   Ning Liu et al., "Low-Dose Naltrexone Plays Antineoplastic Role in
       Cervical Cancer Progression Through Suppressing PI3K/AKT/mTOR
       Pathway," *Translational Oncology* 14, no. 4 (April 2021): 101028,
       https://doi.org/10.1016/j.tranon.2021.101028

641   Ning Liu et al., "Low-Dose Naltrexone Plays Antineoplastic Role in
       Cervical Cancer Progression Through Suppressing PI3K/AKT/mTOR
       Pathway," *Translational Oncology* 14, no. 4 (April 2021): 101028,
       https://doi.org/10.1016/j.tranon.2021.101028

642   Wai M Liu et al., "Naltrexone at Low Doses Upregulates a Unique Gene
       Expression Not Seen with Normal Doses: Implications for its use in
       Cancer Therapy," *International Journal of Oncology* 49, no. 2 (August
       2016): 793-802, https://doi.org/10.3892/ijo.2016.3567

643   Alshimaa Aboalsoud et al., "The Effect of Low-Dose Naltrexone on
       Solid Ehrlich Carcinoma in Mice: The Role of OGFr, BCL2, and
       Immune Response," *International Immunopharmacology* 78 (January
       2020): 106068, https://doi.org/10.1016/j.intimp.2019.106068

644   Wai M Liu et al., "Naltrexone at Low Doses Upregulates a Unique Gene
       Expression Not Seen with Normal Doses: Implications for its Use in
       Cancer Therapy," *International Journal of Oncology* 49, no. 2 (August
       2016): 793-802, https://doi.org/10.3892/ijo.2016.3567

645   Mingxing Ma et al., "Low-Dose Naltrexone Inhibits Colorectal
       Cancer Progression and Promotes Apoptosis by Increasing M1-Type

Macrophages and Activating the Bax/Bcl-2/Caspase-3/PARP Pathway," *International Immunopharmacology* 83 (June 2020): 106388, https://doi.org/10.1016/j.intimp.2020.106388

646 Alshimaa Aboalsoud et al., "The Effect of Low-Dose Naltrexone on Solid Ehrlich Carcinoma in Mice: The Role of OGFr, BCL2, and Immune Response," *International Immunopharmacology* 78 (January 2020): 106068, https://doi.org/10.1016/j.intimp.2019.106068

647 Mingxing Ma et al., "Low-Dose Naltrexone Inhibits Colorectal Cancer Progression and Promotes Apoptosis by Increasing M1-Type Macrophages and Activating the Bax/Bcl-2/Caspase-3/PARP Pathway," *International Immunopharmacology* 83 (June 2020): 106388, https://doi.org/10.1016/j.intimp.2020.106388

648 Rachel Cant, Angus G Dalgleish and Rachel L Allen, "Naltrexone Inhibits IL-6 and TNFα Production in Human Immune Cell Subsets following Stimulation with Ligands for Intracellular Toll-Like Receptors," *Frontiers in Immunology* 8 (July 2017): 809, https://doi.org/10.3389/fimmu.2017.008

649 Jingjuan Meng et al., "Low Dose Naltrexone (LDN) Enhances Maturation of Bone Marrow Dendritic Cells (BMDCs)," *International Immunopharmacology* 17, no. 4 (December 2013): 1084-9, https://doi.org/10.1016/j.intimp.2013.10.012

650 Jarred Younger, Luke Parkitny and David McLain, "The Use of Low-Dose Naltrexone (LDN) as a Novel Anti-Inflammatory Treatment for Chronic Pain," *Clinical Rheumatology* 33, no. 4 (April 2014): 451-9, https://doi.org/10.1007/s10067-014-2517-2

651 Wai M Liu et al., "Naltrexone at Low Doses Upregulates a Unique Gene Expression Not Seen with Normal Doses: Implications for its Use in Cancer Therapy," *International Journal of Oncology* 49, no. 2 (August 2016): 793-802, https://doi.org/10.3892/ijo.2016.3567

652 Wai M Liu et al., "Naltrexone at Low Doses Upregulates a Unique Gene Expression Not Seen with Normal Doses: Implications for its Use in Cancer Therapy," *International Journal of Oncology* 49, no. 2 (August 2016): 793-802, https://doi.org/10.3892/ijo.2016.3567

653 Stan Sonu, Sharon Post and Joe Feinglass, "Adverse Childhood Experiences and the Onset of Chronic Disease in Young Adulthood," *Preventative Medicine* 123 (June 2019): 163-70, https://doi.org/10.1016/j.ypmed.2019.03.032

654 Shunsuke Chikuma, "CTLA-4, an Essential Immune-Checkpoint for T-Cell Activation," *Current Topics in Microbiology and Immunology* 410 (2017): 99-126, https://doi.org/10.1007/82_2017_61

655 Yoshiyuki Nakamura, "Biomarkers for Immune Checkpoint Inhibitor-

Mediated Tumor Response and Adverse Events," *Frontiers in Medicine* (May 2019): https://doi.org/10.3389/fmed.2019.00119

Epilogue

656   Bernard Bihari et al., "Low Dose Naltrexone in the Treatment of Acquired Immune Deficiency Syndrome," Poster presentation at the IV international AIDS conference, Stockholm, Sweden, (June 1988), https://issuu.com/ldnim/docs/low_dose_naltrexone_in_the_treatmen

657   Jan M. Keppel Hesselink and David J. Kopsky, "Enhancing Acupuncture by Low Dose Naltrexone," *Acupuncture in Medicine* 29, no.2, (June 2011): 127-130, https://doi.org/10.1136/aim.2010.003566

658   Jarred Younger, Luke Parkitny and David McLain, "The Use of Low-Dose Naltrexone (LDN) as a Novel Anti-Inflammatory Treatment for Chronic Pain," *Clinical Rheumatology* 33, no. 4, (February 2014): 451-459, https://doi.org/10.1007/s10067-014-2517-2

659   Burton M. Berkson, Daniel M. Rubin and Arthur J. Berkson, "The Long-Term Survival of a Patient with Pancreatic Cancer with Metastases to the Liver After Treatment with the Intravenous A-Lipoic Acid/Low-Dose Naltrexone Protocol," *Integrative Cancer Therapies* 5, no. 1, (March 2006): 83-89, https://doi.org/10.1177/1534735405285901

660   Burton M. Berkson, Daniel M. Rubin and Arthur J. Berkson, "Revisiting the ALA/N (A-Lipoic Acid/Low-Dose Naltrexone) Protocol for People with Metastatic and Nonmetastatic Pancreatic Cancer: A Report of 3 New Cases," *Integrative Cancer Therapies* 8, no. 4, (December 2009): 416-422, https://doi.org/10.1177/1534735409352082

661   Karlo Toljan and Bruce Vrooman, "Low-Dose Naltrexone (LDN)— Review of Therapeutic Utilization," *Medical Sciences* 6, no. 4, (September 2018): 82, https://doi.org/10.3390/medsci6040082

662   Guttorm Raknes and Lars Småbrekke, "A Sudden and Unprecedented Increase in Low Dose Naltrexone (LDN) Prescribing in Norway. Patient and Prescriber Characteristics, and Dispense Patterns. A Drug Utilization Cohort Study," *Pharmacoepidemiology and Drug Safety* 26, no. 2, (September 2016): 136-142, https://doi.org/10.1002/pds.4110

Index

ACA 111, 120, 121, 155
ACE-2 receptor 36
ACE2 receptor 188, 189, 193
acetylation 31
ACTH 111, 119, 120, 151, 152
ACTH, Cortisol, and Stress 151
acupuncture and LDN 214
ADH 111, 118, 119, 131, 161, 165, 168
adrenal insufficiency 46
Adverse Childhood Experiences 15, 293
AGA 111, 116, 117, 164
Aging 58, 59, 60, 76, 229, 230
akinesis 26
ALA 201
Allergies 14, 220
allergy 12, 13, 15, 93, 117, 164
amino acids 20, 136, 137, 143
AMPs 35, 37, 48, 49, 55
amyloidosis 190
amyotrophic lateral sclerosis 28
andropause 18
angiotensin-converting enzyme 36
Angus Dalgleish 225
Anhedonia 14
anticancer action 203
anti-depressant 10, 11
antidepressants 18, 75, 123
antigenic drift 24
antigenic shift 24
anti-inflammatory diet 15, 51, 56
anti-NMDA receptor 28
Antioxidants 74
antiviral therapeutics 21
antiviral therapies 39
anxiety 11, 14, 16, 17, 19, 97, 99, 100, 108, 125, 126, 127, 128, 133, 148, 150, 206, 207
Anxiety 219
Apigenin 56

aquaporin-4 28
ARDS 45, 190
arthralgia 82
asthma 13
Astragalus 56, 61
atherosclerosis 12, 65, 68, 83
attention deficit disorder (ADD) 16
Attenuating TLR4 with LDN 48
autoantibody 30, 46
autoimmune disease 28, 38, 80, 82, 83, 84, 85, 86, 88, 89, 90, 91, 92, 93, 94, 96, 97, 98, 99, 100, 101, 112, 113, 122, 125, 128, 133, 140, 161, 167, 205
autoimmune thyroiditis 209, 210, 212, 214
autoimmunity 11, 12, 13, 14, 37, 38, 46, 51, 65, 90, 109, 121, 122, 129, 130, 132, 136, 140, 144, 145, 146, 147, 149, 152, 157, 159, 160, 208, 226, 230
Autoimmunity Workup 46
autonomic nervous system 99, 100, 102
Autophagy 67, 69, 245, 246, 247, 248
B19V 41, 42
Bacterial and Fungal Co-Infections 45
BAD 202, 203
Barr body 38
BAX 202, 203
BAX:BCL2 202
BCL2 202, 292, 293
beta-defensin 2 35
biochemical change 11
Biomarker C4a 113
Biomarkers 120, 149
biomarker tests 110, 111
bipolar 11, 100, 127
Blood Brain Barrier 14
BPC-157 133, 134, 135, 137, 140, 143, 144, 145, 148, 149, 150, 151, 152, 158, 159, 162, 164, 166

ABOUT THE EDITOR

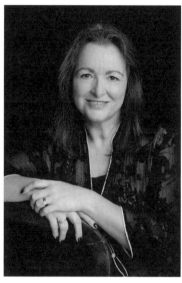

Photo by Julia Holland

Linda Elsegood is the founder of the UK charity LDN Research Trust, established in 2004. She has Multiple Sclerosis (MS), and Low Dose Naltrexone (LDN) significantly impacted her life. She wanted to help other people, not only with MS but all autoimmune diseases, cancers, mental health issues, etc. In the last 18 years, the charity has helped over a million people worldwide.

NOTES

NOTES

NOTES

NOTES